MRCOG Part 2

550 MCQs, EMQs and SAQs

MRCOG Part 2

550 MCQs, EMQs and SAQs

Rekha Wuntakal MBBS MD(O&G) DNB DFFP MRCOG

Specialist Registrar in Obstetrics and Gynaecology,
Barking, Havering and Redbridge University Hospital NHS Trust;
Honorary Research Fellow, Whipps Cross University Hospital,
Barts Health NHS Trust, London, UK

Edited by

Tony Hollingworth MBChB PhD MBA FRCS(Ed) FRCOG

Consultant in Obstetrics and Gynaecology,
Whipps Cross University Hospital,
Barts Health NHS Trust, London, UK

David Redford MB FRCS FRCOG

Consultant in Obstetrics and Gynaecology,
Royal Shrewsbury Hospital, Shrewsbury, UK

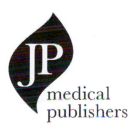

JP
medical
publishers

London • St Louis • Panama City • New Delhi

© 2013 JP Medical Ltd.
Published by JP Medical Ltd
83 Victoria Street, London, SW1H 0HW, UK
Tel: +44 (0)20 3170 8910   Fax: +44 (0)20 3008 6180
Email: info@jpmedpub.com   Web: www.jpmedpub.com

ISBN: 978-1-907816-50-5

British Library Cataloguing in Publication Data
A catalogue record for this book is available from the British Library

Library of Congress Cataloging in Publication Data
A catalog record for this book is available from the Library of Congress

JP Medical Ltd is a subsidiary of Jaypee Brothers Medical Publishers (P) Ltd, New Delhi, India

Publisher: Richard Furn
Commissioning Editor: Hannah Applin
Senior Editorial Assistant: Katrina Rimmer
Design: Designers Collective Ltd

Typeset, printed and bound in India.

Preface

The MRCOG examination is made up of two parts. This book provides a revision aid for the Part 2 exam. It presents 250 MCQs, 250 EMQs and 50 SAQs, all mapped to the syllabus topics. The EMQ and SAQ answers are supplemented with explanatory notes and further reading. The SAQs are in the current style used in the MRCOG Part 2 examination, with fully worked answers that are accompanied by the marking scheme, to give trainees a thorough understanding of how the SAQs are marked in the real exam.

The aims of the book are to help trainees to work through a wealth of questions, understand the exam format and focus on topics of weakness. Any exam can seem daunting in the lead up to it. It is important to read widely and cover all aspects of the specialty. Answering practice questions is a vital part of the revision process.

We hope that this book will prove useful in your preparations for the MRCOG Part 2 exam.

Rekha Wuntakal
Tony Hollingworth
David Redford
October 2012

Dedication

Dedicated to my mother, Akkamma, my brothers Sateesh and Manjunath, my sister Neelu and all my teachers in the UK

Rekha Wuntakal

Contents

Contents

Section C: SAQs

Revision advice

Introduction and syllabus

The aim of the MRCOG exam is to set a standard for the competent and safe practice of Obstetrics and Gynaecology. The exam is made up of two parts, MRCOG Part 1 and MRCOG Part 2. The MRCOG Part 1 deals with the basic sciences relevant to the specialty, which must be passed before taking the MRCOG Part 2.

The MRCOG Part 2 is divided into two parts, namely the written, which aims to test knowledge, and the Objective Structured Clinical Examination (OSCE), which tests the application of knowledge. The written exam is composed of three types of questions: short answer questions (SAQs), extended matching questions (EMQs) and multiple choice questions (MCQs). The exam is aimed at the level of an ST5 trainee in Obstetrics and Gynaecology, and 'blue printed' to ensure the whole of the syllabus is covered by the written and OSCE components.

The MRCOG Part 2 exam is a test of knowledge in Obstetrics and Gynaecology. The modules in the syllabus include teaching and appraisal, information and technology, clinical governance and research, core surgical skills, postoperative care, surgical procedures, antenatal care, maternal medicine, fetal medicine, puerperium, management of labour and delivery, gynaecological problems, subfertility, early pregnancy care, women's sexual and reproductive health, gynaecology oncology and urogynaecology. A thorough description of the topics covered in each of these modules is available on the Royal College of Obstetricians and Gynaecologists' (RCOG) website (http://www.rcog.org.uk).

Format of the paper

The MRCOG Part 2 written exam is held twice a year, in March and September. It comprises SAQs, EMQs and MCQs. Only candidates who pass the written exam can proceed to the OSCE exam.

The entire written paper is 375 minutes in duration. The timetable starts with the SAQ Paper, comprising four questions to be answered within 105 minutes. This is followed by a short break of 30 minutes. The next section is EMQ and MCQ Paper 1, which comprises 45 EMQs and 120 MCQs to be answered within 135 minutes. This is followed by a 45-minute lunch break. After lunch, EMQ and MCQ Paper 2 begins, which comprises 45 EMQs and 120 MCQs to be answered within 135 minutes.

The time is evenly divided between the EMQ and MCQ Papers 1 and 2. However, for each Paper, the RCOG suggest that candidates spend 85 minutes answering the EMQs and 50 minutes answering the MCQs. The marks are divided as follows: SAQs – 30%, EMQs – 40%, MCQs –30%.

The RCOG website provides details about the written exam format, with set examples of SAQs, EMQs and MCQs. We have matched the RCOG format in this book.

How to prepare for the exam

The best time to sit the MRCOG Part 2 is while working at the level of an ST4 or ST5 trainee in Obstetrics and Gynaecology. Without realising it, the necessary knowledge will be gathered relating to the syllabus topics by discussing cases with senior colleagues (senior registrars and consultants), attending consultant ward rounds, obstetrics and gynaecology outpatients, and attending organised departmental and regional teaching sessions. However, a theoretical base is important to ensure that trainees understand why they are doing what they are doing when undertaking a particular task. The role of textbooks is essential to acquire this knowledge and to succeed in the exam.

Start planning for the exam at least 12 months before the exam date, especially if your clinical experience (post-registration training) has to be assessed for approval to sit for the exam (the application for assessment of training for entry to the MRCOG Part 2 exam is available via RCOG website). Applications must reach the RCOG examination department by the preceding 1 October for the March exam or the preceding 1 April for the September exam. Doctors in training posts can sit the MRCOG Part 2 two years after passing the MRCOG Part 1, while doctors in Trust posts (clinical fellows) can sit the exam following four years of experience in obstetrics and gynaecology (MRCOG Part 2 regulations are also available on the RCOG website).

Start preparing and reading for the exam at least six months before the exam date and use the initial month or two to gain momentum to study faster. By this stage, you should have gathered all the necessary revision aids, including relevant textbooks, guidelines (RCOG, NICE, family planning) and exam revision books. Sign up to recommended exam revision websites and work through as many questions as many times as possible, in order to learn and memorise the topics. When doing this, you will be surprised at the amount of information you process and take in.

An effective method for exam study is to ensure that information is quickly and readily accessible. Organise yourself and take the time to learn about the exam: what it is like, the type of questions likely to be encountered and the exam format. Make a list of common topics and repeated themes from the syllabus and past papers. Then three months before the exam, attend an MRCOG Part 2 theory course to speed up revision and develop knowledge further. Write down the important topic-based points in a small notebook or make revision cards. These can be used to revise topics in a short period of time several times over when the exam is approaching.

Plan ahead, make notes and revise common topics and themes, reading EMQs, MCQs, SAQs and past papers. Practice answering a wealth of questions before the exam to acquire the necessary knowledge and identify any gaps in learning. The main emphasis is on reading the question and answering each one carefully. A week of study leave before the exam is ideal for revision purposes and make sure you are not on call the day before the exam. Take note of the time and place of your exam, and arrive on time to avoid the added pressure of running late (remember you will not be allowed to sit for the exam if you arrive late).

To ensure success in the exam, it is important to develop and expand knowledge beyond the basics of the syllabus. A brief list of RCOG recommended textbooks and guidelines is given below:

MRCOG and Beyond series: http://www.rcog.org.uk/catalog/rcog-press/mrcog-and-beyond

RCOG Green-top Guidelines (all): http://www.rcog.org.uk/guidelines

Non-RCOG guidelines, e.g. The Faculty of Sexual & Reproductive Healthcare: www.fsrh.ord

NICE guidelines in obstetrics and gynaecology (all): http://www.nice.org.uk

The Obstetrician & Gynaecologist, published four times a year. The MRCOG Part 2 SAQs are set six months prior to the set date for the exam. Therefore, read the issues covering at least three years prior to this period.

Luesley DM and Baker PN. Obstetrics and gynaecology: an evidence-based text for MRCOG (2nd edn). London: Hodder Arnold, 2010.

To help save time when preparing for the MRCOG exam and to encourage trainees to broaden knowledge on each topic, we have provided further reading (current key textbooks and journal articles) after every answer or groups of answers.

SAQs, EMQs and MCQs

Short answer questions (SAQs)

The exam comprises four SAQs and you will get approximately 26 minutes to answer each one. Each SAQ is divided into three- or four-part questions and marks are divided according to complexity. It is important to note that the writing space for each answer is limited (two sides of A4-size paper) and paper is not replaced in the event of mistakes. Therefore, spend the first two to four minutes planning the answer by logical thinking rather than impulsive writing. Write down the key words from the question and plan each component of the essay answer in order of priority so that you do not miss any important marks when writing the final answer onto the main sheet (do not just write everything you know, be specific to the question that is asked). You can write the plan on the coloured paper provided in the exam. Then start writing the actual answer, which should be written on the basis of the essay plan. The systematic approach described in this book will help to ensure that important facts and vital information, which need to be reproduced in the exam, are not forgotten. This method is recommended when practising SAQs prior to the exam and during the actual exam, to help score the maximum marks. The RCOG recommends that the answers should be written in the given space for each subdivision of the question. If you write anything outside this given space, you will be wasting time and will not gain any marks. The examiner will ignore written text in the non-designated areas.

The exam is a test of knowledge and clinical experience in Obstetrics and Gynaecology at ST5 level or Year 3 specialist registrars (the best care to patients with the best available evidence after considering the resources and setting). If you are not certain about an answer, consider a patient you have discussed with a senior colleague or have managed in the past, in order to answer the question.

Marks are awarded for legible writing, concise answers and good coherent English. Read and understand the question before proceeding to plan the answer. Familiarise yourself with the different terminologies used to frame the questions. These include the words 'discuss' (write in detail), 'debate' (list pros and cons), 'evaluate' (put a value on something), 'justify' (proving something to be reasonable or right for that particular scenario or patient), 'critically appraise the treatment' (treat as well as appraise the treatment) and 'appraise' (to assess the value of something).

Answer all the questions. You are likely to fail the exam if you fail to answer one of the SAQs or if you answer a SAQ incorrectly. Spend an equal amount of time answering each question and try not to leave difficult questions to the end, when you will not have time to think intelligently and quickly. Most examiners suggest answering the questions in numerical order. Do not spend a disproportionate amount of time on one question.

Examiners discuss the answers with other examiners before they start marking papers. Marks can be deducted for unsafe or dangerous statements regarding patient care or management. So be careful, do not write something of which you are not really sure.

Extended matching questions (EMQs)

Papers 1 and 2 consist of 90 EMQs. Each EMQ presents up to five stems with 10–14 options. To answer the EMQ, match the stem (typically a statement or clinical scenario) with one of the 10–14 options available. The options are presented in alphabetical order and not all the options may be used. However, a single option may be used more than once. The questions are of a more practical nature than scientific, and the main focus is on the MRCOG Part 2 syllabus. Therefore you are likely to fail if you do not have the necessary knowledge or clinical experience before sitting the exam.

When answering EMQs, formulate an answer in your head before going through the 10–14 options and then look for the right answer. This will save time and avoid confusion. Sometimes you may not be sure between two similar options. In this case, choose the most likely option. If you do not know the answer, start eliminating the options one by one until you get a suitable option which seems like a close fit. Occasionally, you may not have any clue about the answer or lack appropriate knowledge about the topic. If this is the case, relax and take a logical approach to make an educated guess. There is no negative marking for EMQs.

Finally, remember to read each question carefully. The question may seem familiar but it may not be exactly the question you read before, for instance the framing of the question may be different.

Multiple choice questions (MCQS)

Papers 1 and 2 consist of 240 MCQs. To answer MCQs, a good theoretical knowledge of obstetrics and gynaecology is required. Each MCQ is made up of five stems (statements), which must each be answered true or false. Marks are given for answering stems correctly. However, there is no negative marking or penalty if any option is answered incorrectly. Remember to answer all the questions.

Make sure you do not leave any questions unanswered as it is difficult to come back later owing to time constraints. If you have time at the end, it is worth going back and reading through the difficult questions to check they are answered correctly. It is important not to get any answers out of sync.

Taking the exam

Finally, remember this is your exam. Take a calm and collected approach, and be positive.

Ability is what you're capable of doing. Motivation determines what you do. Attitude determines how well you do it.

Lou Holtz

Good luck for the exam!

Rekha Wuntakal

Section A

MCQs

Chapter 1

Adolescent gynaecology

1. **With regards to complete androgen insensitivity syndrome:**
   A   Phenotypically they have male appearance
   B   The karyotype in this condition is 46XY
   C   The breast development is normal
   D   It is inherited as Y-linked trait
   E   There is insensitivity to androgens secreted by the testis

2. **A woman with Mayer–Rokitansky–Küster–Hauser syndrome:**
   A   Has a female genotype
   B   Has a male phenotype
   C   May have associated renal abnormalities
   D   Has normal development of secondary sexual characteristics
   E   May have associated skeletal abnormalities

3. **The following are causes of delayed puberty:**
   A   Constitutional
   B   Coeliac disease
   C   Turner syndrome
   D   Congenital hypogonadotrophic hypogonadism
   E   Cystic fibrosis

4. **Precocious puberty:**
   A   Is defined as onset of puberty after 10 years
   B   Is associated with encephalitis
   C   Is associated with McCune–Albright syndrome
   D   Has been associated with exogenous administration of oestrogens
   E   Is associated with Cushing disease

5. **The following are true with regards to normal puberty in females:**
   A   The first physical sign of puberty in females is growth of pubic hair
   B   Adrenarche precedes gonadarche by approximately 3 years
   C   Most girls begin to menstruate when their bone age is between 12 and 13 years
   D   The apocrine glands in the axilla start to function at the time when axillary hair is appearing
   E   Breast development usually occurs at around 10.0–12.5 years of age

6. **The following are causes of primary amenorrhoea:**
    A   Familial
    B   Kallman syndrome
    C   Hyperprolactinaemia
    D   Androgen insensitivity syndrome
    E   Thyroid dysfunction

Answers

1. **A False.** Individuals are phenotypically normal and external genitalia appear female.

   B True. In view of the 46XY karyotype, removal of gonadal tissue is suggested at or after puberty to prevent malignant transformation (seen in 5% of cases).

   C True. There is absence of axillary and pubic hair.

   D False. It is inherited as an X-linked trait (the androgen receptor is located on the short arm of the X chromosome).

   E True. The testis is present and secretes androgens. The defect is at the receptor level (partial or complete insensitivity) and male secondary sexual features therefore fail to develop.

   Critchley HOD, Horne A, Munro K. Chapter 16: Amenorrhoea and oligomenorrhoea, and hypothalamic–pituitary dysfunction. In: Shaw RW, Luesley D, Monga A (eds). Gynaecology (4th edn). Edinburgh: Churchill Livingstone, 2011.
   Balen A. Chapter 14: Disorders of puberty. In: Shaw RW, Luesley D, Monga A (eds). Gynaecology (4th edn). Edinburgh: Churchill Livingstone, 2011.

2. **A True.** The incidence is approximately 1 in 5000 female births and affected babies have a normal female genotype 46XX.

   B False. The woman has a normal female phenotype.

   C True. Renal abnormalities (double ureter, horseshoe-shaped kidney) are seen in 15–40% of cases.

   D True. Due to the presence of normal functioning ovaries, the secondary sexual characteristics are well developed in females. However, the uterus is absent or is rudimentary, with associated vaginal agenesis (or short vagina with blind ending).

   E True. Skeletal abnormalities are seen in 10–20% of cases.

   Balen A. Chapter 14: Disorders of puberty. In: Shaw RW, Luesley D, Monga A (eds). Gynaecology (4th edn). Edinburgh: Churchill Livingstone, 2011.
   Critchley HOD, Horne A, Munro K. Chapter 16: Amenorrhoea and oligomenorrhoea, and hypothalamic–pituitary dysfunction. In: Shaw RW, Luesley D, Monga A (eds). Gynaecology (4th edn). Edinburgh: Churchill Livingstone, 2011.

3. **A True.** Constitutional delay in growth is the most common cause of delayed puberty.

   B True. Malabsorption can lead to delayed puberty.

   C True. Most commonly due to 45XO, which is associated with streak non-functioning gonads (hypergonadotrophic hypogonadism). Spontaneous menstruation may occur only when there is mosaicism (45XO/45XX) but it eventually results in premature ovarian failure. When performing genetic analysis one should specifically look for the presence of a Y chromosome. Its presence increases the risk of women developing gonadoblastoma, and therefore streak gonads should be removed.

D True. Usually due to gonadotrophin deficiency, e.g. Kallman syndrome (which manifests with amenorrhoea plus anosmia).

E True. Women with chronic disease may present with amenorrhoea, e.g. in tuberculosis or chronic renal failure.

Balen A. Chapter 14: Disorders of puberty. In: Shaw RW, Luesley D, Monga A (eds). Gynaecology (4th edn). Edinburgh: Churchill Livingstone, 2011.

4. **A False.** Precocious puberty is defined as puberty before 8 years of age in females and 9 years in males.

   B True. Precocious puberty is also associated with hydrocephalus, brain tumours, radiation therapy and trauma.

   C True. McCune–Albright syndrome occurs sporadically and mainly results from spontaneous activation of gonadotrophin receptors (gonadotrophin-independent activation) and increased sex steroid hormone secretion. Bone (polyostotic fibrous dysplasia) and skin (café au lait spots) are usually affected. It can also be associated with hyperparathyroidism and hyperthyroidism. Gonodatrophin levels are low.

   D True. This is usually iatrogenic.

   E True. Precocious puberty is also associated with congenital adrenal hyperplasia, female hormone-secreting ovarian tumours and adrenal tumours.

   Balen A. Chapter 14: Disorders of puberty. In: Shaw RW, Luesley D, Monga A (eds). Gynaecology (4th edn). Edinburgh: Churchill Livingstone, 2011.

5. **A False.** Breast development is the first sign of puberty in girls.

   B True. Adrenarche (growth of pubic hair) is due to adrenal androgens and usually precedes gonadarche. The sequence of events during puberty includes linear growth, breast development, adrenarche, gonadarche and menarche (occurs at 11–16 years in most women in the UK).

   C False. Most girls menstruate when their bone age is between 13 and 14 years.

   D True. The same applies to the pubic region.

   E True.

   Balen A. Chapter 14: Disorders of puberty. In: Shaw RW, Luesley D, Monga A (eds). Gynaecology (4th edn). Edinburgh: Churchill Livingstone, 2011.

6. **A True.**

   B True. Kallman syndrome is a rare syndrome occurring in 1 in 50,000 girls. It is inherited as an autosomal dominant or X-linked recessive disorder. The abnormality is due to failure of migration of GnRH neurones from the nasal pit to the hypothalamus and also due to the inability to activate pulsatile GnRH secretion. Pregnancy has been achieved with ovulation induction in these women.

   C True.

   D True.

   E True.

Amenorrhoea can be primary or secondary. Primary amenorrhoea is a delay in puberty. Investigations are usually initiated by the age of 14 years in the absence of secondary sexual features and menstrual period or when there is no menstruation within 4 years of the onset of adrenarche and thelarche.

The other causes of primary amenorrhoea include nutrition, excessive exercise, excessive weight loss (anorexia nervosa), imperforate hymen, congenital absence of uterus or vagina, Turner syndrome, hyperprolactinaemia, ovarian failure, polycystic ovary syndrome and tumours.

Critchley HOD, Horne A, Munro K. Chapter 16: Amenorrhoea and oligomenorrhoea, and hypothalamic–pituitary dysfunction. In: Shaw RW, Luesley D, Monga A (eds). Gynaecology (4th edn). Edinburgh: Churchill Livingstone, 2011.

Chapter 2

Antenatal care

1. **With regards to pregnancy-induced hypertension (PIH) and pre-eclampsia/eclampsia during pregnancy:**
   A The incidence of PIH is 14% in primigravidas
   B The incidence of PIH is approximately 6% in multigravidas
   C The incidence of PIH is increased with twin pregnancy
   D The risk of hypertensive disorder in a subsequent pregnancy is 33%
   E The risk of developing chronic hypertension is on average 23%

2. **With regards to pre-eclampsia/eclampsia and recurrence of pre-eclampsia in subsequent pregnancies:**
   A The incidence of pre-eclampsia in women carrying twins is approximately 25%
   B The incidence of recurrence of eclampsia is approximately 10%
   C Multiparous women with no history of previous pre-eclampsia have a 1% risk of developing pre-eclampsia in subsequent pregnancies
   D Multiparous women who had previous pre-eclampsia in one pregnancy, have a 15% risk of developing pre-eclampsia in subsequent pregnancies
   E Multiparous women who had previous pre-eclampsia in their previous two pregnancies, have a 30% risk of developing pre-eclampsia in subsequent pregnancies

3. **With regards to pre-eclampsia and recurrence of pre-eclampsia in subsequent pregnancies:**
   A The overall recurrence rate of pre-eclampsia in subsequent pregnancies is around 18%
   B For women who had pre-eclampsia in their first pregnancy, the risk of developing pre-eclampsia is approximately 15% in their second pregnancy
   C For women who had pre-eclampsia in their previous two pregnancies, the risk of developing pre-eclampsia is 32% in subsequent pregnancies
   D The rate of recurrence of pre-eclampsia is approximately 10% if a primigravida had pre-eclampsia at term in a previous pregnancy
   E The recurrence of pre-eclampsia is almost 40% if a woman had pre-eclampsia in a previous pregnancy before 30 weeks of gestation

4. **With regards to eclampsia during pregnancy:**
   A The incidence of eclampsia is 1 in 10,000 pregnancies
   B The incidence of recurrent eclampsia is approximately 10%
   C Eclampsia carries a risk of 2% maternal mortality
   D The risk of neonatal death is 34 in 1000 live births

E   Thirty-eight per cent of eclampsia cases occur before hypertension and proteinuria are documented

5. **With regards to haemolysis, elevated liver entymes and low platelets (HELLP) syndrome:**

A   The incidence of HELLP is 2% of those with pre-eclampsia/eclampsia
B   The rate of recurrent HELLP syndrome in subsequent pregnancies is 4%
C   HELLP syndrome is associated with 2–4% maternal mortality
D   Women who had HELLP syndrome in a previous pregnancy have a 55% risk of developing pre-eclampsia in subsequent pregnancies
E   Burr cells and polychromasia on peripheral smear are indicative of haemolysis

6. **With regards to thrombotic thrombocytopenic purpura (TTP) during pregnancy:**

A   It is characterised by aplastic anaemia
B   It may present with seizures
C   It may present with fever
D   The peripheral blood smear shows fragmented red blood cells
E   The peripheral blood smear shows reticulocytosis

7. **With regards to haemolytic uremic syndrome (HUS) during pregnancy:**

A   Renal failure is less severe in HUS than TTP
B   Thrombocytopenia and bleeding are more marked in HUS compared to TTP
C   HUS is associated with neurological symptoms but is less severe than TTP
D   HUS is characterised by microangiopathic haemolytic anaemia
E   A history of viral infection usually precedes the HUS disease

8. **With regards to acute fatty liver of pregnancy (AFLP):**

A   It is a fatal disease if not timely treated
B   It may progress to fulminant hepatic failure rapidly
C   Serum antithrombin III levels are increased
D   Blood glucose levels are very high
E   It may present with disseminated intravascular coagulation

9. **Complications of HELLP syndrome are:**

A   Acute renal failure
B   Hepatic rupture
C   Massive hepatic necrosis
D   Subcapsular liver haematoma
E   Placental abruption

10. **With regards to herpes simplex virus (HSV):**

A   Caesarean section should be considered if the primary herpes infection occurs within 6 weeks of delivery
B   Caesarean section is recommended if recurrent herpes occurs within 6 weeks of delivery
C   Herpes infection in the neonates is usually caused by primary herpes infection in the mother

D Caesarean section should be undertaken in women with active genital herpes presenting 4 hours following rupture of membranes

E In women developing primary genital herpes during pregnancy, oral acyclovir can be used for treatment during pregnancy

11. **With regards to anti-D administration and rhesus (Rh) isoimmunisation:**

A The sensitisation occurs in about 15% of rhesus (RhD)-negative women during pregnancy

B The standard dose which is normally given following delivery will cover a feto-maternal haemorrhage (FMH) of 50 mL

C Anti-D is required following medical termination of an 8-week missed miscarriage of RhD-negative women

D The National Institute of Health and Clinical Excellence (NICE) recommends 1500 IU of anti-D immunoglobulin to sensitised RhD-negative women at 28 and 34 weeks of pregnancy

E Intramuscular anti-D injection is best given into the gluteal region

12. **With regards to women with type 2 diabetes mellitus during pregnancy:**

A It can be associated with hypoglycaemic episodes during the first trimester

B It is associated with increased risk of miscarriage

C It is associated with a 50-fold increase in the incidence of congenital abnormalities compared to the general population

D It is associated with increased risk of pre-eclampsia

E It is associated with increased risk of postoperative infection

13. **With regards to the transfusion of red blood cells, blood products and platelets in pregnant women:**

A When there are no irregular antibodies in the blood, group-specific compatible blood can be provided within 10 minutes plus transport time

B In an extreme situation or if the blood group is unknown, O RhD-positive red cells should be given

C Cryoprecipitate and fresh frozen plasma (FFP) should ideally be of the same group as the recipient

D Anti-D prophylaxis is essential if a RhD-negative woman receives RhD-positive FFP or cryoprecipitate

E RhD-negative women can receive RhD-positive platelets

14. **With regards to varicella during pregnancy:**

A The incubation period of the virus is 8–10 days

B Varicella zoster IgG is effective when given up to 20 days after contact

C Women who are exposed to chickenpox should have a blood test for varicella IgG to confirm this before receiving any treatment

D The risk of fetal varicella before 20 weeks of gestation is around 2%

E The risk of spontaneous miscarriage is significantly high if varicella develops in the first trimester of pregnancy

15. **The following coagulation factors are increased during pregnancy:**

    A   Factor II
    B   Factor VII
    C   Factor VI
    D   Factor X
    E   Factor VIII

16. **With regards to maternal thrombocytopenia:**

    A   During pregnancy, the most frequent cause is gestational thrombocytopenia (GT)
    B   The second common cause of thrombocytopenia during pregnancy is immunity related
    C   Immune causes account for 20% of maternal thrombocytopenia
    D   Fetus is affected if maternal platelet count is less than 100×10^9/L and the diagnosis is GT
    E   Maternal platelet count returns to normal within 6 hours of delivery

17. **With regards to megaloblastic anaemia of pregnancy:**

    A   It has a recognised association with sub-acute combined degeneration of the spinal cord
    B   It can be excluded if the mean corpuscular volume is less than 90 μm^3
    C   It is associated with an increased incidence of pre-eclampsia
    D   It responds to treatment with pyridoxine
    E   It is more common in multiple than in singleton pregnancies

18. **Characteristic features of megaloblastic anaemia of pregnancy include:**

    A   The fall in haemoglobin level is more rapid when compared to microcytic anaemia
    B   A prompt response to hydroxycobalamin
    C   An associated histamine fast achlorhydria
    D   It resolves spontaneously after delivery
    E   Circulating antibodies to gastric parietal cells

19. **With regards to immune thrombocytopenia and pregnancy:**

    A   It accounts for 50% of maternal thrombocytopenia
    B   Thrombotic thrombocytopenia purpura is the most common cause of immune thrombocytopaenia
    C   Vaginal delivery is allowed if platelet count is more than 50×10^9/L
    D   Epidural anaesthesia can be given if the platelet count is more than 50×10^9/L and less than 80×10^9/L
    E   High dose intravenous immunoglobulin can be used in treatment

20. **With regards to iron metabolism:**

    A   About 30% of total body iron is usually incorporated in haemoglobin
    B   Iron storage is generally in macrophages
    C   Haemosiderin accounts for 65% of storage iron in the body
    D   The ferritin molecule contains iron in ferrous state
    E   Ferritin is a protein

21. **The following conditions during pregnancy increase the risk of placental abruption:**
    A Spontaneous rupture of membranes at term
    B Pre-eclampsia
    C Precipitate labour
    D Fetal growth restriction
    E Previous postpartum haemorrhage

22. **With regards to phaeochromocytoma:**
    A Adrenaline is the predominant hormone secreted by this tumour
    B Ninety per cent of tumours are located outside the adrenal glands
    C Paroxysmal flushing of the skin is a characteristic feature
    D Treatment with beta adrenergic blocking agents is adequate for care during pregnancy
    E The condition is responsible for 10% of cases of eclampsia in the UK

23. **With regards to thyroid hormones:**
    A Plasma concentrations of T4 are equal to those of T3
    B Thyrotrophin-releasing hormone is a decapeptide
    C Thyroid-stimulating hormone (TSH) stimulates both synthesis and release of hormones by the thyroid gland
    D TSH is secreted by the posterior pituitary gland
    E Negative feedback by T4 and T3 acts chiefly on posterior pituitary

24. **With regards to thyrotoxicosis during pregnancy:**
    A TSH excess is the most common cause of thyrotoxicosis
    B Antibodies with TSH receptor stimulating properties are frequently found
    C Relatively little colloid is seen on histological examination of the thyroid gland
    D Thyroid gland activity may be patchy
    E Maternal thyroid hormones cross placenta and hence cause fetal thyrotoxicosis

25. **With regards to carbimazole therapy:**
    A Carbimazole therapy can cause agranulocytosis
    B Rashes are a common side effect
    C It enhances the binding of iodine to tryptamine
    D Combination with thyroxine administration is routinely used during pregnancy
    E It should be used at regular intervals during the day to achieve a consistent therapeutic effect

26. **With regards to hyperthyroidism in pregnant women:**
    A Radioactive iodine treatment can be used in the second trimester following organogenesis
    B Thyroid surgery is absolutely contraindicated during pregnancy
    C Hyperthyroidism may be associated with fetal goitre

    D   The serum concentration of thyroid hormone binding globulins are decreased during pregnancy

    E   Propylthiouracil is not secreted in breast milk

27. **Systemic lupus erythematosus (SLE):**

    A   Is an autoimmune disease

    B   Has bad prognosis in women with pre-existing renal disease during pregnancy

    C   Increases the risk of fetal loss

    D   Increases the risk of pre-eclampsia

    E   Increases the risk of structural fetal abnormalities

28. **The criteria for diagnosis of antiphospholipid antibody syndrome (APAS) include:**

    A   The history of current or past arterial thrombosis

    B   The history of current or past venous thrombosis

    C   The presence of antiphospholipid antibodies on a single occasion

    D   The presence of lupus anticoagulant on more than one occasion at least 6 weeks apart

    E   Previous history of miscarriage due to blighted ovum on two occasions

29. **With regards to fetal macrosomia during pregnancy:**

    A   It is defined as the estimated fetal weight greater than the 50th centile

    B   It is associated with high maternal blood glucose levels after meals

    C   It is associated with increased risk of shoulder dystocia

    D   It is an indication for induction of labour in non-diabetic women

    E   It is an indication for early delivery in diabetic women

30. **With regards to diabetic ketoacidosis:**

    A   It is associated with increased risk of fetal loss

    B   It is more common in women with gestational diabetes

    C   It is associated with fetal heart rate abnormalities which is shown on cardiotocograph (CTG)

    D   It is associated with fetal hypoxia

    E   It is associated with increased maternal morbidity

31. **Dating scans during the first trimester of pregnancy have the following uses:**

    A   To determine chorionicity in twin pregnancies

    B   To identify fetal abnormalities like anencephaly

    C   To measure nuchal translucency

    D   To determine viability

    E   To measure the number of fetuses

32. **With regards to sickle cell disease in pregnancy:**

    A   The fetus has a 50% chance of having sickle cell disease if the mother and father are carriers

    B   Prenatal diagnosis is possible in the first trimester by undertaking chorionic villous biopsy

C   Pulmonary hypertension in these women increases the risk of maternal morbidity and maternal mortality

D   A tricuspid regurgitant jet velocity >2.5 m/s on echocardiography is associated with increased risk of pulmonary hypertension

E   Women with sickle cell disease during pregnancy are at risk of developing pyelonephritis

33. **In pregnancy, smoking increases the risk of:**

A   Placental abruption

B   Placenta praevia

C   Bleeding in early pregnancy

D   Bleeding in late pregnancy

E   Premature delivery

34. **With regards to prolactin-producing adenomas and pregnancy:**

A   In women with prolactinomas during pregnancy, measuring prolactin levels is reliable for monitoring tumour regression

B   Prolactinomas may enlarge during pregnancy and cause symptoms

C   It is better to avoid pregnancy until treated and cured

D   Breastfeeding is not contraindicated

E   Prolactin levels can be difficult to interpret in breastfeeding mothers

35. **With regards to iron deficiency anaemia and pregnancy:**

A   The first laboratory change in iron deficiency anaemia is low serum ferritin

B   Transferrin receptor gives a true reflection of tissue iron deficiency

C   Serum transferrin receptor increases in iron deficiency anaemia

D   The rise in serum transferrin receptor precedes the reduction in mean corpuscular volume (MCV)

E   The rise in serum transferrin receptor precedes the reduction in erythrocyte protoporphyrin

36. **With regards to megaloblastic anaemia during pregnancy:**

A   Vitamin B12 deficiency is the most common cause of megaloblastic anaemia during pregnancy

B   It is rarely due to folate deficiency during pregnancy

C   The cause of megaloblastic anaemia is dietary folate deficiency in one-third of all pregnant women in the world

D   Premature delivery decreases the risk of folate deficiency in the neonate when the mother is deficient in folate

E   Dietary deficiency is still the commonest cause because folate is rapidly destroyed by cooking

37. **The following situations precipitate sickling crisis in women with sickle cell disease during pregnancy:**

A   Lower respiratory tract infection

B   Dehydration

C   Acidosis

    D   Hypoxia

    E   Oxytocin use in labour

38. With regards to inflammatory bowel disease and pregnancy:

    A   The presence of active disease at conception almost doubles the rate of miscarriage

    B   Relapse is more common in the third trimester although it may occur at any time

    C   The disease should be optimised before pregnancy and contraception should be advised if the disease is active

    D   A daily oral intake of 0.5 mg folic acid is recommended if the terminal ileum is involved

    E   Caesarean section should be reserved for obstetric indications

39. With regards to listeriosis:

    A   It is usually self-limiting during pregnancy

    B   It is caused by gram–positive organisms

    C   It is more common in the third trimester of pregnancy

    D   It may present with flu-like symptoms

    E   It is more severe in immunocompromised women

40. With regards to diabetes mellitus in pregnancy:

    A   It increases the risk of fetal organomegaly including the brain

    B   It increases the risk of aneuploidy in the fetus

    C   It increases the risk of miscarriage in women with well-controlled type 2 diabetes

    D   It increases the risk of hyperglycaemia in the neonate

    E   The insulin used to treat diabetes crosses the placenta easily

41. With regards to rhesus blood group and antibodies:

    A   The presence of 'e' antigen determines whether an individual is rhesus positive or negative

    B   The primary response to fetal D antigen exposure is mainly formation of IgM antibodies

    C   Fetomaternal haemorrhage is the commonest cause of maternal sensitisation

    D   The longer the interval between exposures the higher the quantity of antibody produced and risk of severe fetal disease

    E   ABO antigens are strongly expressed by fetal red cells at 4 weeks

42. With regards to rhesus isoimmunisation and anti-D immunoglobulin administration:

    A   The sensitisation occurs in about 5% of Rh-negative women during pregnancy

    B   The standard dose which is normally given following delivery will cover a fetomaternal haemorrhage of 100 mL

    C   Anti-D should be administered following medical termination of an eight-week missed miscarriage of Rh-negative women

D   NICE recommends 1000 IU of anti-D immunoglobulin to non-sensitised Rh-negative women at 28 and 34 weeks of pregnancy

E   Intramuscular anti-D injection is best given in the deltoid area

43. With regards to gestational diabetes:

A   It recurs in subsequent pregnancies (30–40%)

B   Maternal hyperglycaemia in gestational diabetes is not associated with fetal acidaemia

C   Women generally are asymptomatic and develop gestational diabetes in the second or third trimester

D   Random blood glucose and glycosylated haemoglobin tests during pregnancy are regarded to have a high sensitivity for a screening test for gestational diabetes (GDM)

E   GDM in mother is not associated with increased birth weight of the baby

44. With regards to SLE disease flare:

A   Pregnancy decreases the likelihood of disease flare

B   Flare is more likely to occur if there has been active disease more than 12 months prior to getting pregnant

C   Flare is less likely to occur in the immediate postpartum period

D   Kidney involvement (nephropathy) may manifest for the first time during pregnancy

E   Prophylactic steroids given during pregnancy prevent the disease flare-up

45. The following haematological and laboratory findings are associated with disease activity in SLE during pregnancy:

A   Megaloblastic anaemia

B   Decreased erythrocyte sedimentation rate (ESR)

C   Increased in complement levels

D   Increase in C-reactive protein levels

E   Thrombocythemia

46. The following antiepileptic drugs and anomalies are correctly matched:

A   Sodium valproate – cleft palate

B   Carbamazepine – neural tube defect

C   Phenytoin – neural tube defect

D   Lamotrigine – isolated cleft palate

E   Phenytoin – cardiac defects

Answers

1. A True.

    B True.

    C True.

    D True.

    E True.

    Hypertensive disorders are seen in 7–10% of all pregnancies. Out of these, PIH-related disorders (pre-eclampsia/eclampsia) account for 70% and chronic hypertension accounts for 30% of hypertensive disorders in pregnancy. The incidence is higher in young primigravidas compared to multiparous woman and increases with age (over 35 years). The incidence is higher in women who carry twins and women who also have a past history of PIH.

    The American College of Obstetricians and Gynaecologists (ACOG) classifies hypertensive disorders as follows: (a) PIH (pre-eclampsia/eclampsia); (b) chronic hypertension preceding pregnancy (any cause); and (c) chronic hypertension (any cause) with superimposed pre-eclampsia and eclampsia.

    PIH is defined as hypertension occurring after 20 weeks of pregnancy in the absence of proteinuria or any other feature of pre-eclampsia; pre-eclampsia is defined as elevation in blood pressure ($\geq$140/90 mmHg) after 20 weeks of pregnancy with proteinuria (300 mg/L or more protein in a 24-h urine collection), with or without oedema. The main pathology of PIH is vasospasm and endothelial injury. It can affect almost every organ in the body, depending on the severity of pre-eclampsia.

    In a normal pregnancy there is an expansion of total blood volume by 50% by the end of the second trimester. There is more expansion of the plasma compared to red cell mass, leading to physiological anaemia. In PIH there is a 16% reduction in the plasma volume. In the absence of haemorrhage women are well compensated, but in the presence of haemorrhage there is further shrinkage of intravascular volume and this would be detrimental if not timely replaced.

    The following changes occur in pre-eclampsia as a result of vasospasm:

    *   increase in peripheral vascular resistance (in normal pregnancy it decreases by 25%)
    *   decrease in renal perfusion by 20%
    *   decrease in renal GFR by 32%
    *   decrease in uteroplacental perfusion by 2– to 3–fold (as a low resistance, low pressure and high flow spiral artery system is converted to a high resistance, high pressure and low flow spiral artery system)
    *   it is associated with high levels of fibronectin, low antithrombin levels and low α-2 antiplasmin levels reflecting the endothelial damage, clotting and fibrinolysis
    *   periportal haemorrhagic necrosis in the periphery of the liver lobule causes elevation of liver enzymes
    *   cerebral vasospasm causing cerebral irritation and seizures

The most common causes of death in women with pre-eclampsia are cerebral haemorrhage and adult respiratory distress syndrome (ARDS).

James D, Steer PJ, Weiner CP, Gonik B, Crowther C, Robson S (eds). High Risk Pregnancy: Management Options (4th edn). St Louis: Saunders, 2011.
Nelson-Piercy C. Handbook of Obstetric Medicine (4th edn). London: Informa Healthcare, 2010.

2. A **True.**

   B **True.**

   C **True.**

   D **True.**

   E **True.**

Mild pre-eclampsia affects up to 10% of primiparous women and severe pre-eclampsia occurs in 1% of women. Following the development of hypertension after 20 weeks, the chances of developing pre-eclampsia is 15%. This risk is related to the gestational age at presentation of PIH. The earlier the hypertension occurs, the higher the risk of developing pre-eclampsia (40% before 30 weeks and 7% after 38 weeks). PIH tends to recur in subsequent pregnancies and the incidence increases with past history of hypertensive disorders in previous pregnancies. Some women may remain hypertensive permanently following PIH or pre-eclampsia during pregnancy.

James D, Steer PJ, Weiner CP, Gonik B, Crowther C, Robson S (eds). High Risk Pregnancy: Management Options (4th edn). St Louis: Saunders, 2011.
Nelson-Piercy C. Handbook of Obstetric Medicine (4th edn). London: Informa Healthcare, 2010.

3. A **True.**

   B **True.**

   C **True.**

   D **True.**

   E **True.**

Pre-eclampsia is a pregnancy-related multisystem disorder with variable manifestations. It is common in (**Table 2.1**):

- women in their first pregnancies
- teenage pregnancies
- older women
- women with new partners
- twin pregnancies
- hydropic babies
- hydatidiform moles
- long birth interval
- women with medical disorders (pre-existing hypertension, renal disease, diabetes, SLE)
- inherited and acquired thrombophilia (antiphospholipid antibody syndrome)
- women with a family history of pre-eclampsia (mother or sister)

Table 2.1   Pregnancy-induced hypertension (PIH), pre-eclampsia, eclampsia and HELLP syndrome

PIH and pre-eclampsia/eclampsia during pregnancy

The incidence of PIH is approximately 14% in primigravidas

The incidence of PIH is approximately 6% in multigravidas

The incidence of PIH is approximately 30% in twin pregnancies

The risk of hypertensive disorder in subsequent pregnancies is approximately 33%

The risk of developing chronic hypertension is on average 23%

Pre-eclampsia in subsequent pregnancies

The incidence of pre-eclampsia in primigravida is approximately 4%

The incidence of pre-eclampsia in multigravida is approximately 2%

The longer the interval between the first and second pregnancy, the higher the risk of recurrence

Multiparous women with no history of previous pre-eclampsia have a 1% risk of developing pre-eclampsia in subsequent pregnancies

Multiparous women who had pre-eclampsia in a previous pregnancy have a 15% risk of developing pre-eclampsia in subsequent pregnancies

Multiparous women who had pre-eclampsia in two previous pregnancies have a 30% risk of developing pre-eclampsia in subsequent pregnancies

Recurrence of pre-eclampsia in subsequent pregnancies

The overall recurrent rate of pre-eclampsia in subsequent pregnancies is approximately 18%

For women who had pre-eclampsia in their first pregnancy, the risk of developing pre-eclampsia in their second pregnancy is approximately 15%

For women who had pre-eclampsia in two previous pregnancies, the risk of developing pre-eclampsia in subsequent pregnancies is approximately 32%

The earlier in gestation a woman develops pre-eclampsia, the higher the rate of recurrence of pre-eclampsia

The rate of recurrence of pre-eclampsia is approximately 10% if a primigravida had pre-eclampsia at term in her previous pregnancy

The recurrence of pre-eclampsia is almost 40% if a woman had pre-eclampsia in a previous pregnancy before 30 weeks of gestation

Eclampsia during pregnancy

The incidence of eclampsia is approximately 5 in 10,000 pregnancies

The incidence of recurrent eclampsia is approximately 10%

Eclampsia carries a risk of approximately 2% maternal mortality

The risk of neonatal death is 34 in 1000 live births

Thirty-eight per cent of instances of eclampsia occur before hypertension and proteinuria are documented

HELLP syndrome

The incidence of HELLP is 4–12% of those with pre-eclampsia/eclampsia

The rate of recurrent HELLP syndrome is 6%

The maternal mortality is 2–4% with HELLP syndrome

Women who had HELLP syndrome in a previous pregnancy have a 55% risk of developing pre-eclampsia in subsequent pregnancies

James D, Steer PJ, Weiner CP, Gonik B, Crowther C, Robson S (eds). High Risk Pregnancy: Management Options (4th edn). St Louis: Saunders, 2011.

Nelson-Piercy C. Handbook of Obstetric Medicine (4th edn). London: Informa Healthcare, 2010.

The classical signs include hypertension, proteinuria and oedema. The complications of pre-eclampsia include eclampsia, HELLP syndrome, pulmonary oedema (mortality 10%), placental abruption, cortical blindness (usually recovers following delivery), cerebral haemorrhage (associated with persistent raised systolic blood pressure of >160 mmHg and hence should not be ignored), disseminated intravascular coagulation, renal failure and hepatic failure.

There is a risk of recurrence of pre-eclampsia in subsequent pregnancies. Although the pathology is not completely known, possible theories have been described. One of the theories is inadequate invasion of the trophoblast into the myometrium past the spiral arteries. As a result the elastic media does not expand and makes it very sensitive to chemical substances. This causes decreased blood flow to the fetus and hence causes fetal growth restriction. The first part of this trophoblastic invasion occurs earlier in the pregnancy and the second wave of trophoblastic invasion occurs around 16 weeks of gestation. It is advocated that low-dose aspirin is started as early as fetal viability is confirmed in women with a previous history of early onset pre-eclampsia. Uterine artery Doppler sonography can be performed to identify notches as their presence indicates an increase in the risk of recurrent pre-eclampsia and fetal growth restriction.

4. A False.

B True.

C True.

D True.

E True.

The incidence of eclampsia reported in the UK is 4.9 in 10,000 pregnancies. It is defined as the occurrence of seizures (not caused by any coexistent neurological disease) in a woman with pre-eclampsia. However, 38% of cases occur in women before proteinuria or hypertension is documented. Overall, 38% of eclampsia occurs during the antepartum period, 18% during the intrapartum period and 44% during the postpartum period.

The main principles of management of eclampsia include:

- airway, breathing, circulation (ABC)
- control of seizures ($MgSO_4$ loading and maintenance dose)
- control of hypertension (use intravenous hydrallazine or labetalol if necessary as per unit protocol)
- stabilisation (important before delivery)
- delivery (mode of delivery depends on the gestational age and the urgency of delivery)

James D, Steer PJ, Weiner CP, Gonik B, Crowther C, Robson S (eds). High Risk Pregnancy: Management Options (4th edn). St Louis: Saunders, 2011.
Royal College of Obstetricians and Gynaecologists. Green-top Guideline No. 10A. Management of Severe Pre-Eclampsia/Eclampsia. London: RCOG Press, 2006 (reviewed 2010).
Magowan B. Churchill's Pocketbook of Obstetrics and Gynaecology (3rd edn). Edinburgh: Churchill Livingston, 2005.

5. A False.

    B False.

    C True.

    D True.

    E True.

HELLP is a complication of severe pre-eclampsia and is characterised by haemolysis, elevated liver enzymes and low platelets. It affects 4–12% of those with pre-eclampsia/eclampsia and is more common in multigravida. It may occur antepartum in 70% of patients and postpartum in 30% of patients. The overall recurrence rate in subsequent pregnancies is 20–25%.

These women may present with nausea, vomiting, epigastric or right upper quadrant pain or tenderness, raised blood pressure, proteinuria and oedema.

The laboratory criteria for diagnosis of HELLP syndrome include:

*   Haemolysis – the blood film shows burr cells, schistocytes and polychromasia. Raised bilirubin (>1.2 mg/dL) or lactate dehydrogenase (LDH) (>600 IU/L) confirms the diagnosis.
*   Elevated liver enzymes – alanine aminotransferase (AST) rises first, followed by LDH. It is associated with hepatic cell damage and parenchymal necrosis. In severe cases, HELLP syndrome is associated with bleeding extending into the subcapsular region leading to haematoma and rupture and intraperitoneal bleeding. This is associated with severe right upper quadrant pain.
*   Low platelet count (<100,000 mm^3).

The risk of placental abruption, disseminated intravascular coagulation and renal failure increases. The management principles are similar to managing a woman with severe pre-eclampsia. She should be stabilised first and then delivered. The mode of delivery depends on the gestational age and severity of HELLP.

The transfusion of blood and blood products may be necessary to correct coagulation and hypovolaemia. The recovery following delivery may be long for some women, and it should be closely monitored clinically and by doing blood tests (platelets, liver function tests [LFTs] and renal function tests [RFTs]) until the platelets are >100,000 mm^3.

James D, Steer PJ, Weiner CP, Gonik B, Crowther C, Robson S (eds). High Risk Pregnancy: Management Options (4th edn). St Louis: Saunders, 2011.
Magowan B. Churchill's Pocketbook of Obstetrics and Gynaecology (3rd edn). Edinburgh: Churchill Livingstone, 2005.

6. A False.

    B True.

    C True.

    D True.

    E True.

TTP is one of the differential diagnoses for severe pre-eclampsia during pregnancy. It is characterised by fever, neurologic symptoms (seizures, syncope, headache, paresis, visual symptoms and altered consciousness), renal abnormalities, thrombocytopenia and microangiopathic haemolytic anaemia. The cerebral symptoms are more marked than renal symptoms. The peripheral blood smear shows signs of haemolysis (fragmented red blood cells and reticulocytosis) and thrombocytopenia. This leads to elevation of the indirect serum bilirubin and lactate dehydrogenase. Serum urea and creatinine are also elevated. The treatment for this condition is plasmapheresis.

James D, Steer PJ, Weiner CP, Gonik B, Crowther C, Robson S (eds). High Risk Pregnancy: Management Options (4th edn). St Louis: Saunders, 2011.
Nelson-Piercy C. Handbook of Obstetric Medicine (4th edn). London: Informa Healthcare, 2010.

7. **A False.**

   B False.

   C True.

   D True.

   E True.

HUS is more common in children but may occur during pregnancy and the postpartum period. There is usually a history of viral infection or gastrointestinal infection. Pre-eclampsia is a differential diagnosis. HUS is characterised by microangiopathic haemolysis, thrombocytopenia, renal failure and neurological symptoms. In HUS, the neurological symptoms are less severe and renal failure is more marked and severe compared to TTP. Thrombocytopenia and bleeding are less severe than TTP.

The treatment for this condition is plasma exchange like TTP.

James D, Steer PJ, Weiner CP, Gonik B, Crowther C, Robson S (eds). High Risk Pregnancy: Management Options (4th edn). St Louis: Saunders, 2011.
Nelson-Piercy C. Handbook of Obstetric Medicine (4th edn). London: Informa Healthcare, 2010.

8. **A True.**

   B True.

   C False.

   D False.

   E True.

The estimated incidence of AFLP in the UK is 1 in 21,900 total births. Most patients are primiparous, Caucasian and under 35 years old. The gestational age at diagnosis and delivery is approximately 36 weeks (range 27–40 weeks) of gestation. It is a fatal condition if not recognised or treated. Women may present with vomiting, liver dysfunction, fulminant hepatic failure, jaundice, disseminated intravascular coagulopathy, encephalopathy, uterine and gastrointestinal bleeding. A high index of suspicion and early intervention are necessary for a better outcome. The treatment is delivery and supportive treatment in the intensive care unit.

The Swansea criteria for diagnosis of AFLP are that the six or more of the following are required in the absence of another cause:

- vomiting
- abdominal pain
- polydipsia/polyuria
- encephalopathy
- elevated bilirubin >14 µmol/L
- hypoglycaemia <4 µmol/L
- elevated urea >340 µmol/L
- leucocytosis >11 × 10^9/L
- ascites or bright liver on ultrasound scan
- elevated transaminases (alanine aminotransferase) >42 IU/L
- elevated ammonia >47 µmol/L
- renal impairment: creatinine >150 µmol/L
- coagulopathy: prothrombin time >14 s or activated partial thromboplastin time >34 s
- micro-vesicular steatosis on liver biopsy

The differential diagnoses include severe pre-eclampsia with liver involvement and HELLP syndrome.

James D, Steer PJ, Weiner CP, Gonik B, Crowther C, Robson S (eds). High Risk Pregnancy: Management Options (4th edn). St Louis: Saunders, 2011.
Nelson-Piercy C. Handbook of Obstetric Medicine (4th edn). London: Informa Healthcare, 2010.
Knight M, Nelson-Piercy C, Kurinczuk JJ, Spark P and Brocklehurs P; UK Obstetric Surveillance System. A prospective national study of acute fatty liver of pregnancy in the UK. Gut 2008;57:951–956.
Kingham JG. Swansea criteria for diagnosis of acute fatty liver of pregnancy. Gut 2010 Oct 11

9. A True.

B True.

C True.

D True.

E True.

HELLP affects 4–12% of women with pre-eclampsia and eclampsia and is more common in multiparous women. Women can present with nausea, vomiting, epigastric pain and right upper quadrant tenderness. There is elevation of the serum AST, a liver enzyme, followed by a rise in serum lactate dehydrogenase. A peripheral blood smear shows polychromasia and burr cells consistent with haemolysis. Complications of HELLP include liver failure, renal failure, subcapsular haematoma, rupture of subcapsular haematoma with intraperitoneal bleeding, placental abruption and disseminated intravascular coagulation. Management is by stabilising the woman's condition (especially coagulation and hypertension) and delivery. The incidence of recurrent HELLP in subsequent pregnancies is approximately 20–25%.

James D, Steer PJ, Weiner CP, Gonik B, Crowther C, Robson S (eds). High Risk Pregnancy: Management Options (4th edn). St Louis: Saunders, 2011.
Nelson-Piercy C. Handbook of Obstetric Medicine (4th edn). London: Informa Healthcare, 2010.
Magowan B. Churchill's Pocketbook of Obstetrics and Gynaecology (3rd edn). Edinburgh: Churchill Livingstone, 2005.

10. A **True.**

 B **False.**

 C **True.**

 D **False.**

 E **True.**

Maternal herpes can be transmitted to the fetus in the perinatal period. Neonatal infection rates are highest when the matenal infection is a primary episode and a virus is transmitted to the fetus during its transit through the birth canal. The risk of viral shedding and disseminated neonatal infection is very high and therefore caesarean section should be considered if the mother develops primary herpes within 6 weeks of delivery.

In a case of recurrent herpes, the risk to the fetus is small (3% risk with vaginal delivery) because of the passive immunity acquired from the mother, other than in a situation where there are active herpetic lesions on the genitalia during delivery. Vaginal delivery may therefore be considered if there are no active lesions and this must be balanced with the risks to the mother having a caesarean section. It should be clearly discussed and documented in the notes. Treatments are mainly supportive, in the form of pain relief and prevention of secondary infection. However, oral acyclovir (200 mg five times daily for 5 days) can be used for treatment in women with primary genital HSV and for prophylaxis in the later weeks of pregnancy to prevent recurrent herpes at delivery.

If a woman presents to the labour ward more than 4 hours following spontaneous rupture of the membranes, there is no benefit in doing a caesarean section. These women should be counselled appropriately.

Royal College of Obstetricians and Gynaecologists. Green-top Guideline No. 30. Management of Genital Herpes in Pregnancy. London: RCOG Press, 2007.

11. A **False.**

 B **False.**

 C **True.**

 D **False.**

 E **False.**

Sensitisation can occur at any time during pregnancy but is more common in the third trimester and during childbirth. It occurs in about 1% of RhD-negative women during pregnancy. NICE recommends 500 IU of anti-D immunoglobulin to non-sensitised RhD-negative women at 28 and 34 weeks of gestation or 1500 IU at 28 weeks of gestation or between 28 and 30 weeks of gestation (this depends on the product). It should be given to women following any sensitising event before delivery (e.g. external cephalic version, abdominal trauma, antepartum haemorrhage) and after medical or surgical termination (the risk of sensitisation with an unrecognised event is 10%). The administration of anti-D immunoglobulin injection is recommended for RhD-negative women following delivery. However, anti-D immunoglobulin should not be given to women who are already sensitised and have developed antibodies.

The standard dose (500 IU), which is normally given following delivery, will neutralise a fetomaternal haemorrhage (FMH) of 4 mL (Studies have shown that approximately 99% of women have an FMH of <4 mL at delivery. Of the cases where the FMH is >4 mL, 50% will have occurred during normal delivery.) For each millilitre of FMH in excess of 4 mL, a further 125 IU of anti-D immunoglobulin is necessary.

The conditions that are associated with a large FMH include:

- traumatic deliveries including caesarean section
- manual removal of the placenta
- stillbirths and fetal deaths
- abdominal trauma during the third trimester
- twin pregnancies (at delivery)
- unexplained hydrops fetalis

A Kleihauer screening test should be performed within 2 hours of delivery to identify RhD-negative women with a large FMH who require additional anti-D immunoglobulin.

A minimum dose of 250 IU is recommended for prophylaxis following sensitising events up to 19+6 weeks of gestation. For all events at or after 20 weeks of gestation, a minimum dose of 500 IU of anti-D immunoglobulin should be given and a test to identify feto-maternal haemorrhage >4 mL red cells should be performed; additional anti-D immunoglobulin should be given as required.

The intramuscular injection of anti-D immunoglobulin is best given into the deltoid muscle as injections into the gluteal region often only reach the subcutaneous tissues and absorption may be delayed. Women who have a bleeding disorder should receive anti-D immunoglobulin via the subcutaneous or intravenous route. Consent should be obtained and recorded in the case notes.

To work effectively, prophylactic anti-D immunoglobulin should be given at the earliest opportunity after the sensitising event but always within 72 h. When it is not given before 72 h, all effort should still be made to administer the anti-D immunoglobulin injection within 9–10 days; it is believed to provide some protection.

Miscarriage

- Anti-D immunoglobulin should be given to all non-sensitised RhD-negative women who have a spontaneous complete or incomplete miscarriage at or after 12+0 weeks of gestation.
- Anti-D immunoglobulin is not required for spontaneous miscarriage before 12+0 weeks of gestation, provided there is no instrumentation of the uterus.
- Anti-D immunoglobulin should be given to non-sensitised RhD-negative women undergoing surgical evacuation of the uterus, regardless of gestation.
- Anti-D immunoglobulin should be considered for non-sensitised RhD-negative women undergoing medical evacuation of the uterus, regardless of gestation.

Threatened miscarriage

- Anti-D immunoglobulin should be given to all non-sensitised RhD-negative women with a threatened miscarriage after 12+0 weeks of gestation. In women in whom bleeding continues intermittently after 12+0 weeks of gestation, anti-D immunoglobulin should be given at 6-weekly intervals.
- Anti-D immunoglobulin should be considered in non-sensitised RhD-negative women if there is heavy or repeated bleeding or associated abdominal pain as gestation approaches 12+0 weeks.

Exceptional circumstances

- In the event that RhD-positive platelets are transfused, prophylaxis against Rh alloimmunisation should be given.
- Anti-D immunoglobulin should be given to RhD-negative women of reproductive capacity who inadvertently receive a transfusion of RhD-positive blood.
- The dose should be calculated on the basis that 500 IU of anti-D immunoglobulin will suppress immunisation by 4 mL of RhD-positive red blood cells.
- Exchange transfusion may be necessary for large volumes of transfused blood.

ABO incompatibility

- Sensitisation risk is affected by the ABO blood group of the fetus, with a lower risk if it is incompatible with the mother's ABO type. It depends on the volume of feto-maternal transfusion of blood and the magnitude of the mother's immune response. The risk of sensitisation is highest in the first pregnancy and decreases with each subsequent pregnancy. Sensitisation is an irreversible process.

Royal College of Obstetricians and Gynaecologists. Green-top Guideline No. 22. The Use of anti-D Immunoglobulin for Rhesus D Prophylaxis. London: RCOG Press, 2011.
National Institute for Health and Clinical Excellence. Routine antenatal anti-D prophylaxis for women who are rhesus D negative (Technology Appraisal Guidance 156). NICE, 2008.

12. A True.

    B True.

    C False.

    D True.

    E True.

Diabetes during pregnancy is associated with increased risk of miscarriage (common in women with high HbA1C around the time of conception or the beginning of pregnancy), congenital malformations (3- to 5-fold), infections (all infections are common including genitourinary and postoperative wound infections), macrosomia (mainly related to poor diabetic control), shoulder dystocia (due to macrosomic babies), stillbirth (pathology unknown), pre-eclampsia (common in women with known renal disease or hypertension prior to pregnancy) and caesarean section. Most of these complications are related to hyperglycaemia which is toxic to the developing fetus.

On the other hand, hypoglycaemia could be dangerous to the mother; it is reported to be the most common cause of maternal deaths in diabetic women, directly or indirectly. It can occur in the first trimester because of increased vomiting, renal clearance, reduced gluconeogenesis, strict glycemic control and reduced awareness. During hypoglycaemic episodes, the insulin dose needs to be reduced and women should be given concentrated glucose solutions for emergency use. NICE advocates prescribing glucagon injection to women who have diabetes and are on insulin. Also, families and partners should be taught on how to administer glucagon.

Diabetic ketoacidosis is a medical emergency and is common in women with type 1 diabetes. It is usually diagnosed when the following are found:

- raised blood glucose
- raised urinary ketones
- reduced bicarbonate in blood

If unidentified, diabetic ketoacidosis could be life-threatening. The main aims of management are identification and prompt treatment with intravenous glucose supplementation, insulin sliding scale, potassium replacement and aggressive hydration.

Lambert K, Germain S. Pre-existing type 1 and type 2 diabetes during pregnancy. Obstet Gynaecol Reprod Med 2010; 20:353–358.

13. A True.

B False. O Rh negative red blood cells should be given.

C True.

D False.

E False.

Red cells

When there are irregular antibodies detected during pregnancy or on a previous occasion, blood must be cross-matched, as obtaining compatible blood may take several hours.

FFP and cryoprecipitate

FFP and cryoprecipitate should not be given on clinical suspicion alone unless there is a delay in obtaining blood results. In the bleeding woman with disseminated intravascular coagulation (DIC), a combination of FFP, platelets and cryoprecipitate is indicated.

The FFP and cryoprecipitate should ideally be of the same group as the recipient. If unavailable, FFP of a different ABO group is acceptable.

No anti-D prophylaxis is required if a RhD-negative woman receives RhD-positive FFP or cryoprecipitate.

Platelet

The platelet count should not be allowed to fall below 50×10^9/L in the acutely bleeding patient. A platelet transfusion trigger of 75×10^9/L is recommended to provide a margin of safety.

The platelets should ideally also be group compatible. RhD-negative women should receive RhD-negative platelets.

Royal College of Obstetricians and Gynaecologists. Green-top Guideline No. 47. Management of women who decline blood and blood products during pregnancy. London: RCOG Press, 2007.

14. A False.

    B False.

    C True.

    D True.

    E False.

The incubation period of chickenpox is 7–21 days. If the woman is not immune, it is important to perform the blood test for varicella IgG before considering giving varicella zoster immunoglobulin (VZIG) injection. For those who develop chickenpox in the first trimester, the risk of miscarriage is not increased. The risk of fetal abnormalities is 2% if the pregnant woman develops chickenpox before 20 weeks of gestation. The overall risk is higher to the fetus earlier on in the pregnancy but higher to the mother later on in the pregnancy, e.g. pneumonia (mortality 10%). The newborn baby is at risk of severe fetal varicella syndrome if the mother develops chickenpox 5 days before and 2 days after delivery (because passive immunity is not transferred to the baby).

Royal College of Obstetricians and Gynaecologists. Green-top Guideline No. 13. Chicken pox in pregnancy. London: RCOG Press, 2007.

15. A **True.** Plasma fibrinogen is markedly increased (it almost doubles in late pregnancy compared to non-pregnant women) during pregnancy, while plasma fibrinolytic activity is decreased (it remains low during labour and normalises within 1 hour after delivery of placenta). The latter is thought to be due to the effect of placental derived plasminogen activator inhibitor type 2.

    B **True.**

    C **False.**

    D **True.**

    E **True.**

During pregnancy, there is little change in antithrombin III levels while there is a fall in protein S and rise in protein C levels from the second trimester onwards.

Letsky E, Murphy MF, Ramsay JE, Walker I. Haemorrhagic Disease and Hereditary Bleeding Disorders. London: RCOG Press, 2005.

16. A **True.** GT is a diagnosis of exclusion. Although its pathogenesis is unclear, it is thought to be due to haemodilution and increased non-immune platelet destruction. The platelet count starts to fall in the second trimester and there is a more pronounced drop at the time of delivery. The platelet count in this condition is in the range of $70–150 \times 10^9/L$.

   B False.

   C False. Immune causes account for only 4%.

   D False. GT has no clinical impact on mother or fetus.

   E False. Maternal platelet count returns to normal within 6 weeks of delivery.

   The overall incidence of maternal thrombocytopenia is 6–7%. GT of pregnancy is the most common cause of maternal thrombocytopenia (74%), followed by hypertensive disorders (21%, pre-eclampsia and HELLP) and immune causes (4%).

   Idiopathic autoimmune thrombocytopenia is the most common immune-related cause of thrombocytopenia, followed by drug-related and some associated with human immunodeficiency virus (HIV) infection.

   DIC is a rare cause of thrombocytopenia and is usually due to pre-eclampsia, placental abruption, amniotic fluid embolism or retention of dead fetus.

   Letsky E, Murphy MF, Ramsay JE, Walker I. Haemorrhagic disease and Hereditary Bleeding Disorders. London: RCOG Press, 2005.
   Myers B. Thrombocytopenia in pregnancy. The Obstetrician and Gynaecologist 2009; 11:177–183.

17. **A True.**

   B False. In the early stages, the only signs may be megaloblasts in the bone marrow and the presence of hypersegmented neutrophil polymorph nucleus in the peripheral blood.

   C False. There is no association with pre-eclampsia.

   D False. The condition responds to treatment with folic acid and vitamin B12.

   E True.

   Folic acid is necessary for both cell growth and division. The more active an organ in its growth and reproduction, the more dependent it is on the turnover and supply of folic acid coenzymes. Hence, epithelial linings and bone marrow are at risk. The need for folic acid increases during pregnancy to meet the demands of the fetus, placenta, maternal red cell mass and maternal organs which hypertrophy. Folic acid is actively transferred to the fetus through the placenta even when there is maternal deficiency. Also, plasma clearance by the kidneys is more than doubled early in the pregnancy (8 weeks of gestation) but this does not contribute to major loss.

   Megaloblastic anaemia during pregnancy is almost invariably due to folic acid deficiency. The WHO recommends oral intake of 800 μg folic acid during pregnancy and 600 μg during lactation to meet the requirements of pregnancy. Megaloblastic anaemia due to dietary deficiency of folic acid occurs in about one third of all pregnant women in the world despite intake of natural foods. This is attributed to loss of folic acid while cooking.

   Fetuses are also at risk of megaloblastic anaemia especially when they are born prematurely and the mother is deficient in folic acid. Folic acid deficiency is associated with neural tube defects, cleft palate and harelip.

Folic acid supplementation in UK

- Standard dose: folic acid (400 µg) preconception and up to 12 weeks of gestation.
- Higher dose: folic acid (5 mg) for women who are diabetic and are on antiepileptic medication.
- Folic acid (5 mg) should also be taken by obese women (joint RCOG–CMACE guideline, 2010).

James D, Steer PJ, Weiner CP, Gonik B, Crowther C, Robson S (eds). High Risk Pregnancy: Management Options (4th edn). St Louis: Saunders, 2011.

Royal College of Obstetricians and Gynaecologists. Periconceptional folic acid and food fortification in the prevention of neural tube defects. SAQ Paper 4. RCOG, 2003.

18. A **True.**

B **False.** A prompt response to hydroxycobalamin is a feature of B12 deficiency. Megaloblastic anaemia of pregnancy is mostly due to folic acid deficiency.

C **False.** It is a feature of B12 deficiency.

D **False.**

E **False.** It is a feature of B12 deficiency.

The diagnosis of true folic acid deficiency during pregnancy is difficult. Red cell folic acid levels are thought to give a better indication of overall body tissue levels than serum folic acid levels. However, by the time these changes occur, there may be a delay as the turnover of red cells is slow. Megaloblastic anaemia can be suspected when the improvement in anaemia is not achieved after adequate iron therapy.

In a non-pregnant woman, the hallmark of megaloblastic anaemia is macrocytosis (identified by raised MCV in the blood film). During pregnancy, this may be the norm and can be masked by iron deficiency. There will be hypersegmentation of neutrophil polymorph nucleus but this can be seen in pure iron deficiency. During pregnancy, the diagnosis may be made purely on morphological grounds.

James D, Steer PJ, Weiner CP, Gonik B, Crowther C, Robson S (eds). High Risk Pregnancy: Management Options (4th edn). St Louis: Saunders, 2011.

19. A **False.**

B **False.** The most common cause is due to idiopathic autoimmune thrombocytopenia. The other causes are related to drugs and HIV infection.

C **True.**

D **False.** Epidural anaesthesia should be avoided if the platelet count is less than 80×10^9/L as this can cause epidural haematoma due to risk of bleeding.

E **True.**

Immune thrombocytopenia

The British Committee for Standards in Haematology on behalf of the British Society for Haematology recommend the following steps in managing women with immune thrombocytopenia.

If the platelet count is >50 × 10⁹/L, it is advisable to monitor the platelet count every 2 weeks. If the platelet count is <50 × 10⁹/L (risk of bleeding), it is suggested to increase the platelet count to >50 × 10⁹/L for vaginal delivery and >80 × 10⁹/L for caesarean section. The therapeutic options to raise the platelet count include (a) corticosteroids (to reduce antibody synthesis and inhibit destruction of antibody coated platelets in reticuloendothelial system) and (b) intravenous immunoglobulin.

Steroids are usually used in the third trimester for short periods to raise the platelet count before delivery if necessary. If there is a need for high dose or prolonged therapy with steroids, intravenous immunoglobulin should be considered (the response rate is 80% and the duration of response is 2–3 weeks).

It is difficult to predict the fetal platelet count from the maternal platelet count. During labour, invasive procedures such as fetal blood sampling, application of fetal scalp electrode and use of ventouse delivery should be avoided. Caesarean section is recommended only for obstetric indications. Cord blood should be taken to measure the baby's platelet count.

Letsky E, Murphy MF, Ramsay JE, Walker I. Haemorrhagic Disease and Hereditary Bleeding Disorders. London: RCOG Press, 2005.
Myers B. Thrombocytopenia in pregnancy. The Obstetrician and Gynaecologist 2009; 11:177–183.

20. A **False.** 80% of total body iron is usually incorporated in haemoglobin.

   B **True.**

   C **False.**

   D **False.** The ferritin molecule contains iron in ferric state.

   E **True.**

The steps in iron deficiency include depletion of iron stores, reduction in the serum iron, followed lastly by a decrease in the circulating haemoglobin. Serum iron with the total binding iron capacity (TIBC is normally one-third saturated with iron) is an estimation of transferrin saturation. A serum iron level less than 12 μmol/L, serum ferritin level less than 12 μg/L and TIBC saturation of less than 15% indicate iron deficiency during pregnancy. Ferritin is not affected by ingestion of iron and reflects the iron stores accurately. Erythroblast protoporphyrin rises when there is deficient supply of iron to the red blood cells.

James D, Steer PJ, Weiner CP, Gonik B, Crowther C, Robson S (eds). High Risk Pregnancy: Management Options (4th edn). St Louis: Saunders, 2011.

21. A **False.** Prolonged premature rupture of membranes increases the risk of placental abruption.

   B **True.**

   C **True.**

   D **False.**

   E **False.**

The incidence of placental abruption is 0.5–1.8%.

The following conditions are associated with increased risk of placental abruption:

- raised serum alpha fetoprotein
- cocaine abuse
- cigarette smoking
- advanced maternal age
- high parity
- thrombophilia
- abdominal trauma
- sudden uterine decompression

The risk of recurrent abruption is 8–17% after one abruption and 25% following two abruptions. The incidence of precipitate labour is 2% in women with spontaneous labours. It is defined as expulsion of the fetus within 3 hours of the commencement of contractions. Labours of 3 hours or less in duration are strongly associated with placental abruption but not with major maternal and fetal morbidity.

Letsky E, Murphy MF, Ramsay JE, Walker I. Haemorrhagic Disease and Hereditary Bleeding Disorders. London: RCOG Press, 2005.
National Institute for Health and Clinical Excellence. NICE guideline on induction of labour (CG70). NICE, 2008.
Magowan B. Churchill's Pocketbook of Obstetrics and Gynaecology (3rd edn). Edinburgh: Churchill Livingstone, 2005.

22. A **False.** It is noradrenaline.

   B **False.** Only 10% of tumours are located outside the adrenal glands.

   C **False.** Paroxysmal pallor of the skin is a characteristic feature.

   D **False.** Both alpha and beta-blocker drugs are necessary for the initial treatment of phaeochromocytoma followed by the continued use of beta-blockers.

   E **False.**

   Phaeochromocytoma is a rare tumour of the adrenal gland. It arises from chromaffin cells of the adrenal medulla or sympathetic nervous tissue. During pregnancy, the tumour is located in the adrenal medulla in 90% of the cases. It is associated with high maternal and fetal mortality (50%) if undiagnosed. Conversely, early diagnosis and treatment during pregnancy decrease maternal and fetal mortality to <5 and 15% respectively. During pregnancy, women can present with a hypertensive crisis or congestive cardiac failure. They can also present with paroxysmal palpitations, high blood pressure, headache, abdominal pain and blurring of vision. Hence, phaeochromocytoma mimics pre-eclampsia. Early presentation during pregnancy (<20 weeks gestation) and the absence of proteinuria and oedema may help to establish a possible differential diagnosis. The other differential diagnosis is thyrotoxicosis.

   Extremely high blood pressures following delivery or anaesthesia should raise suspicion of phaeochromocytoma. It can be diagnosed by imaging (ultrasound, computed tomography [CT] scan or magnetic resonance imaging [MRI]) and 24-h urine collection for catecholamine and its metabolites. If diagnosed early in the pregnancy, surgical removal can be accomplished before 24 weeks. If diagnosed later in the pregnancy, it is advised to delay surgery until term, when delivery can be performed by caesarean section, although removal of the tumour at the same time as caesarean section is controversial.

James D, Steer PJ, Weiner CP, Gonik B, Crowther C, Robson S (eds). High Risk Pregnancy: Management Options (4th edn). St Louis: Saunders, 2011.

23. A False. Plasma concentration of T4 exceeds that of T3.

B False. Thyrotrophin-releasing hormone is a tripeptide.

C True.

D False. Thyroid-stimulating hormone (TSH) is secreted by the anterior pituitary gland. The other hormones secreted by the anterior pituitary include follicle-stimulating hormone (FSH), luteinising hormone (LH), growth hormone (GH), prolactin and adrenocorticotropic hormone (GH and prolactin are secreted by acidophils and rest by basophils). FSH, LH and TSH are glycoproteins and the rest are polypeptides. The posterior pituitary secretes oxytocin and vasopressin and is made up of axons from supraoptic and paraventricular nuclei of the hypothalamus; the anterior pituitary has special vascular connections called portal hypophyseal vessels.

E False. Negative feedback by T4 and T3 acts mainly on the anterior pituitary.

Many physiological changes occur in relation to thyroid hormones during pregnancy. Some of these are hypermetabolic changes and hence can mimic thyroid disease. Careful assessment and interpretation of the results of investigation is important to avoid making a wrong diagnosis.

The thyroid gland is regulated by both pituitary and hypothalamus. Thyrotropin-releasing hormone (synthesised in hypothalamus) stimulates both synthesis and release of TSH from the anterior pituitary. TSH in turn stimulates the synthesis and release of thyroid hormones (T4 and T3) from the thyroid gland. T4 contributes to 80% of thyroid secretion while T3 contributes to only 20%. However, T3 is the biologically active form of thyroid hormone and is primarily derived from the peripheral conversion of T4. Both hormones have a negative feedback effect on the pituitary secretion of TSH.

The first change during pregnancy is elevation of thyroxine binding globulin (TBG) which leads to increases in the total T4 and T3 serum levels. However, there is no change in the amount of free circulating T3 and T4 levels.

James D, Steer PJ, Weiner CP, Gonik B, Crowther C, Robson S (eds). High Risk Pregnancy: Management Options (4th edn). St Louis: Saunders, 2011.

24. A False. TSH excess is a rare cause of thyrotoxicosis.

B True.

C True.

D True.

E False.

Thyroid disorders are common in women of reproductive age (women are generally more affected than men). Some of the symptoms caused by these disorders mimic normal physiological changes during pregnancy and can be easily overlooked.

The incidence of hyperthyroidism is 1 in 2000 pregnancies. The most common cause of hyperthyroidism is Graves' disease (90%) which is an autoimmune disorder associated with thyroid-stimulating antibodies in the circulation. This disease can improve during pregnancy due to immunosuppressive effects but is frequently aggravated during the postpartum period. One should therefore be observant especially during the postpartum period for signs of thyrotoxicosis. The signs and symptoms include palpitation, increased appetite, heat intolerance, increase in resting pulse rate, tachycardia and systolic flow murmurs (infiltrative dermopathy and ophthalmopathy are typically present in Graves' disease). The serious complications of untreated hyperthyroidism include cardiac failure and thyroid storm (25% maternal mortality).

Maternal thyroid hormones do not cross the placenta. However, thyroid-stimulating antibodies and drugs used in the treatment of hyperthyroidism (propylthiouracil, carbimazole and iodine) cross the placenta and can alter fetal thyroid physiology. The use of radioactive iodine should be avoided during pregnancy as the fetal thyroid gland concentrates iodine at a significantly higher rate than the maternal thyroid gland and can cause permanent damage to the gland (hypothyroidism).

James D, Steer PJ, Weiner CP, Gonik B, Crowther C, Robson S (eds). High Risk Pregnancy: Management Options (4th edn). St Louis: Saunders, 2011.

25. **A True.** There is therefore the need to monitor symptoms and also the white blood cell count.

 B True.

 C False.

 D False.

 E False.

Medical therapy with propylthiouracil and carbimazole (both cross placenta) are equally safe and effective during pregnancy for treating hyperthyroidism. The response to treatment is usually seen 1 week following initiation of therapy but may take 4–6 weeks for complete effect. The serum T4 levels should be measured closely to avoid maternal hypothyroidism and lowest possible dose of the drugs should be used for medical therapy.

The side effects (seen in 2–3% of patients) of these drugs include pruritus, skin rash, agranulocytosis, granulocytopaenia, nausea, vomiting and diarrhoea. The development of agranulocytosis warrants complete cessation of therapy with these drugs.

The above drugs can block the fetal thyroid gland leading to development of fetal goitre (10% of all cases) and are dose-related. Transient and self-limiting neonatal hypothyroidism is seen in 1–5% of patients treated with these drugs. On the other hand, neonatal thyrotoxicosis (10%) can develop in women with Graves' disease due to circulating thyroid-stimulating antibodies stimulating the fetal thyroid.

James D, Steer PJ, Weiner CP, Gonik B, Crowther C, Robson S (eds). High Risk Pregnancy: Management Options (4th edn). St Louis: Saunders, 2011.

26. A False. The treatment modalities for hyperthyroidism include:

- thioamides (propylthiouracil, methimazole and carbimazol)
- beta-blockers
- iodides
- radioactive iodine
- surgery

The mainstay of treatment during pregnancy is medical therapy with thioamides. Radioactive use is absolutely contraindicated as it permanently destroys the fetal thyroid gland causing fetal goitre and fetal hypothyroidism.

B False. Thyroid surgery is indicated for the following women:

- women with retrosternal extension of goitre causing pressure symptoms
- women not responding to medical therapy
- women who are intolerant to medical therapy
- women with severe complication where further therapy cannot be continued
- women with suspected malignancy in the thyroid gland

C True. Maternal therapy with thioamides (blocks fetal thyroid gland as they cross the placenta) is associated with fetal goitre in 10% of all cases.

D False. Thyroxine binding globulins are increased during pregnancy.

E False. Propylthiouracil is secreted in breast milk.

James D, Steer PJ, Weiner CP, Gonik B, Crowther C, Robson S (eds). High Risk Pregnancy: Management Options (4th edn). St Louis: Saunders, 2011.

27. A True. SLE shows raised antinuclear antibodies and anti-double stranded DNA levels.

B True. The prognosis is poor in women with impaired renal function. There is an increase in perinatal and maternal mortality in women who have disease flare-ups (e.g. SLE nephritis) during pregnancy.

C True. There is an increase in the risk of fetal loss, especially in women who have raised anticardiolipin antibodies.

D True. SLE flare-ups (associated with hypertension and proteinuria) are usually difficult to differentiate from pre-eclampsia. The presence of blood and casts in the urine, low serum C3 and C4 complement levels, high anti-DNA levels and systemic signs of SLE would be indicative of SLE more than pre-eclampsia. The indications to deliver early during pregnancy include fetal compromise, hypertension and deterioration in renal function.

E False. SLE does not increase the risk of structural abnormalities. However, SLE can cause congenital heart block in the fetus in the presence of anti-Ro and anti-La antibodies.

Nelson-Piercy C. Handbook of Obstetric Medicine (4th edn). London: Informa Healthcare, 2010.

28. A True.

B True.

C **False.**

E **True.**

E **False.**

At least one of the clinical and one of the laboratory criteria should be met to make a diagnosis of APAS. The criteria for its diagnosis are listed below.

Laboratory criteria

- The presence of anticardiolipin antibodies or lupus anticoagulant on more than one occasion at least 6 weeks apart.

Clinical criteria

- Arterial or venous thrombosis.
- Pregnancy-associated bad outcomes include: one or more unexplained loss of a morphologically normal fetus (>10 weeks of gestation); one or more pre-term births less than 34 weeks of gestation as a result of severe placental insufficiency, pre-eclampsia and eclampsia; three or more consecutive miscarriages (<10 weeks of gestation).

Nelson-Piercy C. Handbook of Obstetric Medicine (4th edn). London: Informa Healthcare, 2010.

29. A **False.** Macrosomia is defined as the estimated fetal weight greater than the 90th centile when measured on ultrasound scan. It occurs in 25–40% of diabetic women.

    B **True.** It is associated with maternal poorly controlled gestational diabetes or diabetes.

    C **True.** Maternal and fetal morbidity are increased with shoulder dystocia. Caesarean section is indicated if the estimated fetal weight exceeds 4.5 kg in diabetic women and >5 kg in non-diabetic women (ACOG recommendation).

    D **False.** Early induction of labour for fetal macrosomia in non-diabetic women has not been shown to improve fetal outcome or reduce the risk of caesarean section.

    E **True.** Macrosomia in diabetic women is suggestive of poor control of diabetes. It is also associated with hypertrophic fetal cardiomyopathy (in diabetic women) and may lead to fetal death. Therefore early delivery is indicated (38 weeks).

    The incidence of fetal macrosomia increases in women suffering from diabetes during pregnancy. This is reflected by an increase in muscle mass, adipose deposition and organomegaly. However, this has no effect on the brain growth and hence the head circumference remains within the normal range. This disproportionate growth predisposes to a difficult vaginal delivery including shoulder dystocia. The risks to the newborn baby include birth injuries, hypoglycaemia (BM <4 occurs during the first 12 hours of life due to a rapid drop in plasma glucose levels), respiratory distress syndrome (the exact aetiology is unknown; however, hyperglycaemia and hyperinsulinaemia inhibit surfactant production in the fetal lungs), hypocalcaemia (which occurs due to failure in the increase of parathyroid hormone secretion following birth) and hypomagnesaemia.

James D, Steer PJ, Weiner CP, Gonik B, Crowther C, Robson S (eds). High Risk Pregnancy: Management Options (4th edn). St Louis: Saunders, 2011.
American College of Obstetricians and Gynaecologists. www.acog.org//publications.cfm

30. **A True.**

   B False. Diabetic ketoacidosis is more common in women with type 1 diabetes.

   C True. Aggressive treatment of diabetic ketoacidosis during pregnancy may undo fetal distress so do not rush to the theatre until the mother is metabolically stable. The treatment is adequate hydration to replace intravascular volume, insulin sliding scale to reduce maternal glucose levels and correction of electrolyte and acid base imbalance.

   D True.

   E True.

Nelson-Piercy C. Handbook of Obstetric Medicine (4th edn). London: Informa Healthcare, 2010.

31. **A True.** It is important to determine the chorionicity earlier on in the pregnancy. A monochorionic pregnancy is associated with higher complications than a dichorionic one. There are also implications for genetic diagnosis. In monochorionic pregnancies, invasive testing (e.g. amniocentesis) of one fetus is enough to identify the abnormality for both the twins; in dichorionic pregnancies, both the twins have to be tested separately to identify abnormality. The risks for monochorionic twin pregnancies include twin-to-twin transfusion, discordancy and death of one twin. Twin-to-twin transfusion can rarely be identified earlier in the pregnancy and has a poor prognosis.

   B True. Both anencephaly and neural tube defects can be identified at this stage.

   C True. Nuchal translucency (NT) is done from 11–13+6 weeks of pregnancies. It is used to assess the risk of trisomies as a part of first trimester screening and combined screening for trisomies. Increased NT is also associated with increased risk of congenital heart defects, triploidy and Turner syndrome.

   D True. Viability reassures.

   E True. Singleton pregnancy has fewer problems than twin pregnancies or triplets.

Jurkovic D, Valentin L, Vyas S. Gynaecological Ultrasound in Clinical Practice: Ultrasound imaging in the management of gynaecological conditions. London: RCOG Press, 2009.
Magowan B. Churchill's Pocketbook of Obstetrics and Gynaecology (3rd edn). Edinburgh: Churchill Livingstone, 2005.

32. **A False.** The fetus has a 25% chance of having sickle cell disease if both parents are carriers.

   B True. Prenatal diagnosis is possible by undertaking chorionic villous biopsy in the first trimester and amniocentesis in the second trimester.

   C True. Women with sickle cell disease and pulmonary hypertension should be advised not to conceive in view of increased mortality rate.

   D True. The presence of pulmonary hypertension increases the risk of maternal mortality, and therefore echocardiography should be performed if this was not done within the last year.

E True. Women with sickle disease are at an increased risk of developing infections (e.g. urinary tract infection, chest infection and pneumococcal pneumonia). For the prevention of the latter, they are offered a vaccine against pneumococcus and given antibiotic prophylaxis with penicillin V 250 mg orally daily due to a non-functioning spleen. Influenza vaccine should be offered if not given within the last year.

Royal College of Obstetricians and Gynaecologists. Green-top Guideline No. 61. Management of sickle cell disease in pregnancy. London: RCOG Press, 2011.

33. **A True.**

    B True.

    C True.

    D True.

    E True.

Smoking increases the perinatal mortality by nearly one third. It is associated with:

- an increased risk of miscarriage
- fetal growth restriction
- risk of pre-term labour (<32 weeks)
- pre-term premature rupture of membranes
- fetal loss: sudden infant death syndrome (27% of deaths due to sudden infant death syndrome are associated with smoking)
- lower intelligent quotient.

Recently, passive smoking has been shown to significantly affect birth weight.

Duncan KR and Johnson P. Smoking in Pregnancy. Personal assessment in continuing education. Reviews, questions and answers. Volume 3. London: RCOG Press, 2003:62–64.

34. **A False.**

    B True.

    C True.

    D True.

    E True.

The anterior pituitary consists of three types of cells: (a) chromophobes – these normally do not secrete any hormone and are known as resting cells; (b) acidophils – these secrete prolactin and growth hormone; and (c) basophils – these secrete TSH, ACTH and gonadotrophins (LH and FSH).

The paraventricular and supraoptic nuclei synthesise oxytocin and vasopressin. The axons of these nuclei pass on to the posterior pituitary.

James D, Steer PJ, Weiner CP, Gonik B, Crowther C, Robson S (eds). High Risk Pregnancy: Management Options (4th edn). St Louis: Saunders, 2011.

35. **A True.** Serum ferritin reflects the storage iron.

    B True. Serum transferrin levels reflect the tissue iron. Transferrin receptor, a transmembrane protein, binds transferrin bound iron and transports it to the inside of the cell. Any decrease in the iron supply results in an increase in the transferrin receptor. This truly reflects tissue iron.

C True. It is increased by three-fold.

D True. This test will be useful to identify iron deficiency anaemia during pregnancy and also differentiate from those with low serum ferritin due to mobilisation of storage iron or those with low haemoglobin concentration due to haemodilution.

E False. The rise in transferrin receptor precedes the rise in erythrocyte protoporphyrin.

James D, Steer PJ, Weiner CP, Gonik B, Crowther C, Robson S (eds). High Risk Pregnancy: Management Options (4th edn). St Louis: Saunders, 2011.

36. **A False.** Vitamin B12 deficiency is rarely implicated during pregnancy.

B False. Megaloblastic anaemia during pregnancy is almost always due to folic acid deficiency.

C True.

D False. Premature delivery increases the risk of folic acid deficiency in the neonate when the mother is deficient in folic acid.

E True. The World Health Organization (WHO) recommends folic acid supplementation during prenatal period and during lactation.

A peripheral blood film may be helpful to make the diagnosis. Outside pregnancy, macrocytosis is the hallmark of megaloblastic haematopoiesis and is first recognised as increased MCV on peripheral blood smear. Hypersegmentation of the neutrophil polymorph nucleus is a significant finding during pregnancy because normally there is a shift to left. However, hypersegmented neutrophils can be seen in pure iron deficiency. Therefore the overall clinical picture should be used to identify folic acid deficiency during pregnancy and is mostly based on morphological laboratory tests.

James D, Steer PJ, Weiner CP, Gonik B, Crowther C, Robson S (eds). High Risk Pregnancy: Management Options (4th edn). St Louis: Saunders, 2011.

37. **A True.**

B True.

C True.

D True.

E False.

Sickle cell crisis can be precipitated by infection, dehydration, hypoxia, acidosis and hypothermia. Deaths are usually reported to be due to a massive sickle cell crisis following an acute infection leading to pulmonary embolus. Therefore, the principles of management are: screen and treat infection, always ensure adequate hydration, avoid hypoxia (supplement with additional oxygen), avoid acidosis and prolonged labour.

James D, Steer PJ, Weiner CP, Gonik B, Crowther C, Robson S (eds). High Risk Pregnancy: Management Options (4th edn). St Louis: Saunders, 2011.
Royal College of Obstetricians and Gynaecologists. Green-top Guideline No. 61. Management of sickle cell disease in pregnancy. London: RCOG Press, 2011.

38. **A True.**

    B False. Relapse is more common in the first trimester and puerperium.

    C True.

    D False. A daily intake of 5 mg folic acid is recommended during pregnancy. Vitamin B12 supplementation is also required if the terminal ileum is involved.

    E True.

    Inflammatory bowel disease is common in developed countries and refers to ulcerative colitis and Crohn's disease. Women with severe disease may be underweight and malnourished, present with amenorrhoea and may be infertile.

    James D, Steer PJ, Weiner CP, Gonik B, Crowther C, Robson S (eds). High Risk Pregnancy: Management Options (4th edn). St Louis: Saunders, 2011.

39. **A True.** Listeriosis manifests with flu-like symptoms and is often mistaken for influenza or a urinary tract infection.

    B True. Listeriosis is caused by *Listeria monocytogenes* which is a non-spore-forming facultative anaerobe, gram positive (bacilli) and beta haemolytic organism. It has a predilection for pregnant women, the immunocompromised and neonates. Women usually give history of flu-like illness which may be mistaken for other infections. The main portal of entry is via the gastrointestinal tract (GI) and sporadic outbreaks can occur due to contamination of food. Information should be given to pregnant women to avoid soft cheese, pâté and the consumption of raw milk.

    C True. Although listeriosis can occur in early pregnancy, the most common time of occurrence is the third trimester. It is associated with decreased cell-mediated immunity and the placenta is thought to be a site of comparative immunosuppression and facilitates spread of infection to the fetus.

    D True. Two thirds of women present with flu-like illness during pregnancy due to bacteraemia. Maternal cases of endocarditis, meningitis and respiratory failure have been reported during pregnancy. Infection in early pregnancy may result in fetal loss within 4 – 7 days. Infection in late pregnancy may cause amnionitis, meconium staining of amniotic fluid, early onset neonatal listeriosis or late onset neonatal listeriosis. In early onset, neonatal listeriosis (intrauterine transmission) will present at birth or a few days later. The baby shows features of disseminated granulomas involving the liver and other organs, including the placenta. This is called granulomatosis infantisepticum. In late onset neonatal listeriosis (horizontal or nosocomial transmission), the common manifestation is meningitis following an uncomplicated pregnancy. The drugs of choice for treatment are ampicillin and penicillin G.

    E True.

James D, Steer PJ, Weiner CP, Gonik B, Crowther C, Robson S (eds). High Risk Pregnancy: Management Options (4th edn). St Louis: Saunders, 2011.

40. **A False.** Diabetes mellitus increases the risk of fetal organomegaly except the brain.

B False. Diabetes should be considered during serum screening for chromosomal anomalies when associated with low maternal serum alpha fetoprotein, beta human chorionic gonadotropin and oestriol. The risk of aneuploidy is not increased with diabetes.

C False. In women with well-controlled diabetes, the risk of miscarriage is not increased unless maternal diabetes is long standing with vascular complications.

D False. It is associated with increased risk of neonatal hypoglycaemia, hypomagnesaemia, hypocalcaemia, neonatal jaundice and respiratory distress syndrome.

E False. Insulin does not cross the placenta. It is glucose which crosses the placenta by facilitated diffusion. Therefore maternal hyperglycaemia causes fetal hyperglycaemia and beta cell hyperplasia in the pancreas with resultant fetal hyperinsulinaemia. This leads to fetal organomegaly as insulin and growth hormone have a similar structure. This eventually results in increased fetal aerobic and anaerobic metabolism, with hypoxia and lactic acidosis. Fetal hypoxia stimulates medullary and extramedullary haematopoiesis causing polycythaemia.

Nelson-Piercy C. Handbook of Obstetric Medicine (4th edn). London: Informa Healthcare, 2010.

41. **A False.** The presence or absence of D antigen site determines whether an individual is Rh positive or Rh negative. The incidence of Rh-negative genotype is 15% in Caucasians and 7–8% in Afro-Caribbeans.

B True. Maternal red cell alloimmunisation results from exposure to foreign red blood cell antigens. The primary immune response to this antigen is IgM formation which occurs over 6 weeks to 12 months and is usually weak. The secondary response is IgG antibody formation which is usually rapid. IgG crosses the placenta while IgM antibodies do not. Therefore the first pregnancy is usually not affected (unless this was the first exposure) by maternal antibodies.

C True. The second most common cause of rhesus sensitisation is blood transfusion.

D True. Second and subsequent exposures to fetal D antigen cause formation of IgG. The longer the interval between exposures, the greater the quantity of antibody formed and the stronger the binding with fetal red blood cells, and therefore there is increased risk of severe fetal disease. These coated red blood cells are ultimately destroyed in the reticuloendothelial system, leading to severe anaemia and hydrops in the fetus (it is not complement mediated, unlike other causes of haemolysis).

E False. Fetal erythropoiesis begins as early as day 21 in the fetal yolk sac and subsequently relocates to the liver and eventually the bone marrow by 16 weeks of gestation (this is reflected by a decreasing number of circulating erythroblasts). ABO antigens are weakly expressed in fetal red cells whereas Rh antigens are strongly expressed in the fetus as early as the fourth week of pregnancy or by 30 days of gestation.

Royal College of Obstetricians and Gynaecologists. Green-top Guideline No. 22. The Use of anti-D Immunoglobulin for Rhesus D Prophylaxis. London: RCOG Press, 2011.
James D, Steer PJ, Weiner CP, Gonik B, Crowther C, Robson S (eds). High Risk Pregnancy: Management Options (4th edn). St Louis: Saunders, 2011.

42. **A False.** The sensitisation occurs in about 1% of Rh-negative women during pregnancy.

    B False. The standard dose which is normally given following delivery will cover only 4 mL of fetomaternal haemorrhage.

    C True. The administration of anti-D immunoglobulin injection is recommended to Rh-negative women following delivery. A Kleihauer test may be helpful to determine if any extra fetomaternal haemorrhage has occurred and identifies the need for additional anti-D dose. Anti-D immunoglobulin should be given after any sensitising event before delivery (e.g. external cephalic version, abdominal trauma, antepartum haemorrhage) and after abortion/surgical or medical.

    D False. NICE recommends 500 IU of anti-D immunoglobulin to non-sensitised Rh-negative women at 28 and 34 weeks of pregnancy or a single dose of 1500 IU at or between 28 and 30 weeks of gestation.

    E True. Intramuscular anti-D immunoglobulin is best given into the deltoid muscle as injections into the gluteal region often only reach the subcutaneous tissues and absorption may be delayed.

    For effective immunoprophylaxis, anti-D immunoglobulin should be given at the earliest after the sensitising event but always within 72 hours. When it is not given before 72 hours, all effort should still be made to administer the anti-D immunoglobulin, as a dose given within 9–10 days may still provide some protection. Anti-D is not given to women who are sensitised.

    Royal College of Obstetricians and Gynaecologists. Green-top Guideline No. 22. The Use of anti-D Immunoglobulin for Rhesus D Prophylaxis. London: RCOG Press, 2011.
    National Institute for Health and Clinical Excellence. Routine antenatal anti-D prophylaxis for women who are rhesus D negative (Technology Appraisal Guidance 156). NICE, 2008.

43. **A True.**

    B False.

    C True.

    D False.

    E False.

    Pregnancy is a state of physiological insulin resistance and relative glucose tolerance. With increasing gestation, glucose tolerance decreases as a result of an increase in anti-insulin hormones secreted by the placenta (cortisol, human placental lactogen and glucagon). This leads to changes in carbohydrate metabolism as a result of decrease in insulin sensitivity. Therefore women with gestational diabetes usually manifest in the second or third trimester.

    Strict glycaemic control is the key to good obstetric outcome. Women with a lesser degree of impaired glucose tolerance may not have worse perinatal outcome. Any amount of hyperglycaemia is associated with increased fetal weight and incidence of fetal macrosomia especially when the mean maternal blood glucose is >7.2 mmol/L.

Maternal hyperglycaemia is associated with fetal acidaemia and is detrimental to the fetus. Maternal ketoacidosis is associated with high fetal mortality (20–40%). Random blood glucose and glycosylated haemoglobin tests done during pregnancy are regarded to have a low sensitivity for a screening test for gestational diabetes (GDM) or impaired glucose tolerance (IGT).

Nelson-Piercy C. Handbook of Obstetric Medicine (4th edn). London: Informa Healthcare, 2010.

44. A False. Pregnancy increases the likelihood of flare of SLE.

B False. The disease flare is more likely if the disease has been active within 6 months prior to the conception although it may be difficult to predict.

C False. SLE flares are more likely in the immediate postpartum period.

D True. The risk increases with the increasing basal level of creatinine, although some women may have uncomplicated pregnancies with moderate renal impairment.

E False. Therefore, routine use of steroids to prevent a flare is not recommended either during antepartum or postpartum period.

Obstetrically SLE increases the risk of the following complications:

- spontaneous miscarriage
- fetal growth restriction
- premature delivery
- pre-eclampsia
- intrauterine death of fetus

These are mainly related to the presence of anticardiolipin antibodies or lupus anticoagulant or the presence of active disease (or disease complications like lupus nephritis and hypertension) at the time of conception or later in the pregnancy.

Nelson-Piercy C. Handbook of Obstetric Medicine (4th edn). London: Informa Healthcare, 2010.

45. A False. The anaemia is normocytic normochromic anaemia.

B False. ESR is increased in SLE due to increase in the immunoglobulin levels

C False. C3 and C4 complement levels are decreased.

D False. C-reactive protein is normal in SLE.

E False. SLE causes thrombocytopenia and neutropenia.

Anti-double stranded DNA (dsDNA) antibodies are linked to SLE and anti-histone antibodies are linked to drug induced lupus. Anti-dsDNA antibodies are highly specific for SLE and are present in 70% of the cases (seen in only 0.5% of the people without SLE). Its presence has been correlated with disease activity in SLE. The increasing levels are directly proportional to the risk of developing an exacerbation of SLE during pregnancy and also the risk of premature delivery. It is also associated with increased fetal loss. Antiphospholipid antibodies are present in 40% of SLE patients. Anti-Ro and Anti-La antibodies are present in 30% of the patients.

Renal involvement is quite common in the course of disease and usually associated with proteinuria (presentation in 70% of cases), haematuria or pyuria (40%) and renal casts (one third of patients). Renal biopsy is important for diagnosis and treatment as well as assessing prognosis. About 40% will have diffuse proliferative glomerulonephritis (a severe lesion with a 10-year survival rate of 60%). The presentation includes hypertension, proteinuria, nephrotic syndrome, haematuria, pyuria, renal casts, decreased serum complement levels and increased immune complexes in the circulation. In focal proliferative glomerulonephritis, all the features are less severe than diffuse proliferative nephritis including renal insufficiency.

Lupus nephritis (associated with hypertension, proteinuria and multiple organ dysfunctions) is difficult to differentiate from pre-eclampsia. The main differentiating features include active urinary sediment (cellular casts and haematuria) and renal biopsy. The other features include elevated anti-dsDNA levels and decreased complement levels.

James D, Steer PJ, Weiner CP, Gonik B, Crowther C, Robson S (eds). High Risk Pregnancy: Management Options (4th edn). St Louis: Saunders, 2011.
Nelson-Piercy C. Handbook of Obstetric Medicine (4th edn). London: Informa Healthcare, 2010.

46. A False. Sodium valproate is associated with neural tube and cardiac defects.

B True. Carbamazepine is also associated with orofacial clefts.

C False. Orofacial clefts and cardiac defects.

D True. Lamotrigine is a weak inhibitor of dihydrofolate reductase and therefore may interfere with folate metabolism. Sodium valproate and lamotrigine carries a dose-dependent teratogenic effect.

E True.

The risk of teratogenicity for one drug is 5–7%. (There is a clear spectrum with valproate and phenytoin having the highest risk, carbamatepine being intermediate, and lamotrigine and other newer drugs having the lowest risk.) Teratogenicity increases to 10–15% with two or more drugs. The combination of all three drugs (carbamazepine, sodium valproate and phenytoin) will increase the risk to 50%.

Antiepileptic drugs and effects

- carbamazepine and sodium valproate – neural tube defect
- phenytoin, carbamazepine and phenobarbitone – orofacial clefts
- phenytoin, phenobarbitone and sodium valproate – congenital cardiac defects

Fetal anticonvulsant syndrome

- Is associated with anticonvulsant use during pregnancy
- Associated with dysmorphic features such as low set ears, broad nasal bridge, irregular teeth and V-shaped eyebrows
- Hypoplastic nails and distal digits
- Hypertelorism and hypoplasia of midface

Nelson-Piercy C. Handbook of Obstetric Medicine (4th edn). London: Informa Healthcare, 2010.
Holmes LB, Baldwin EJ, Smith CR, Habecker E, Glassman L, Wong SL, Wyszynski DF. Increased frequency of isolated cleft palate in infants exposed to lamotrigine during pregnancy. Neurology 2008; 70:2152–2158.

Chapter 3

Benign gynaecology

1. **The following findings warrant a referral to colposcopy clinic:**
   A   One smear test showing borderline changes in squamous cells
   B   One smear test showing severe dyskaryosis
   C   One smear test showing glandular neoplasia
   D   One smear test showing borderline in endocervical cells
   E   Three smear tests showing inadequate samples

2. **The following smear results require referral to colposcopy:**
   A   Smear showing wart virus infection
   B   Squamous metaplasia
   C   Inflammatory changes
   D   Endometrial cells in women <40 years old
   E   Actinomyces in smear

3. **With regards to cervical glandular intraepithelial neoplasia (CGIN):**
   A   It is 100 times more common than cervical intraepithelial neoplasia (CIN)
   B   Cervical screening programme is specifically designed to detect glandular abnormalities
   C   It is associated with CIN in almost 50% of the cases
   D   Histological evaluation fails to confirm glandular lesions in 50% of the cases where cervical smear is reported as endocervical glandular abnormalities
   E   The aetiology is totally different for CGIN and CIN

4. **With regards to the management of premenstrual syndrome (PMS):**
   A   Microgynon (ethinylestradiol/levonorgestrel IUS) is preferable to Yasmin (ethinylestradiol/drospirenone)
   B   Both the physical and the psychological symptoms of PMS have not shown to improve with the use of selective serotonin reuptake inhibitors (SSRIs)
   C   Continuous back-to-back treatment with a combined oral contraceptive pill (COCP) has been shown to be more effective than the standard cyclical treatment
   D   Complementary therapies such as vitamin B supplements and reflexology have no substantial evidence base and therefore should not be tried
   E   Cognitive behavioural therapy should be considered routinely as a treatment option for women with severe PMS

5. **With regards to cervical smears:**
   A   All pregnant women should be offered a cervical smear
   B   It should be done on day 1 of the menstrual period

C   Women with Chlamydia infection should be offered a cervical smear
D   The cervical smear should be done at one-month postnatal if indicated
E   All virgin women should have a cervical smear

6. **With regards to the management of endometriosis:**

A   Suppression of ovarian function for 6 months with gonadotropin-releasing hormone analogues has shown to reduce pain associated with endometriosis
B   Ablation of uterine nerve is as effective as ablation of endometriotic lesions with laser for reducing endometriosis-related pain
C   Endometrioma is an indication for oophorectomy in young woman
D   Endometriosis-associated pain can be reduced by removing the entire lesions in severe and deeply infiltrating disease
E   Levonorgestrel IUS is an effective treatment in controlling endometriosis-associated pain

7. **With regards to polycystic ovary disease:**

A   It is associated with oligoovulation
B   It is associated with insulin resistance
C   It is associated with increased follicle-stimulating hormone (FSH): luteinising hormone (LH) ratio
D   It is associated with oligomenorrhoea
E   It is associated with dysmenorrhoea

8. **The following are effective in reducing the menstrual blood loss in women with dysfunctional uterine bleeding (DUB):**

A   Anti-fibrinolytics
B   Prostaglandin synthetase inhibitors
C   Oral medroxyprogesterone acetate from days 16–25 of menstrual cycle
D   Combined oral contraceptive pill (COCP)
E   Copper intrauterine contraceptive device (IUCD)

9. **With regards to hirsutism:**

A   It is idiopathic in most cases
B   It can be due to late onset congenital adrenal hyperplasia
C   It can be due to androgen insensitivity syndrome
D   It can be due to polycystic ovary syndrome (PCOS)
E   It can be due to adrenal tumours

10. **PCOS is associated with:**

A   Increased hip circumference
B   Insulin resistance
C   Clitoromegaly
D   Increased serum oestrogen levels
E   Decreased corticosteroid binding globulin

11. **With regards to testosterone in women:**

A   It is in the range of 5–7 nmol/L
B   It is produced only in the adrenal gland in women

    C   Eighty per cent of it is bound to albumin

    D   Approximately 78% is derived from peripheral conversion of androstenedione

    E   It is derived both from the ovaries and adrenal glands in equal amounts in women

12. With regards to thyroid hormone:

    A   Its deficiency leads to anovulation

    B   The circulating thyroid hormone is bound to proteins

    C   Oestrogen decreases the thyroxine binding capacity

    D   T3 levels in the circulation directly reflects thyroid secretion

    E   T4 levels play a major role in thyroid-stimulating hormones (TSH) regulation

13. The following are risk factors for venous thromboembolism (VTE) in hospitalised patients:

    A   Antithrombin deficiency

    B   Increased body mass index (BMI) >40

    C   Nephrotic syndrome

    D   Trauma to the pelvis

    E   Homocystinaemia

14. With regards to androgens in women:

    A   Androstenedione has androgenic activity with androgenic effects on tissues

    B   Dehydroepiandosterone DHEA has androgenic activity with androgenic effects on tissues

    C   Testosterone is converted to biologically active dihydrotestosterone by 5 alpha reductase

    D   Testosterone is metabolised to androstenedione and then excreted as androsterone and etiocholanolone

    E   The main ovarian androgen is testosterone

15. The following are indications for surgical treatment of prolactin producing macroadenomas:

    A   Women not responding to medical drug therapy

    B   Women with non-functioning adenoma

    C   Women not compliant with medical therapy due to side effects

    D   Women who wish to breastfeed

    E   Women with good response to medical therapy, with significant tumour shrinkage and planning for pregnancy in the future

16. With regards to the treatment of endometriosis:

    A   COCP and danazol are equally effective in alleviating the endometriosis-associated pain

    B   There is a risk of virilisation of the female fetus if women conceive while on danazol

    C   There is a risk of virilisation of the female fetus if women conceive while on gestrinone

    D   Aspiration of the endometrioma is associated with a high recurrence rate

    E   Pelvic clearance is considered in women with debilitating symptoms where fertility is not an issue

17. **With regards to transvaginal ultrasound scan for ovarian cyst:**
    A   The absence of a crescent sign indicates the benign nature of the cyst
    B   The presence of multiple septae within the cyst indicates the benign nature of the cyst
    C   Increased colour flow Doppler into the septa or papillary projection is indicative of malignancy
    D   The risk of malignancy index (RMI) is used to assess the risk of malignancy of ovarian cyst in premenopausal and postmenopausal women
    E   Septae <3 mm and papillary projections <3 mm favours the benign nature of the cyst

Answers

1. A **False.**

    B **True.**

    C **True.**

    D **True.**

    E **True.**

Three smears tests reported as having borderline abnormalities in squamous cells and one smear test reported as borderline nuclear changes in endocervical cells should be referred for colposcopy. The latter indicates borderline glandular changes in endocervical cells and is often associated with cervical glandular intraepithelial neoplasia. One smear test showing moderate or severe dyskaryosis should be referred for colposcopy as the incidence of high grade CIN is 50% and 75%, respectively. Women with a report of glandular neoplasia should be referred to a colposcopy clinic urgently and should be seen in the colposcopy clinic within 2 weeks of referral to the clinic. These women may have an underlying cervical or endometrial malignancy and are associated with CIN in 50% of cases.

NHS Cervical Screening Programme guideline recommendations for referral to colposcopy clinic

- Three inadequate samples: The smear is inadequate for interpretation in the laboratory to give any definitive diagnosis. This could be due to a poorly prepared smear or it may not contain the right type of cells (not representative of transformation zone). The rate of inadequate smears has been significantly reduced with the introduction of liquid-based cytology (LBC).
- Three smear tests reported as borderline nuclear changes in the squamous cells: The smear is interpreted as borderline either when it is difficult to differentiate between human papillomavirus (HPV) changes or mild dyskaryosis or where it is difficult to differentiate benign or reactive changes from significant degrees of dyskaryosis.
- One smear test reported as borderline nuclear change in endocervical cells: This indicates borderline glandular changes in endocervical cells. Glandular changes in the endocervical cells are often associated with CIN and an underlying malignancy (adenocarcinoma) must not be overlooked.
- One smear report of mild dyskaryosis.
- One smear report of moderate and severe dyskaryosis.
- One smear test reported as possible invasion.
- One test reported as glandular neoplasia.
- Suspicious-looking cervix.

NHS Cervical Screening Programme. Colposcopy and Programme Management. Guidelines for the NHS Cervical Screening Programme (2nd edn). Publication No 20. NHSCSP, 2010. http://www.bsccp.org.uk/docs/public/pdf/nhscsp20.pdf

Wuntakal R and Hollingworth T. Chapter 3: Management of abnormal Pap smears. In: Rajaram S, Maheswari A, Chitrathara (eds). Cervical Cancer: Contemporary Management. New Delhi: Jaypee Brothers Medical Publishers, 2011.

2. A False.

    B False.

    C False.

    D False.

    E False.

    An incidental finding of Actinomyces-like organisms in the cervical smear is not an indication for referral to colposcopy. They are common in women fitted with a long-standing copper IUCD and are usually harmless. Symptomatic women with pelvic infection need coil removal and antibiotic therapy (penicillin group of drugs) while asymptomatic women do not necessarily require any treatment.

    NHS Cervical Screening Programme. Colposcopy and Programme Management. Guidelines for the NHS Cervical Screening Programme (2nd edn). Publication No 20. NHSCSP, 2010. http://www.bsccp.org.uk/docs/public/pdf/nhscsp20.pdf

3. A False.

    B False.

    C True.

    D True.

    E False.

    Glandular abnormalities of the cervix are relatively rare and account for only 0.05% of cytological abnormalities (100 times less common than CIN). The aetiological factors for CGIN and CIN are the same. HPV 18 accounts for the majority of the cases of CGIN.

    Most cases are found accidentally as the cervical screening programme is not designed to detect glandular abnormalities and moreover routine smears have poor specificity for glandular lesions.

    Cervical screening is not designed to pick up glandular abnormalities other than by chance (first challenge). The second challenge is the interpretation of features on colposcopy as there are no definitive specific features described to accurately diagnose CGIN, unlike CIN. The final challenge is treating these abnormalities in view of possible skip lesions (multifocal lesions) higher up in the endocervical canal. Over and above all these problems, follow-up can be less than perfect as cytology is much better at detection of squamous lesions compared to glandular lesions. However, the risk of recurrence is estimated at approximately 14% even when the treatment margins are negative for disease as the lesions may be higher up in the canal.

    A histological assessment of the cervix is recommended in the presence of glandular abnormality. These are often associated with CIN but also with an underlying adenocarcinoma in almost 40% of cases and therefore warrant further evaluation rather than just a repeat cytology. In view of this an excision treatment (knife cone biopsy or laser cone) is recommended rather than a punch biopsy to confirm the diagnosis and exclude an occult invasive adenocarcinoma. A hysteroscopy and endometrial biopsy, with or without a transvaginal scan, should be performed if any doubt or in the presence of normal colposcopy to rule out abnormality higher up in the genital tract.

Treatment ranges from conservative (cylindrical cone of 25 mm deep has been shown to be curative in most women) to hysterectomy in those who have completed their family. This is after thorough discussion and counselling. On follow-up, in addition to conventional LBC, regular endocervical cytology with a brush and colposcopy should be performed. If any symptoms or signs are suggestive of uterine disease a hysteroscopy and endometrial biopsy are performed.

Teale G and Jordan J. Chapter 7: Lower genital tract intraepithelial neoplasia. In: Shafi MI, Luesley DM, Jordan JA (eds), Handbook of Gynaecological Oncology. Edinburgh: Churchill Livingstone, 2001: 151–160.
NHS Cervical Screening Programme. Colposcopy and Programme Management. Guidelines for the NHS Cervical Screening Programme (2nd edn). Publication No 20. NHSCSP, 2010. http://www.bsccp.org.uk/docs/public/pdf/nhscsp20.pdf
The British Society for Colposcopy and Cervical Pathology. www.bsccp.org.uk
Wuntakal R and Hollingworth T. Chapter 3: Management of abnormal Pap smears. In: Rajaram S, Maheswari A, Chitrathara (eds). Cervical Cancer: Contemporary Management. New Delhi: Jaypee Brothers Medical Publishers, 2011.

4. A **False.**

    B **False.**

    C **False.**

    D **False.**

    E **True.**

Cognitive behavioural therapy should be offered to everybody and could be extremely effective, even with severe cases of PMS.

SSRIs have been shown to be effective in improving physical and psychological symptoms. This group of drugs can be used either continuously or in the luteal phase, and both have been shown to be beneficial.

COCPs have not been shown to be of benefit in relieving PMS symptoms. It is proposed that mineralocorticoid activity of the progestogen (in second generation pills) may regenerate PMS symptoms, Yasmin however, contains drospirenone which has anti-mineralocorticoid and anti-androgenic progestogen and helps in the relief of some of the symptoms of PMS. There is no evidence to support continuous rather than cyclical use of COCPs.

The evidence for use of complementary therapy is limited. It is considered appropriate to try those therapies which have not been shown to be detrimental, while our understanding of the aetiology of PMS remains poor.

Royal College of Obstetricians and Gynaecologists. Green-top Guideline No. 48. Management of Premenstrual Syndrome. London: RCOG Press, 2007.

5. A **False.**

    B **False.**

    C **False.**

D False.

E False.

Supplementary cervical screening is not warranted in the following situations provided the woman is in the cervical screening age and has undergone screening within the previous 3–5 years (age dependent):

- women taking a COCP
- following insertion of an IUCD
- women taking or starting hormone replacement therapy
- Following pregnancy, antenatal, postnatal, or after termination unless a previous cytology is abnormal
- women presenting with vaginal discharge
- women who have multiple sexual partners
- women with pelvic infection or pelvic inflammatory disease
- women with genital warts
- women who smoke heavily

It is difficult to interpret smear results if the test is taken during pregnancy or the menstrual period. The smears are usually also reported as inadequate (few cells picked up on smear) when taken too early during the postnatal period due to hypo-estrogenic effects. Therefore a cervical smear should be taken at a later date during the postnatal period (3 months postnatal) if smear is indicated and possibly avoided during the menstrual period. The incidence of cervical cancer in women who are virgins is very low.

NHS Cervical Screening Programme. Colposcopy and Programme Management. Guidelines for the NHS Cervical Screening Programme (2nd edn). Publication No 20. NHSCSP, 2010. http://www.bsccp.org.uk/docs/public/pdf/nhscsp20.pdf
NHS Cervical Screening Program. Taking Samples for Cervical Screening. A Resource Pack for Trainers. Publication No. 2. NHSCSP, 2007.

6. **A True.** Recurrence of symptoms is common following cessation of treatment.

   B False.

   C False.

   D True.

   E True.

In women with symptoms suggestive of endometriosis, a trial of hormonal therapy (progestogen, danazol or GnRH analogues) can be given to reduce menstrual blood flow, before proceeding to diagnostic laparoscopy and management. Although hormonal therapy is a treatment option for endometriosis, there is insufficient evidence of benefit to justify its use either before or after surgery. Levonorgestrel IUS is an effective method for endometriosis-associated symptoms, with symptom control maintained for up to 3 years.

The use of a GnRH agonist with 'add-back' (oestrogen and progestogen) therapy protects against bone mineral density loss at the lumbar spine during treatment and for up to 6 months after treatment.

Laparoscopic ablation of endometriotic lesions has shown to reduce endometriosis-associated pain compared to diagnostic laparoscopy. Uterine nerve ablation in itself has not been shown to be effective in reducing endometriosis-related pain. It should be reserved for women who have failed to respond to other therapies.

Ovarian endometrioma is not an indication for oophorectomy. However, laparoscopic ovarian cystectomy is recommended if an endometrioma is >3 cm in diameter or there is a deeply infiltrating lesion, to exclude a rare association of malignancy. In women having in vitro fertilisation (IVF) treatment ovarian endometrioma should be removed if >4 cm as this may reduce the risk of infection, improve access to follicles, and possibly improve ovarian response and prevent endometriosis progression. The woman should be thoroughly counselled regarding the risks of reduced ovarian function following surgery.

Royal College of Obstetricians and Gynaecologists. Green-top Guideline No. 24. Investigation and Management of Endometriosis. London: RCOG Press, 2006.

7. **A** True.

  B True.

  C False.

  D True.

  E False.

Polycystic ovary syndrome (PCOS)

PCOS is characterised by:

- anovulatory infertility
- oligomenorrhoea
- hyperandrogenism – hirsutism and/or acne

Twenty per cent of women of reproductive age demonstrate ultrasound evidence of PCOS while 10% of women have biochemical or clinical signs of anovulation or hyperandrogenism. Women with these phenotypes are also associated with metabolic conditions such as type 2 diabetes and an increased risk of cardiovascular disease and endometrial hyperplasia or cancer.

Differential diagnosis

One should exclude:

- congenital adrenal hyperplasia
- adrenal gland tumours
- Cushing syndrome

Criteria for diagnosis

The European Society of Human Reproduction and Embryology (ESHRE) need the presence of two out of the following three criteria:

- oligo- or anovulation
- clinical and/or biochemical signs of hyperandrogenism

- polycystic ovaries and exclusion of other aetiologies (congenital adrenal hyperplasia, androgen-secreting tumours, Cushing syndrome)

LH levels and PCOS

FSH and LH:FSH levels are raised in women with PCOS. Interestingly, increased LH levels are found in only 60% of patients, whereas LH:FSH ratios are increased in 95% of patients. The effect of LH on fertility has been investigated, with the hypothesis that high LH could impair oocyte maturity and fertilisation, reduce fertility and increase miscarriage risk. However, some studies negate this and that is why LH levels are not considered necessary for PCOS diagnosis.

Anti-Müllerian hormone (AMH) and PCOS

AMH is a special protein released by cells that are involved in the growth of the ovum every month. Its levels correlate with the number of antral follicles found on the ovary every month. The higher the antral follicle count, the higher the serum AMH levels. Women with PCOS typically have higher antral follicle and therefore higher AMH levels. AMH is now used in many clinics as a potential diagnostic marker for PCOS and an indicator of ovarian reserve in older women.

Main problems in diagnosis

- Biochemical abnormalities are seen in those with regular cycles and normal ultrasound scans who present with hirsutism or acne.
- Women with normal BMI who present with oligomenorrhoea often have abnormal biochemical and ultrasound results.
- There is a significant variation in the clinical and biochemical pictures seen.
- It is important that patients are diagnosed properly in order to treat the metabolic complications of PCOS.

Relation with body mass index

- PCOS has been associated with obesity; however, the condition still affects those with normal body mass index.
- There is evidence that exercise and weight control increases fertility in a significant number of obese anovulatory PCOS patients.
- For women with a normal body mass index, there is no evidence of improvement with exercise and diet. However, adverse lipid profiles are seen in normal weight PCOS patients, and therefore there may be benefit from screening for long-term risk, by measuring fasting blood glucose, lipids and triglycerides.

Treatment

- Lifestyle modifications (exercise and weight loss).
- Symptomatic management, e.g. regularise period, treat hirsutism and acne.
- Ovulation induction agents for women who want to conceive (e.g. clomiphene citrate: ovulation rate of 70–85% and pregnancy rate of 40–50%). The limitation is short-term use as there is possible risk of ovarian cancer when used for more than 12 months.
- Metformin (promotes resumption of menstruation, increases rate of spontaneous ovulation and enhances ovulatory response to clomiphene citrate). Metformin is not currently licensed for the treatment of ovulatory disorders in the UK.

- Laparoscopic ovarian drilling.
- IVF if other methods of fertility treatment fail.

Role of laparoscopic ovarian drilling and advantages

- clomiphene-resistant PCOS
- as effective as gonadotrophin therapy
- ovulation occurs in 80% of the patients while 40–69% get pregnant
- serum LH, androgens and sex hormone binding globulin (SHBG) normalise in more than 60%
- has a low miscarriage rate (14%)
- no risk of multiple pregnancy or ovarian hyperstimulation syndrome (OHSS)
- no need for intensive monitoring

Disadvantages

- short-lasting effect of treatment (6–12 months)
- expensive procedure
- operative and anaesthetic complications

Pregnancy complications in women with proven PCOS

- gestational diabetes (13% vs. 5% in normal individuals)
- pregnancy-induced hypertension
- increased risk of miscarriage (30–40%)

Royal College of Obstetricians and Gynaecologists. Green-top Guideline No. 33. Long Term Consequences of Polycystic Ovary Syndrome. London: RCOG Press, 2007.
Rotterdam ESHRE/ASRM-Sponsored PCOS Consensus Workshop Group. Revised 2003 consensus on diagnostic criteria and long-term health risks related to polycystic ovary syndrome. Fertil Steril 2004; 81:19–25.
Clark AM, Ledger WL, Galletly C, Tomlinson L, Blaney F, Wang X, Norman RJ. Weight loss results in significant improvement in pregnancy and ovulation rates in anovulatory obese women. Hum Reprod 1995; 10:2705–2712.

8. **A True.**

   B True.

   C False.

   D True.

   E False. Copper IUCD increases bleeding while levonorgestrel IUS decreases menstrual blood loss.

National Insititue of Health and Clinical Excellence (NICE)

Heavy menstrual bleeding (HMB) can be defined as excessive menstrual blood loss which interferes with a woman's physical, social, emotional and/or material quality of life.

Facts in the UK

- One in 20 women aged 30–49 years consults her general practitioner with HMB.
- Once referred to a gynaecologist, surgical intervention is highly likely.
- One in five women in the UK will have a hysterectomy before the age of 60 years.

- In at least half of those who undergo hysterectomy, HMB is the main presenting problem.
- About half of all women who have a hysterectomy for HMB have a normal uterus removed.
- Only 58% of women receive medical therapy for HMB before referral to a specialist.

Indications for imaging (ultrasound)

- failure of pharmaceutical treatment
- Vaginal examination reveals a pelvic mass of unknown origin
- the uterus is palpable abdominally

Drug therapy

Tranexamic acid

- is an antifibrinolytic agent
- dose 1 g three times daily (tds)
- second line drug for treatment of DUB with a regular cycle (levonorgestrel IUS is the first line treatment)
- reduces blood loss by 50%
- preserves fertility
- side effects: thrombosis, dizziness, headache and gastrointestinal upset
- stop the drug if there is no improvement after three cycles

Mefenamic acid

- prostaglandin synthetase inhibitor
- dose 500 mg tds
- second line drug for treatment of DUB
- reduces blood loss by 30–40%
- preferred in women with dysmenorrhoea
- preserves fertility
- side effects: mainly gastrointestinal
- stop the drug if there is no improvement after three cycles

Long cycle progestogens (days 5–25)

- pseudodecidual change and endometrial atrophy
- effective method
- norethisterone 5 mg tds or medroxyprogesterone acetate 10 mg tds
- reduces blood loss by 90%
- side effects: acne and weight gain

Luteal phase progestogens (days 16–25)

- causes endometrial atrophy
- norethisterone 5 mg tds or medroxyprogesterone acetate 10 mg tds
- blood loss increased (–4%)
- not recommended
- side effects: acne and weight gain

COCP

- causes endometrial atrophy
- effective method
- dose depends on the preparation
- reduces blood loss by 50%
- provides contraception
- side effects: systemic and thrombosis

Danazol

- synthetic androgen with anti-oestrogenic, anti-progestogenic and anti-gonadotrophic actions
- directly suppresses endometrium
- dose 200 mg daily
- reduces blood loss by 85%
- side effects: weight gain and androgenic effects (acne, hirsutism, musculoskeletal pains, seborrhoea, hot flushes and breast atrophy). Almost all side effects are reversible once the drug is stopped except voice changes
- can cause virilisation of a female fetus and hence women should be advised to use barrier contraception while taking this drug to avoid pregnancy
- need to use contraception
- side effect profile precludes its use

Gestrinone

- 19-nortestosterone derivative, androgen with anti-oestrogenic, anti-progestogenic, anti-gonadotrophic actions
- dose 2.5 mg twice weekly
- reduces blood loss by 85%
- side effects similar to danazol but less severe
- information is limited
- not licensed for treatment of menorrhagia
- can virilise female fetus if the woman conceives while on this drug

GnRH analogues

- acts by pituitary down regulation
- recommended for short-term use
- may be used for short-term use for intractable menorrhagia
- may be used prior to myomectomy to shrink the fibroids
- may be used prior to transcervical resection of fibroids to shrink the fibroids
- may be used prior to transcervical resection of endometrium to suppress endometrial growth
- dose depends on the preparation
- frequency depends on the dose
- injected subcutaneously
- reduces blood loss by 100%
- side effects: vasomotor symptoms and osteoporosis

Levonorgestrel IUS

- causes endometrial atrophy
- levonorgestrel (20 µg) is released daily
- reduces blood loss by 85–90%
- first time treatment
- provides contraception
- side effects: expulsion, perforation and breakthrough bleeding

Community setting

- When the first pharmaceutical treatment proves ineffective, a second can be considered rather than immediate referral to surgery. However, following the failure of the second line drug therapy, the patient should be referred to a gynaecologist.

NICE guideline with reference to endometrial ablation

Endometrial ablation should be considered in women:

- where bleeding has a severe impact on quality of life (QOL) and they do not want to conceive in the future
- with HMB who have a normal uterus and with small uterine fibroids (<3 cm in diameter)
- preferentially to a hysterectomy alone when the uterus is no bigger than 10 weeks size and the woman suffers from HMB alone
- women must be advised to avoid subsequent pregnancy and of the need to use effective contraception, if required

NICE: Indications for endometrial biopsy

- persistent inter-menstrual bleeding
- women aged >45 years
- failed medical treatment
- very low haemoglobin

Hysterectomy

- if other treatments fail and the women no longer wishes to retain her uterus or fertility
- if the woman has been fully informed
- if the woman wishes to have amenorrhoea

National Institute for Health and Clinical Excellence. Guideline on Heavy Menstrual Bleeding (CG44). NICE, 2007.

Sen S and Lumsden MA. Chapter 31: Menstruation and menstrual disorder. In: Shaw RW, Luesley D, Monga A (eds). Gynaecology (4th edn). Edinburgh: Churchill Livingstone, 2011.

Letsky E, Murphy MF, Ramsay JE, Walker I. Haemorrhagic Disease and Hereditary Bleeding Disorders. London: RCOG Press, 2005.

9. **A True.** Idiopathic hirsutism may be because of end-organ hypersensitivity. There may be a mild increase in the serum testosterone with normal LH:FSH ratio.

   B True. It is a rare condition and women usually present with amenorrhoea/oligomenorrhoea and virilisation.

   C False.

D True. PCOS is a common condition and the duration of onset is usually years. There is an increase in serum testosterone, and an increased LH with the normal FSH levels. The women usually manifest with oligomenorrhoea/amenorrhoea and/or hirsutism but without signs of virilisation.

E True. It is a rare condition with a typical history of sudden onset of hirsutism (usually months). Women may present with oligomenorrhoea/amenorrhoea and signs of virilisation.

Royal College of Obstetricians and Gynaecologists. Green-top Guideline No. 33. Long Term Consequences of Polycystic Ovary Syndrome. London: RCOG Press, 2007.

10. **A False.** PCOS is associated with increased waist circumference.

B True. PCOS is also associated with hyperinsulinaemia.

C False. Clitoromegaly is a symptom and sign of virilisation which is seen in women with congenital adrenal hyperplasia and androgen secreting adrenal and ovarian tumours. It is not a feature of PCOS.

D True. This is the only condition with amenorrhoea which is associated with increased serum oestrogen levels. This in turn puts these women at high risk of developing endometrial hyperplasia and endometrial cancer.

E False. It is associated with decreased SHBG which is considered a surrogate marker for hyperinsulinaemia.

Royal College of Obstetricians and Gynaecologists. Green-top Guideline No. 33. Long Term Consequences of Polycystic Ovary Syndrome. London: RCOG Press, 2007.

11. **A False.** In women, the range is 0.5–3 nmol/L.

B False. Testosterone is produced both in the ovaries and adrenal gland and also peripherally.

C False. Eighty per cent of testosterone in the circulation is bound to SHBG.

D False. Fifty per cent is derived from peripheral conversion of androstenedione to testosterone: 25% is produced by the ovaries and 25% from the adrenal cortex.

E True. In women, both adrenal glands and ovaries contribute 25% testosterone each to the circulation except at midcycle when the ovarian contribution is said to increase by 10–15%.

The androgens in women are produced both by the ovaries and the adrenal gland. DHEA is mainly derived from the adrenal gland. In men testosterone is produced from Leydig cells in the testis. It is predominantly bound to SHBG. The metabolism of steroid hormones occurs in the kidneys. Androgens are mainly excreted as 17-oxosteroids.

Nelson SM and Grudzinskas JG. Chapter 10: Hormones; their actions and measurements in gynaecological practice. In: Shaw RW, Luesley D, Monga A (eds). Gynaecology (4th edn). Edinburgh: Churchill Livingstone, 2011.

12. **A True.** It is associated with increased gonadotrophin levels.

B True. The circulating thyroid hormone is bound mainly to thyroxine-binding globulin.

C False. Oestrogen increases the thyroxine-binding globulin by increasing its synthesis in the liver.

D False. T3 levels are not a direct reflection of thyroid secretion because of the peripheral source of this hormone.

E True.

Nelson SM and Grudzinskas JG. Chapter 10: Hormones; their actions and measurements in gynaecological practice. In: Shaw RW, Luesley D, Monga A (eds). Gynaecology (4th edn). Edinburgh: Churchill Livingstone, 2011.

13. **A True.**

    B True.

    C True.

    D True.

    E True.

The other risk factors include:

- patient factors: pregnancy, puerperium, immobility, varicose veins, hormone therapy, thrombophilia and previous venous thromboembolism (VTE)
- surgical or disease factors: pelvic surgery, cancer in pelvic organs, cardiac failure, infection, paraplegia, polycythaemia and paroxysmal nocturnal haemoglobinuria.

Letsky E, Murphy MF, Ramsay JE, Walker I. Venous Thromboembolism in Obstetrics and Gynaecology. London: RCOG Press, 2005.

14. **A False.** Androstenedione does not have androgenic activity and is converted to testosterone in the peripheral tissues.

    B False. DHEA does not have androgenic activity and is converted to testosterone in the peripheral tissues.

    C True. Increased activity of this enzyme may result in hirsutism.

    D True. Small amounts are excreted as testosterone glucuronide.

    E True. The main androgen of the adrenal gland is dehydroepiandrosterone sulphate (DHEA-S). Ovaries and adrenals produce androstenedione in equal amounts.

Khan R. Chapter 12: Principles and new developments in molecular biology. In: Shaw RW, Luesley D, Monga A (eds). Gynaecology (4th edn). Edinburgh: Churchill Livingstone, 2011.
Critchley HOD, Horne A, Munro K. Chapter 16: Amenorrhoea and oligomenorrhoea, and hypothalamic–pituitary dysfunction. In: Shaw RW, Luesley D, Monga A (eds). Gynaecology (4th edn). Edinburgh: Churchill Livingstone, 2011.

15. **A True.** Transsphenoidal approach is used for surgical removal of macroadenomas.

    B True. Non-functioning adenomas will not respond to medical therapy.

    C True.

    D False. Breastfeeding is not an indication for surgery and the presence of adenoma is not a contraindication to breastfeeding.

E False. In view of the high risk of developing pressure symptoms (headache and visual field defects), women should be counselled to avoid pregnancy until they have had a good response to drug therapy or surgical removal of macroadenoma.

The commonest causes of increased prolactin levels are pituitary prolactinomas (40–50% of cases) and idiopathic secretion. Drugs account for 1–2% and primary hypothyroidism for 3–5% of cases.

The typical presentation is amenorrhoea/oligomenorrhoea with or without galactorrhoea (there is no correlation of galactorrhoea with either prolactin levels or presence of micro- or macroadenoma). Only 5% have visual field defects (bitemporal hemianopia). Hence women with macroadenomas should have a full visual assessment to exclude bitemporal hemianopia.

The first line of therapy in women with adenomas is a dopamine agonist such as bromocriptine or cabergoline. It causes a fall in prolactin levels and shrinkage in the volume of the tumour within 2 months. This results in the return of ovulation and pregnancy. Transsphenoidal surgery is rarely indicated for prolactinomas in view of the high recurrence rate and possible panhypopituitarism.

Vogiatzi M and Shaw RW. Chapter 17: Ovulation induction. In: Shaw RW, Luesley D, Monga A (eds). Gynaecology (4th edn). Edinburgh: Churchill Livingstone, 2011.
Critchley HOD, Horne A, Munro K. Chapter 16: Amenorrhoea and oligomenorrhoea, and hypothalamic–pituitary dysfunction. In: Shaw RW, Luesley D, Monga A (eds). Gynaecology (4th edn). Edinburgh: Churchill Livingstone, 2011.

16. **A True.** COCP, progestogens, GnRH agonists and danazol are equally effective in alleviating endometriosis-related pain. However, one has to balance the side effects before prescribing them.

    B True. Danazol has androgenic side effects. Therefore women should be advised to use barrier contraception while using this drug.

    C True. Gestrinone has similar actions to danazol but has a better side effect profile than danazol. Therefore, women should be advised to use barrier contraception while using this drug.

    D True. Recurrence is almost 100% with aspiration of the endometriosis. Therefore other methods should be used (cystectomy, excision or deroofing) followed by GnRH agonist therapy.

    E True. Pelvic clearance is also indicated in women with failed drug therapy or failed conservative surgical therapy (suitable for women where fertility is not an issue).

    Royal College of Obstetricians and Gynaecologists. Green-top Guideline No. 24. Investigation and Management of Endometriosis. London: RCOG Press, 2006.

17. **A False.** A crescent sign indicates normal ovarian tissue surrounding the cyst. It indicates the benign nature of the cyst.

    B False. A unilocular and uniform cyst is suggestive of the benign nature of the cyst. A multilocular cyst increases the suspicion of malignancy.

    C True. Round or halo vascularity with the colour Doppler is seen in functional cysts, which are benign.

D True. The higher the RMI, the greater the risk of malignancy.

E True. Septae or papillary projections >3 mm increase the suspicion of malignancy.

Royal College of Obstetricians and Gynaecologists. Green-top Guideline No. 34. Ovarian cysts in postmenopausal women. London: RCOG Press, 2003.
Royal College of Obstetricians and Gynaecologists. Green-top Guideline No. 62. Management of suspected ovarian masses in premenopausal women. London: RCOG Press, 2011.
National Institute for Health and Clinical Excellence. NICE guideline on ovarian cancer: the recognition and initial management (CG122). NICE, 2011.

Chapter 4

Core surgical skills

1. **With regards to safe entry techniques during laparoscopy:**
   A The Veress needle should be inserted through the umbilical incision, angled at 45 degrees to the skin
   B Entry pressure into the abdomen should be more than 11 mmHg when the gas tube is attached to the Veress needle
   C It is important to push the Veress needle further into the abdomen following two audible clicks on insertion into the abdomen
   D It is important to move the Veress needle by lateral movements on obtaining high pressure on the monitor on insertion as it may be touching the omentum in the abdomen
   E The patient should be in Trendelenburg position when inserting a Veress needle through the umbilical incision

2. **Complications during laparoscopy**
   A Fifty per cent of bowel injuries are not recognised at the time of surgery
   B The risk of death is 8 in 100,000 as a result of complications
   C The risk of serious complications is 2 in 10,000 women
   D The risk of bowel injury is much less using Hassan's technique than closed technique.
   E The risk of visceral injury is higher with Veress needle insertion compared to direct trocar entry into the abdomen

3. **With regards to safe entry and closing practice in laparoscopic surgery:**
   A Palmer's entry into the abdomen is recommended in women with multiple previous abdomino-pelvic surgeries
   B If the size of lateral ports is >10 mm, they should be closed with a J-shaped needle
   C If the size of midline ports is >7 mm, they should be closed with a J-shaped needle
   D The laparoscope should point towards the pelvis on first entry into the umbilical port
   E Transillumination should be used to identify the inferior epigastric artery before insertion of the lateral ports

4. **With regards to the surgical management of ectopic pregnancy:**
   A The Royal College of Obstetricians and Gynaecologists (RCOG) recommends salpingectomy on the side of the ectopic pregnancy if the contralateral tube is diseased

B   The RCOG recommends salpingotomy on the side of the ectopic pregnancy if the contralateral tube is healthy

C   Future pregnancy rates are higher when salpingotomy is performed compared to salpingectomy

D   Future pregnancy rates are higher with open salpingectomy compared to laparoscopic salpingectomy

E   The risk of recurrent ectopic pregnancy is more with salpingectomy compared to salpingotomy

5. **With regards to paralytic ileus:**

A   It is associated with good tolerance to oral fluids

B   It is associated with abdominal distension with good bowel sounds

C   It is associated with bowel handling during surgery

D   It is associated with delayed passage of stool or flatus

E   It can be managed conservatively

6. **With regards to bowel obstruction following gynaecological surgery:**

A   It is a very common complication

B   It is usually apparent on the first postoperative day

C   In the presence of peritonism, immediate surgery is necessary

D   Recent reports show closure of the pelvic peritoneum decreases the incidence of bowel obstruction

E   It can be managed conservatively in the absence of peritonism

7. **With regards to bowel injury during gynaecological surgery:**

A   It is uncommon

B   The incidence is <1%

C   In 75% of cases, site of injury is the small bowel

D   Vaginal surgery is associated with a higher rate of bowel injury compared to abdominal surgery

E   It usually manifests on days 2–3 in the postoperative period if it goes unrecognised and unrepaired during surgery

8. **With regards to abdominal incisions:**

A   A vertical midline incision avoids all major nerves and vessels

B   A vertical midline incision gives very good access to subdiaphragmatic areas

C   Transverse muscle-cutting incisions heal more rapidly than vertical incisions

D   Cherney's incision is similar to Pfannenstiel incision except rectus muscles are cut 1 cm from their insertion into the symphysis pubis

E   Maylard's incision involves dividing all layers of the abdominal wall at the same level as the skin incision and also involves division of the inferior epigastric artery

Answers

1. **A False.** The Veress needle should be sharp, with a good spring action. A disposable needle is recommended as it fulfils these criteria. The Veress needle should be inserted through the umbilical incision perpendicular to the skin.

    B False. The entry pressure should be less than 8 mmHg (low pressure).

    C False. Double clicks are usually heard when the Veress traverses the fascia and the peritoneum. Once a double click is achieved and there is loss of resistance, there is no need to push the Veress needle further into the abdomen as it might damage the internal organs (bowel, bladder or vessels).

    D False. It is good practice to avoid excessive lateral movements of the Veress needle on entry into the abdomen as a small visceral injury can be made larger.

    E False. The patient should be flat on the table when inserting the Veress needle through the abdomen as the Trendelenburg position can facilitate the Veress towards the direction of aorta.

    Royal College of Obstetricians and Gynaecologists. Diagnostic laparoscopy. Consent advice No.2. London: RCOG, 2008.
    Magowan B. Churchill's Pocketbook of Obstetrics and Gynaecology (3rd edn). Edinburgh: Churchill Livingston, 2005.
    Royal College of Obstetricians and Gynaecologists. Preventing entry related gynaecological laparoscopic injuries. RCOG guideline No. 49. London: RCOG, 2008.

2. **A False.** Fifteen per cent of bowel injuries are not recognised at the time of surgery and present later.

    B True. Death is often not explained by doctors or included in the consent form.

    C False. The risk of serious complications is 2 in 1000 women.

    D False. Hassan's technique does not reduce the risk of bowel injury but does reduce vascular injury.

    E False. There is no supporting evidence. Direct trocar entry is an acceptable method of entry into the abdomen in experienced hands.

    Hassan's technique

    This is an open technique where the surgeon can see what he or she is doing. After the induction of anesthesia, a 1 cm incision is made on the skin (the site where you want to put the port). Following this, blunt dissection is performed until the underlying fascia is identified. The fascia is elevated with a pair of Kocher clamps and adherent subcutaneous tissue is gently dissected free. It is then incised to permit entry of the trocar into the peritoneal cavity. Two heavy, absorbable sutures are placed on either side of the fascial incision in the same way as an umbilical hernia is repaired. Care must be taken when applying these sutures not to cause injury to the underlying viscera. The Kocher clamps are next removed, and a 10 mm blunt trocar is advanced into the peritoneal cavity. The obturator is removed and the sleeve is secured in position with the previously placed two sutures. The sleeve of the trocar is wrapped with Vaseline gauze to prevent leakage of insufflated gas around the trocar.

Royal College of Obstetricians and Gynaecologists. Diagnostic laparoscopy. Consent advice No.2. London: RCOG Press, 2008.

Magowan B. Churchill's Pocketbook of Obstetrics and Gynaecology (3rd edn). Edinburgh: Churchill Livingston, 2005.

Royal College of Obstetricians and Gynaecologists. Preventing entry related gynaecological laparoscopic injuries. RCOG guideline No. 49. London: RCOG Press, 2008.

3. **A True.** Palmer's entry point is 3 cm below the costal margin in the midclavicular line. Recently, it has been advocated that the ninth intercostal space can be used for this purpose, as a landmark. One should always palpate for any masses or splenomegaly before insertion of the Veress needle and also the stomach should be deflated by using a nasogastric tube if there is any doubt in order to avoid injury to the stomach (case reports).

   B False. If the size of the lateral port is >7 mm, the lateral port sites should be closed with a J-shaped needle to avoid port site hernias.

   C False. If the size of the midline port is >10 mm, the midline port should be closed with a J-shaped needle to avoid port site hernias.

   D False. One should have a direct view at the entry site and also a 360° view all around the port site in order to identify any visceral injury before entering the pelvic region or before starting the procedure. When looking at the liver, one should bear in mind the falciform ligament in the midline in order to avoid damage and bleeding from the ligament.

   E False. Transillumination is usually used to identify the vessels beneath the skin at the port sites. It does not identify the inferior epigastric vessels and therefore should not be used for this purpose.

Royal College of Obstetricians and Gynaecologists. Diagnostic laparoscopy. Consent advice No.2. London: RCOG Press, 2008.

Magowan B. Churchill's Pocketbook of Obstetrics and Gynaecology (3rd edn). Edinburgh: Churchill Livingston, 2005.

Royal College of Obstetricians and Gynaecologists. Preventing entry related gynaecological laparoscopic injuries. RCOG guideline No. 49. London: RCOG Press, 2008.

4. **A False.** The RCOG recommends salpingectomy on the side of the ectopic pregnancy when the contralateral tube is healthy.

   B False. The RCOG recommends salpingotomy on the side of the ectopic pregnancy when the contralateral tube is diseased.

   C False. The pregnancy rates are similar for both salpingotomy and salpingectomy.

   D False. There is no evidence to suggest this fact.

   E False. The risk of recurrent ectopic pregnancy is greater with salpingotomy than with salpingectomy. The general risk of recurrent ectopic pregnancies following an ectopic pregnancy is around 10%. The risk of recurrent ectopic pregnancies following salpingotomy is 20% (double).

Royal College of Obstetricians and Gynaecologists. Green-top Guideline No. 21. Management of tubal pregnancy. London: RCOG Press, 2004.

Magowan B. Churchill's Pocketbook of Obstetrics and Gynaecology (3rd edn). Edinburgh: Churchill Livingston, 2005.

5. **A** **False.** It is associated with poor tolerance to oral fluids.

    B **False.** It is associated with abdominal distension with absent bowel sounds.

    C **True.** Normally bowel sounds return within 24 hours following surgery and failure to do so will indicate paralysis of activity.

    D **True.** This is due to inactivity of the bowel.

    E **True.** There is often an electrolyte imbalance in the form of hypokalaemia. The majority of cases resolve with conservative therapy which includes giving intravenous fluids, no intake of fluids or food by mouth (to rest the bowel) and nasogastric drainage (using nasogastric tubes). In cases that do not resolve other causes should be ruled out. These include pelvic infection in the form of abscess or a haematoma which may need treatment, although this is a rare situation.

    Amer SA. Chapter 9: Postoperative care. In: Shaw RW, Luesley D, Monga A (eds). Gynaecology (4th edn). Edinburgh: Churchill Livingstone, 2011.

6. **A** **False.** Bowel obstruction is rare following gynaecological surgery.

    B **False.** It usually starts manifesting on postoperative day five.

    C **True.** Peritonism may indicate sepsis or any organ injury.

    D **False.** Closure of the pelvic peritoneum during surgery does not decrease either bowel obstruction or postoperative adhesions.

    E **True.** The initial treatment should be nasogastric drainage and intravenous fluids. Some women may have symptoms of vomiting large volumes of fluid, pain and no passage of flatus or faeces and may require surgical management.

    Amer SA. Chapter 9: Postoperative care. In: Shaw RW, Luesley D, Monga A (eds). Gynaecology (4th edn). Edinburgh: Churchill Livingstone, 2011.

7. **A** **True.**

    B **True.** The incidence is 0.3–0.8%.

    C **False.** Abdominal surgery is associated more with increased risk of bowel damage than laparoscopic or vaginal surgery.

    D **True.**

    E **True.** Depending on the site and extent of damage, patients may present with abdominal distention, vomiting, swinging pyrexia, signs of peritonism and shock. Abdominal X-ray may show gas under the diaphragm or distended loops. Computed tomography (CT) scan with contrast may further help to localise the collection.

    Amer SA. Chapter 9: Postoperative care. In: Shaw RW, Luesley D, Monga A (eds). Gynaecology (4th edn). Edinburgh: Churchill Livingstone, 2011.

8. **A** **True.**

    B **False.** It provides good access to the abdomen but not to subdiaphragmatic areas.

    C **True.** All transverse incisions heal more rapidly than vertical incisions.

    D **True.**

E True. Both Cherney's and Maylard's incision provide good access to the pelvis and are useful in gynaecological oncological surgeries.

Abdominal incisions can be vertical (midline or paramedian incision) or transverse incisions.

Vertical incisions

Advantages:

- avoids all major vessels, nerves and muscles and involves only cutting the rectus sheath
- used in gynaecological oncology surgery
- allows quick entry into the abdominal cavity with little blood loss
- easily extended in length to accommodate the operative findings

Disadvantages:

- an increased risk of wound dehiscence
- an increased risk of hernia formation
- delayed healing

Mass closure technique should be used to close a midline incision in view of the above complications. This involves 1 cm deep bites of the rectus sheath, muscle and peritoneum in a continuous closure with sutures placed 1 cm apart.

Transverse incisions

Transverse incisions include Pfannenstiel, Maylard's, Cherney's and Rutherford-Morrison incisions.

Advantages:

- heal better and faster
- better cosmetic results
- less pain
- low incidence of hernia formation

Disadvantages:

- limit access and exploration of the upper abdomen
- are associated with greater blood loss
- are more prone to haematoma formation
- nerve injury can result in paraesthesia of the overlying skin

McIndoe A. Chapter 8: Principles of surgery and management of intraoperative complications. In: Shaw RW, Luesley D, Monga A (eds). Gynaecology (4th edn). Edinburgh: Churchill Livingstone, 2011.

Chapter 5

Drug therapy in obstetrics and gynaecology

1. **With regards to mifepristone:**
   - A   It is a progesterone receptor agonist
   - B   It is an 11β-dimethyl-amino-phenyl derivative
   - C   It has a high affinity for progesterone receptors
   - D   It has a high affinity for glucocorticoid receptors
   - E   It blocks the progesterone receptors in the myometrium and cervix

2. **Mifepristone:**
   - A   Is absolutely contraindicated in women with adrenal insufficiency
   - B   Is absolutely contraindicated in women with mild asthma
   - C   Is absolutely contraindicated in women on anticoagulant therapy
   - D   Is absolutely contraindicated in women with hypertension
   - E   Is absolutely contraindicated in women smokers <25 years age

3. **With regards to antihypertensive drug use during pregnancy:**
   - A   Methyldopa is an α1-agonist
   - B   Methyldopa can cause systemic lupus erythematosus (SLE) like symptoms
   - C   Methyldopa may cause a positive Coomb's test
   - D   Methyldopa may cause a raised serum alanine aminotransferase
   - E   Methyldopa is contraindicated in women with intrauterine fetal growth restriction (IUGR)

4. **With regards to antihypertensive drugs:**
   - A   Sodium nitroprusside can be safely used during all trimesters of pregnancy
   - B   Atenolol can be safely used to treat pre-eclampsia during pregnancy
   - C   Diazoxide can be safely used during pregnancy
   - D   Angiotensin converting enzyme (ACE) inhibitors can be safely used during pregnancy
   - E   Nifedipine can be safely used during pregnancy

5. **With regards to antihypertensive treatment during pregnancy:**
   - A   Labetalol should be used with caution in women with asthma
   - B   Labetalol has a positive effect on fetal lung maturation in women with severe hypertension who are distant from term

    C Intravenous labetalol, when used for treating severe hypertension, causes more reflex tachycardia than hydralazine

    D Intravenous hydralazine causes controlled decrease in blood pressure when administered for treatment of severe hypertension

    E Intravenous nitroglycerine in high doses may result in methemoglobinemia

6. **The following abnormalities and drugs are correctly matched:**

    A Neural tube defects – sodium valproate

    B Ebstein's anomaly – lithium

    C Orofacial defects – carbamazepine

    D Limb defects – thalidomide

    E Vaginal adenosis – diethylstilboestrol

7. **Tranexamic acid:**

    A Is an antifibrinolytic agent

    B Is used as a third line drug for the treatment of menorrhagia

    C Increases endometrial tissue plasminogen activator activity

    D Reduces menstrual blood loss by 90%

    E Can cause dysmenorrhoea

8. **With regards to heparin:**

    A Unfractionated heparin crosses the placenta

    B Low molecular weight heparin (LMWH) increases the risk of fetal haemorrhage

    C Thrombocytopenia is more common with LMWH compared to unfractionated heparin

    D Unfractionated heparin can cause symptomatic osteoporosis

    E LMWH has a better side effect profile compared to unfractionated heparin

9. **With regards to warfarin and pregnancy:**

    A It crosses the placenta

    B It is not a teratogen

    C Epidural anaesthesia can be used if mother is on warfarin

    D Spinal anaesthesia can be used if mother is on warfarin

    E Its use should be avoided after 36 weeks of gestation

10. **With regards to Dextran 70:**

    A It can be safely used in pregnancy

    B It can cause an anaphylactoid reaction in the mother

    C It can cause uterine hypotonus

    D It can cause fetal distress

    E It can cause fetal death

11. **With regards to aspirin:**

    A It is used in pregnancy for thromboprophylaxis in women with previous venous thrombosis

    B In low doses (75 mg) aspirin is safe to use in the second and third trimesters of pregnancy

C   It is effective in the management of recurrent pregnancy loss when no cause is found
D   Aspirin alone significantly reduces the pregnancy loss in women with antiphospholipid antibody syndrome
E   Aspirin plus heparin improve the live birth rate to around 70% in women with antiphospholipid antibody syndrome

12. **With regards to thromboprophylaxis during pregnancy:**
   A   Prophylactic LMWH should be stopped at least 24 hours before giving epidural anaesthesia
   B   Therapeutic LMWH should be stopped at least 48 hours before giving spinal anaesthesia
   C   At least 12 hours should pass after the last prophylactic dose of LMWH and the introduction of an epidural catheter
   D   At least 24 hours should pass after the last prophylactic dose of LMWH and the removal of an epidural catheter
   E   Antenatal thromboprophylaxis with LMWH should be started only after 12 weeks of pregnancy

13. **Regarding the management of acute venous thromboembolism (VTE) during pregnancy:**
   A   Intravenous unfractionated heparin is contraindicated
   B   Subcutaneous unfractionated heparin can be used twice daily after an initial intravenous bolus dose
   C   LMWH is as effective as unfractionated heparin for the initial management of VTE
   D   In pregnancy, unfractionated heparin is preferred to LMWH for the treatment of acute massive VTE
   E   In pregnancy, a twice daily regimen of LMWH is recommended for treatment of VTE rather than a single daily dose

14. **With regards to unfractionated heparin:**
   A   Thrombin time should be monitored to adjust the dose of unfractionated heparin
   B   Activated partial thromboplastin time (APTT) should be performed 6 hours after the loading dose
   C   APTT should be maintained in the therapeutic ratio of 3–5 times the mean control value
   D   If there are problems interpreting APTT during pregnancy, anti-Xa levels may be useful to monitor heparin dose
   E   Blood test for platelet count should be undertaken between days 4 and 8 after the commencement of treatment

15. **Cabergoline:**
   A   Can cause agranulocytosis
   B   Promotes the return of regular menstruation
   C   Has recognised teratogenic effects
   D   Has more side effects than bromocriptine
   E   Is a dopamine antagonist

16. **The following drugs are used in the treatment of hirsutism:**

    A   Cyproterone acetate
    B   Ketoconazole
    C   Progesteogen only pill
    D   Amiodarone
    E   Ciprofloxacin

17. **The following actions of drug mechanisms are correctly matched:**

    A   Tamoxifen – oestrogen antagonist
    B   Ketoconazole – inhibits dopa decarboxylase
    C   Clomiphene – oestrogen antagonist
    D   Combined oral contraceptive pill (COCP) – direct inhibition of ovarian oestrogen production
    E   Desmopressin or 1–deamino–8-D–arginine vasopressin (DDAVP) – increases von Willebrand's factor (VWF)

18. **The following drugs are correctly matched with regards to reduction in menstrual blood loss:**

    A   Tranexamic acid: reduces menstrual blood loss by 90%
    B   Mefenamic acid: reduces menstrual blood loss by 60%
    C   Luteal phase progestogens (days 16–25): reduce menstrual blood loss by 90%
    D   Danazol: reduces menstrual blood loss by 30%
    E   Gonadotropin-releasing hormone analogues: reduce menstrual blood loss by 80%

19. **With regards to iron therapy:**

    A   Oral iron causes a rise in haemoglobin (Hb) by 0.8 g/dL/week
    B   Parenteral iron causes a rise in Hb by 2 g/dL/week
    C   A blood transfusion should be considered if Hb is 6 g/dL at term
    D   Slow release iron preparations have more side effects than conventional preparations like ferrous sulphate
    E   Iron therapy has less effect on cellular enzymes defects than blood transfusion (red cells) used to increase the Hb

20. **The following can be used to treat genital warts during pregnancy:**

    A   Interferon
    B   Cryotherapy
    C   5-fluorouracil
    D   Topical trichloroacetic acid
    E   Podophyllin

21. **Antibiotic prophylaxis during pregnancy is recommended for women with:**

    A   Recurrent urinary tract infections
    B   Renal transplant
    C   Renal tract abnormalities
    D   A first episode of urinary tract infection in the third trimester
    E   2+ blood on urine dipstick

22. **With regards to drug interactions:**
    A Danazol enhances the effect of anticoagulant warfarin by inhibiting its metabolism
    B Metoclopramide antagonises the effect of bromocriptine in treating hyperprolactinaemia
    C Rifampicin accelerates metabolism of COCP and reduce its contraceptive efficacy
    D Broad spectrum antibiotics reduce the contraceptive efficacy of COCP
    E Sulphonamides increase the antifolate effects of phenytoin during pregnancy

Answers

1. A **False.**

    B **True.**

    C **True.**

    D **True.**

    E **True.**

    The most common drugs used in medical management and medically induced abortion in the UK include anti-progesterone, mifepristone and prostaglandin analogues (misoprostol and gemeprost).

    Mifepristone is an anti-progesterone and has a high affinity for progesterone and glucocorticoid receptors. It acts by blocking the progesterone receptors in the decidua, myometrium and cervix and thereby promotes termination of pregnancy.

    Mifepristone alone has a success rate of around 88% and in combination with prostaglandin, the success rate increases to 94–96%.

    Medical management is advised before 9 weeks of gestation (earlier termination increases its effectiveness and results in fewer complications). Mifepristone must be administered in a hospital in the UK. Following this, prostaglandin is administered 36–48 hours later and the patient is kept under observation for 4–6 hours. Women must be warned that 5% will require surgical management, and the continuing pregnancy rate is 0.3% and 7% with the use of gemeprost and misoprostol, respectively.

    Amis S. Medical management of first trimester induced abortion and miscarriage. Personal assessment in continuing education. Reviews, questions and answers. Volume 3. London: RCOG Press, 2003:67–68. Royal College of Obstetricians and Gynaecologists. Green-top Guideline No. 25. Early pregnancy loss. London: RCOG Press, 2006.

2. A **True.**

    B **False.**

    C **True.**

    D **False.**

    E **False.**

    The absolute contraindications include:

    *   porphyria
    *   smokers >35 years of age
    *   known allergy to mifepristone and misoprostol
    *   anaemia
    *   women on long-term glucocorticoid therapy
    *   known haemoglobinopathies
    *   women on anticoagulant therapy

- adrenal insufficiency
- suspected ectopic pregnancy

The relative contraindications include severe hypertension and severe asthma.

Amis S. Medical management of first trimester induced abortion and miscarriage. Personal assessment in continuing education. Reviews, questions and answers Volume 3. London: RCOG Press, 2003:67–68.

3. A False.

   B True.

   C True.

   D True.

   E False.

A methyldopa is an antihypertensive drug which is commonly used in pregnant women to treat raised blood pressure (pregnancy-induced hypertension and pre-eclampsia). It has not been shown to cause any fetal abnormality.

Methyldopa is a centrally acting α2-agonist. It is converted in the adrenergic nerve endings to a false neurotransmitter called alpha methylnoradrenaline, which stimulates α2 receptors in the medulla and reduces sympathetic outflow (centrally acting). The side effects include drowsiness, haemolytic anaemia, elevation of liver enzymes and positive Coomb's test. It can cause SLE -like syndrome and should be therefore avoided in people with SLE.

James D, Steer PJ, Weiner CP, Gonik B, Crowther C, Robson S (eds). High Risk Pregnancy: Management Options (4th edn). St Louis: Saunders, 2011.

4. A False.

   B False.

   C False.

   D False.

   E True.

ACE inhibitors

The use of ACE inhibitors and angiotensin receptor blockers are contraindicated in pregnancy due to significant fetal effects. In the second and third trimesters, use of these medications has been associated with renal dysgenesis, oligohydramnios, calvarial and pulmonary hypoplasia, intrauterine growth restriction, and fetal demise (fetal abnormalities similar to Potter syndrome). First trimester exposure to ACE inhibitors has been shown to be associated with a greater incidence of malformations of the cardiovascular and central nervous system.

Beta-blockers (labetalol)

There is an extensive amount of literature on the use of beta-blockers in pregnancy. The adverse effects of beta-blockers are still under scrutiny with some reports of increased IUGR, hypoglycaemia, bradycardia and hyperbilirubinaemia (in the case of propranolol). Labetalol, a non-selective beta-blocker with vascular alpha-1 receptor blocking capabilities is currently the beta-blocker of choice in pregnancy and has been shown to be safe when administered orally to women with chronic hypertension. However, there are some reports of fetal growth restriction and fetal bradycardia with labetalol. The other side effects are mainly due to beta-blocking effects and include fatigue, lethargy, exercise intolerance, peripheral vasoconstriction, sleep disturbance and bronchoconstriction (therefore possibly avoid its use in women with history of asthma).

Labetalol is used parenterally to treat severe hypertension.

Nifedipine

With regards to calcium channel blockers, nifedipine has been the most widely researched and is now used in pregnancy. The use of long-acting nifedipine has been recommended as short-acting nifedipine is associated with maternal hypotension and fetal distress. Other maternal adverse effects of calcium channel antagonists include tachycardia, palpitations, peripheral oedema, headaches and facial flushing. There has also been concern regarding its use with magnesium sulphate in the treatment of pre-eclampsia and eclampsia. Drug interactions between them were reported to cause neuromuscular blockade, myocardial depression, or circulatory collapse in a few cases. Recently these medications have been used together without increased risk of the above. There is insufficient evidence regarding the use of other calcium channel blockers during pregnancy.

Hydralazine

Hydralazine selectively relaxes arteriolar smooth muscle. It can be used orally, intramuscularly or intravenously. For the acute control of blood pressure it is administered intravenously (the main use of hydralazine).The side effects include maternal tachycardia, headache, nausea, flushing or palpitations. Long-term use of this drug is known to cause pyridoxine-responsive polyneuropathy or immunologic reactions, including a drug-induced lupus syndrome. It can be used in all trimesters of pregnancy and is not known to be teratogenic (although neonatal thrombocytopenia and lupus have been reported). Intravenous hydralazine is associated with more side effects than intravenous labetalol or oral nifedipine (which include maternal hypotension, increase risk of caesarean sections, placental abruptions, low Apgar scores and oliguria).

Sodium nitroprusside

Sodium nitroprusside is a direct nitric oxide (NO) donor. NO activates guanylate cyclase in the vascular smooth muscle and increases intracellular production of 3', 5'- cyclic guanosine monophosphate (cGMP), which in turn stimulates calcium movement from the cytoplasm to the endoplasmic reticulum and reduces the concentration of calcium available to bind with calmodulin. It non-selectively relaxes both arteriolar and venular vascular smooth muscle and hence causes vessel dilatation.

It is only administered by continuous intravenous infusion. It acts immediately and the duration of effect lasts 3 minutes. Metabolism of this drug in the body releases cyanide which is further metabolized to thiocyanate.

The theoretical risk of fetal cyanide intoxication remains unknown. The other side effects include excessive vasodilation and cardioneurogenic syncope (paradoxical bradycardia) in volume-depleted pre-eclamptic women. Due to availability of safer alternatives in pregnancy (parenteral hydralazine, labetalol and oral calcium channel blockers) the use of this drug is not recommended during pregnancy.

James D, Steer PJ, Weiner CP, Gonik B, Crowther C, Robson S (eds). High Risk Pregnancy: Management Options (4th edn). St Louis: Saunders, 2011.

5. A True.

    B True.

    C False.

    D False.

    E True.

Labetalol is an alpha- and beta-receptor blocker and is safe to use during pregnancy (it does not cause fetal anomalies). However, some studies show an increased risk of fetal growth restriction when this drug is used throughout pregnancy, whereas others shows no such association. Overall the benefits of its use during pregnancy outweigh the risks. Its use should be avoided in women suffering from asthma.

Labetalol causes a controlled decrease in blood pressure by reducing the systemic vascular resistance in patients with severe hypertension. When used in a setting to treat severe hypertension, it causes less reflex tachycardia compared to hydralazine. The maximum dose per day is 2400 mg.

Hydralazine decreases mean arterial pressure and systemic vascular resistance while increasing heart rate and cardiac output. When administered parenterally to treat severe hypertension, it causes rapid and profound reduction in blood pressure. This may greatly decrease the blood flow to the fetoplacental unit and cause fetal distress. In order to avoid this, a fluid bolus (Gelofusine 250–500 mL) can be administered before administering hydralazine.

Nitroglycerine is mainly a venous dilator. It reduces preload at small doses and afterload in large doses. It is fast-acting and has a short half-life of 3 minutes. Methemoglobinaemia may result from administration of large doses parenterally (>7 mg/kg/min). Patients who appear cyanotic should be evaluated for its toxicity.

Diazoxide is an antihypertensive and its use during pregnancy has been associated with alopecia and transient neonatal hypoglycaemia.

Diuretics are used to treat pulmonary oedema during pregnancy. The long-term use of thiazide diuretics to treat hypertension during pregnancy can cause transient neonatal thrombocytopaenia, neonatal hyperbilurubinaemia, decrease in maternal blood volume and decrease uteroplacental perfusion.

James D, Steer PJ, Weiner CP, Gonik B, Crowther C, Robson S (eds). High Risk Pregnancy: Management Options (4th edn). St Louis: Saunders, 2011.

6.   **A**   True.

    B   True.

    C   True. Orofacial defects are treated with carbamazepine, phenytoin, phenobarbitone and benzodiazepines.

    D   True.

    E   True.

Anticonvulsant drugs and fetal defects

Almost all anticonvulsant drugs cross the placenta and are teratogenic (primidone, phenytoin, phenobarbitone, carbamazepine and sodium valproate).

The major malformations caused by these drugs include:

- orofacial defects (carbamazepine, phenytoin, phenobarbitone and benzodiazepines)
- congenital heart defects (phenytoin, phenobarbitone and sodium valproate)
- neural tube defects (sodium valproate and carbamazepine)

The risk of fetal abnormality with one drug is 6–7%, with two or more drugs 10–15% and with a combination of valproate, phenytoin and phenobarbitone, the risk increases to 50%. Dose-dependent teratogenicity is known with sodium valproate and lamotrigine.

When women are referred for antenatal care or preconception counselling, one needs to balance the risk of stopping the above drugs versus the risks of teratogenicity. A prompt referral should be made for joint psychiatric and obstetric care and avoid starting certain medications known to be harmful to the developing fetus in women who wish to conceive.

Lithium

- is associated with fetal heart defects (60 in 1000)
- involves the right side of the heart
- possible risk of Ebstein anomaly (1 in 20,000 children): characterised by apical displacement of the septal and posterior trucuspid valve leaflets, leading to atrialization of the right ventricle with a variable degree of malformation and displacement of the anterior leaflet.
- if possible, change the drug before conception
- is secreted in high levels in breast milk
- during pregnancy: check drug levels every 4 weeks to adjust the dose to keep serum levels towards the lower end of the therapeutic range
- intrapartum: maintain fluid balance during labour

The clinical manifestation is at birth if the abnormality is severe. Otherwise it can present at any age (teenagers or adults). The outcome for children presenting after 1 year of age is good. It is more common in Caucasians and is equally distributed between men and women.

Thalidomide

Thalidomide was withdrawn from the market after identification of limb defects in babies born to mothers exposed to this drug in the first trimester. It causes amelia, phocomelia, cardiac defects, deafness, mental retardation and autism.

Diethylstilboestrol (DES)

It is a non-steroidal oestrogen and was used for treating menopausal symptoms, prevention of miscarriage and pre-term birth in the past. Subsequent studies showed that *in utero* exposure to DES caused vaginal adenosis and vaginal clear cell adenocarcinoma in female offspring. It is also known to cause genital tract abnormalities (T-shaped uterus, transverse vaginal and cervical ridges) and infertility.

Nelson-Piercy C. Handbook of Obstetric Medicine (4th edn). London: Informa Healthcare, 2010.
National Institute for Clinical Excellence. Antenatal and postnatal mental health (CG45). NICE, 2007.

7. **A** **True.**

    B **False.** Tranexamic acid is used as a second line therapy in the treatment of menorrhagia.

    C **False.** It is antifibrinolytic and hence decreases endometrial tissue plasminogen activator activity.

    D **False.** It causes a 54% reduction in menstrual blood loss.

    E **False.** The side effects are minimal and can cause nausea, headache and dizziness.

    Letsky E, Murphy MF, Ramsay JE, Walker I. Haemorrhagic Disease and Hereditary Bleeding Disorders. London: RCOG Press, 2005.

8. **A** **False.** Both unfractionated and LMWH do not cross the placenta.

    B **False.** There is no risk of bleeding in the fetus or teratogenesis.

    C **False.** Thrombocytopenia is more common (1–3%) with unfractionated heparin and considerably lower with LMWH. When it occurs, it could be life-threatening as it is caused by idiosyncratic immune mediated reaction and is associated with widespread venous thrombosis (days 5–15 after starting therapy with heparin).

    D **True.** The incidence of osteoporotic fractures is generally around 2% (long-term therapy >5–8 months). The exact mechanism by which heparin causes osteoporosis is unknown (it may be via enzymatic inhibitions involved in bone and mineral metabolism and vitamin D activation). The three proposed mechanisms include (1) inhibition of cytokine (IL-1, IL-6 and IL-11) and tumour necrosis factor (TNF)-induced differentiation of mesenchymal into mature osteoblasts and (2) antagonises insulin-like growth factor (IGF) dependent osteoblastic maturation. (3) decreases cancellous bone volume in a dose-dependent fashion; unfractionated heparin causes significantly more cancellous bone loss that LMWH.

    E **True.** LMWH is used in pregnancy because of its better side effect profile compared to unfractionated heparin: it causes less thrombocytopenia and osteoporosis. Also monitoring with anti-Xa levels (monitoring is required in antithrombin deficiency) is not required provided renal function is normal. Platelet count should be checked 1 week after initiation of therapy.

Letsky E, Murphy MF, Ramsay JE, Walker I. Haemorrhagic Disease and Hereditary Bleeding Disorders. London: RCOG Press, 2005.

9. **A True.**

B False. It crosses the placenta and is a teratogen. It causes fetal embryopathy (4–5%) when used between 6 and 12 weeks of gestation. The abnormalities include midface hypoplasia, short phalanges, short proximal limbs and stippled chondral calcification.

C False. Epidural and spinal anaesthesia are contraindicated if the mother is on warfarin therapy.

D False.

E True. The risk of bleeding increases for both mother and fetus as it reduces vitamin K dependent coagulation factor. Therefore its use should be avoided after 36 weeks of pregnancy.

Vitamin K is used to reverse the effects of warfarin. However, it is not useful in acute situations (e.g. maternal bleeding). Fresh frozen plasma can be used in such situations.

Letsky E, Murphy MF, Ramsay JE, Walker I. Haemorrhagic Disease and Hereditary Bleeding Disorders. London: RCOG Press, 2005.

10. **A False.** Dextran has anticoagulation properties. Its use during or after the operation has been shown to reduce fatal pulmonary thromboembolism. However, its use should be avoided in pregnancy due to risk of anaphylaxis.

B True. It can cause severe allergic reactions. It should be avoided in patients with inadequate cardiac or renal function.

C False. Its use in pregnancy is associated with uterine hypertonus, fetal distress and fetal death.

D True.

E True.

Letsky E, Murphy MF, Ramsay JE, Walker I. Haemorrhagic Disease and Hereditary Bleeding Disorders. London: RCOG Press, 2005.

11. **A False.** Its value in preventing venous thrombosis during pregnancy is still under research.

B True. Aspirin is safe to use in pregnancy and has not been shown to have any adverse pregnancy outcomes.

C False. It is mainly used in women with antiphospholipid antibody syndrome and recurrent pregnancy loss.

D False. Aspirin plus heparin has been shown to significantly decrease the pregnancy loss compared to aspirin alone.

E True. It is therefore recommended therapy in women with history of recurrent miscarriage plus antiphospholipid antibody syndrome. It is suggested to start aspirin (75 mg) as soon as the pregnancy test is positive and heparin as soon as the fetal viability is confirmed on ultrasound scan. Blood tests for platelet count should be arranged weekly for 3 weeks after the commencement of therapy and 4–6 weekly thereafter.

Letsky E, Murphy MF, Ramsay JE, Walker I. Haemorrhagic Disease and Hereditary Bleeding Disorders. London: RCOG Press, 2005.

12. **A False.** Prophylactic LMWH should be stopped at least 12 hours before epidural anaesthesia. The required interval between a prophylactic dose of unfractionated heparin and regional analgesia or anaesthesia is less (4 hours) and there is less concern regarding neuraxial haematomas with unfractionated heparin. However, any use of unfractionated heparin carries a risk of heparin-induced thrombocytopaenia.

B False. Therapeutic LMWH should be stopped at least 24 hours before giving a spinal anaesthesia.

C True.

D False. At least 12 hours should pass after the last prophylactic dose of LMWH and the removal of the epidural catheter.

E False. Antenatal thromboprophylaxis with LMWH should be started early in pregnancy or as soon as the risk is identified.

Women receiving antenatal LMWH should be advised that, if they have any vaginal bleeding or once labour begins, they should not inject any further LMWH. They should be reassessed on admission to hospital and further doses should be prescribed by medical staff.

Letsky E, Murphy MF, Ramsay JE, Walker I. Haemorrhagic Disease and Hereditary Bleeding Disorders. London: RCOG Press, 2005.
Royal College of Obstetricians and Gynaecologists. Green-top Guideline No. 37A. Thrombosis during pregnancy and puerperium, reducing the risk. London: RCOG Press, 2009.

13. **A False.** Unfractionated heparin can be given by continuous intravenous infusion.

B True. Subcutaneous unfractionated heparin is an effective alternative.

C True. The initial results were extrapolated from non-pregnant women and LMWH was found to be as effective as unfractionated heparin in the management of deep venous thrombosis (DVT) and also associated with lower risk of bleeding complications and lower mortality. LMWH is recommended for the initial management of VTE in pregnancy.

D True. Intravenous unfractionated heparin is the traditional method of heparin administration in acute VTE and remains the preferred treatment in massive pulmonary thromboembolism (PTE) because of its rapid effect and extensive experience of its use in this situation.

E True. A single daily dose of LMWH is recommended for treatment of VTE in non-pregnant women; a twice daily dose is recommended in pregnant women because of altered pharmacokinetics.

Routine measurement of peak anti-Xa activity for patients on LMWH for treatment of acute VTE in pregnancy or postpartum is not recommended except in women at extremes of body weight (≤ 50 kg and ≥ 90 kg) or with other complicating factors (e.g. with renal impairment or recurrent VTE) putting them at high risk.

Routine platelet count monitoring should not be carried out (unless unfractionated heparin has been given).

Letsky E, Murphy MF, Ramsay JE, Walker I. Haemorrhagic Disease and Hereditary Bleeding Disorders. London: RCOG Press, 2005.
Royal College of Obstetricians and Gynaecologists. Green-top Guideline No. 37B. Thrombosis and embolism during pregnancy and puerperium, the acute management of. London: RCOG Press, 2007.
Royal College of Obstetricians and Gynaecologists. Green-top Guideline No. 37A. Thrombosis during pregnancy and puerperium, reducing the risk. London: RCOG Press, 2009.

14. **A False.** APTT should be used to monitor and adjust unfractionated heparin dose.

B True. The Royal College of Obstetricians and Gynaecologists (RCOG) recommends measurement of APTT 4–6 hours after the loading dose, 6 hours after any dose change and then at least daily when in the therapeutic range. The therapeutic target APTT ratio is usually 1.5–2.5 times the average laboratory control value.

C False. APTT should be maintained at 1.5–2.5 times the mean laboratory control value and failure to attain this may lead to increased risk of recurrent VTE.

D True.

E True. The first test should be arranged 4–8 days after the commencement of treatment and thereafter should be undertaken monthly to identify heparin-induced thrombocytopenia.

Letsky E, Murphy MF, Ramsay JE, Walker I. Haemorrhagic Disease and Hereditary Bleeding Disorders. London: RCOG Press, 2005.
Royal College of Obstetricians and Gynaecologists. Green-top Guideline No. 37B. Thrombosis and embolism during pregnancy and puerperium, the acute management of. London: RCOG Press, 2007.
Royal College of Obstetricians and Gynaecologists. Green-top Guideline No. 37A. Thrombosis during pregnancy and puerperium, reducing the risk. London: RCOG Press, 2009.

15. **A False.** Agranulocytosis is caused by carbimazole and propylthiouracil.

B True. It also reduces tumour size of prolactinomas. However, the size increases once the treatment is stopped.

C False. It has no known teratogenic effects.

D False. Cabergoline has fewer side effects compared to bromocriptine (postural hypotension, nausea and vomiting).

E False. Cabergoline and bromocriptine are dopamine agonists and used as the first line in the management of hyperprolactinaemia including prolactinomas. Surgical (transsphenoidal excision of the tumour) management is indicated to treat tumours that are resistant to medical therapy.

Bromocriptine and cabergoline are used in the treatment of hyperprolactinaemia and prolactin-producing pituitary adenomas (both microprolactinomas and asymptomatic macroprolactinomas). Bromocriptine use is possibly safe during pregnancy. Women should be advised not to conceive until cured. However, if the woman presents during pregnancy they should be screened to identify recurrence and monitored to recognise exacerbation (this can be done by monitoring symptoms such as headache and visual disturbances). Surgery is indicated in extreme or symptomatic patients. Breastfeeding is not contraindicated in women with prolactinomas.

Cabergoline (an ergot derivative) is a potent dopamine receptor agonist and often used as a first line drug to treat prolactinomas. Its absorption from the gastrointestinal tract is variable and may take 0.5–4 hours. Its therapeutic effect persists for 4 weeks following cessation of therapy. Its use should be avoided during pregnancy.

Other uses

- suppress breast milk during postpartum period (single oral dose 1 mg)
- hyperprolactinaemia
- Parkinson disease
- acromegaly
- other pituitary adenomas

Side effects

- nausea, vomiting, dyspepsia and constipation
- somnolence, insomnia, vertigo, dyskinesia, hallucination and depression
- peripheral oedema, arrhythmias and palpitation

Contraindications

- hypersensitivity to ergot derivatives
- children (no clinical experience in paediatric children)
- severe hepatic dysfunction
- while using drugs such as erythromycin and ketoconazole

Caution

- cardiovascular disease
- hypotension
- gastrointestinal ulcers
- active gastrointestinal bleeding
- Raynaud disease

James D, Steer PJ, Weiner CP, Gonik B, Crowther C, Robson S (eds). High Risk Pregnancy: Management Options (4th edn). St Louis: Saunders, 2011.
Cabergoline. http://en.wikipedia.org/wiki/Cabergoline

16. **A** True.

   B True.

   C False.

   D False.

   E False.

Hirsutism is defined as excessive growth of terminal hair in a male pattern distribution.

Causes of hirsutism

- idiopathic – is due to increased 5 alpha reductase activity in pilosebaceous unit
- exogenous or iatrogenic androgens – testosterone, androgenic progestogens, danazol, gestrinone and anabolic steroids
- adrenal pathology – adrenal adenoma, adult onset congenital adrenal hyperplasia and Cushing syndrome
- ovarian pathology – PCOS, Sertoli-Leydig cell tumours, hilus cell tumours and stromal hyperthecosis
- other drugs – Minoxidil, Phenytoin, Cortisone, Diazoxide and Cyclosporin A (the pattern of hair growth is not androgenic and is described as hypertrichosis)
- luteoma of pregnancy
- other causes – Acromegaly and ectopic production of ACTH hormone

The anti-androgenic drugs used in the treatment of hirsutism include low dose COCP, medroxyprogesterone acetate depot or orally 10 mg daily, dexamethasone (more effective with adrenal cause), flutamide, finasteride, cimetidine and eflornithine hydrochloride (Vaniqa cream).

Anti-androgen drugs

- COCP suppresses luteinising hormone (LH) which in turn decreases ovarian androgen synthesis. It increases serum sex hormone binding globulin (SHBG) levels and therefore decreases free serum testosterone levels. It also has some action on inhibition of 5 alpha reductase enzyme activity.
- Finasteride inhibits 5 alpha reductase activity and therefore blocks the conversion of testosterone to dihydrotestosterone. However, it should be used with caution in women carrying a male fetus.
- Flutamide acts at receptor level and directly on the hair follicle. It is hepatotoxic and causes dry skin. Like finasteride, it should be used with caution in women carrying a male fetus.
- Cyproterone acetate is an androgen receptor antagonist with weak progestogenic activity. It inhibits gonadotrophin secretion and therefore reduces ovarian androgen production. The side effects include mastalgia, loss of libido, weight gain, fluid retention causing oedema, fatigue and feminisation of male fetus (e.g. Dianette – animal studies). Clinical data on fetal outcomes following exposure in humans is limited.
- Spironolactone is an aldosterone antagonist with anti-androgen properties. It increases metabolic clearance and reduces cutaneous 5 alpha reductase activity (by binding to the intracellular androgen receptor and forming a biologically inactive receptor). The side effects include hyperkalaemia and hypotension.
- Eflornithine hydrochloride (Vaniqa cream) inhibits the enzyme (ornithine decarboxylase) in the dermal papillae required for hair growth. It slows hair growth and makes it soft when applied locally twice daily. Its use is recommended for women with facial hair but it can cause acne as it blocks the sebaceous glands.

Barth J. Chapter 26: Hirsutism and virilisation. In: Shaw RW, Luesley D, Monga A (eds). Gynaecology (4th edn). Edinburgh: Churchill Livingstone, 2011.

17. A True. Tamoxifen is an oestrogen antagonist and partial oestrogen agonist. It has anti-oestrogenic effects on the breasts (reduces the risk of recurrent breast cancer in receptor positive patients) and oestrogenic effects on the uterus (therefore can cause endometrial polyps, hyperplasia and cancer).

B False. Ketoconazole is a synthetic imidazole derivative which interferes with the fungal synthesis of ergosterol, a constituent of fungal cell membranes, as well as inhibits certain enzymes such as cytochrome P450 14 alpha-demethylase (it blocks both gonadal and adrenal steroidogenesis). It is mainly used as an antifungal agent but is also effective but rarely used in the management of hirsutism due its side effects (nausea, asthenia and alopecia).

C True. It is used for ovulation induction and can be hostile to sperm due its anti-oestrogen action on cervical mucus.

D False. It decreases ovarian steroidogenesis by inhibiting gonadotrophin (LH) secretion from the pituitary.

E True. DDAVP is a derivative of antidiuretic hormone which is mainly used for the treatment of patients with haemophilia A and VWF deficiency.

Letsky E, Murphy MF, Ramsay JE, Walker I. Haemorrhagic Disease and Hereditary Bleeding Disorders. London: RCOG Press, 2005.
National Institute for Health and Clinical Excellence. NICE guideline on fertility: assessment and treatment for people with fertility problems (CG11). NICE, 2004.
Hughes E, Brown J, Collins JJ, Vanderkerchove P. Clomiphene citrate for unexplained sub fertility in women. Cochrane Database Syst Rev 2000; (2):CD000057.
Magowan B. Churchill's Pocketbook of Obstetrics and Gynaecology (3rd edn). Edinburgh: Churchill Livingstone, 2005.
Hamilton M. Chapter 20: Disorders and investigation of female reproduction. In: Shaw RW, Luesley D, Monga A (eds). Gynaecology (4th edn). Edinburgh: Churchill Livingstone, 2011.
Vogiatzi M and Shaw RW. Chapter 17: Ovulation induction. In: Shaw RW, Luesley D, Monga A (eds). Gynaecology (4th edn). Edinburgh: Churchill Livingstone, 2011.

18. A False.

B False.

C False.

D False.

E False.

Drugs used in the treatment of menorrhagia and reduction in blood loss are:

- Tranexamic acid is antifibrinolytic and reduces menstrual blood loss by 50%.
- Mefenamic acid is a prostaglandin inhibitor and reduces menstrual blood loss by 30–40%.
- COCP causes decrease in LH and steroidogenesis in the ovaries and therefore causes endometrial atrophy. It reduces menstrual blood by 50%.
- Luteal phase progestogens (days 16–25) are not effective and in fact increase blood loss.
- Long cycle progestogens (days 5–25) cause pseudo-decidual change and decrease menstrual blood loss by 90%.

- Danazol is anti-gonadotrophin, anti-oestrogen, anti-progestogen and a weak androgen. It reduces menstrual blood loss by 85%.
- Gonadotropin-releasing hormone analogues cause pituitary down-regulation and reduce menstrual blood loss by almost 100%.

Letsky E, Murphy MF, Ramsay JE, Walker I. Haemorrhagic Disease and Hereditary Bleeding Disorders. London: RCOG Press, 2005.
National Institute for Health and Clinical Excellence. NICE guideline on heavy menstrual bleeding (CG44). NICE, 2007.
Sen S and Lumsden MA. Chapter 31: Menstruation and menstrual disorder. In: Shaw RW, Luesley D, Monga A (eds). Gynaecology (4th edn). Edinburgh: Churchill Livingstone, 2011.

19. A True.

B False. The response to raise Hb (0.8 g/dL/week) is similar whether the iron is given parenterally or orally. Parenteral iron is preferred in women who are not compliant or intolerant to oral iron.

C True. There are no firm criteria for initiating red cell transfusion. The decision to perform a blood transfusion should be made on both clinical and haematological grounds. A transfusion is rarely indicated in the stable patient when Hb is greater than 10 g/dL and is almost always indicated when less than 6 g/dL.

D False. Slow release preparations are more expensive and comparatively have fewer side effects than the conventional oral iron therapy.

E False. Blood transfusion (red cells) used to raise Hb level does not correct the cellular enzyme defects.

The World Health Organization (WHO) recommends that iron supplementation of 30–60 mg per day is given to pregnant women who have enough stores and 120–240 mg per day to those with no stores.

James D, Steer PJ, Weiner CP, Gonik B, Crowther C, Robson S (eds). High Risk Pregnancy: Management Options (4th edn). St Louis: Saunders, 2011.
Royal College of Obstetricians and Gynaecologists. Green-top Guideline No. 47. Blood transfusion in obstetrics. London: RCOG Press, 2008.

20. A False. It is contraindicated during pregnancy.

B True. Laser vaporisation can also be used to treat large lesions.

C False. It is contraindicated during pregnancy.

D True.

E False. It is contraindicated during pregnancy.

Most anogenital warts are caused by human papilloma virus (HPV) types 6 and 11. The maternal implications include discomfort and obstructed labour if the lesions are large (may rarely require caesarean section for delivery) and fetal implications include fetal transmission during the passage through the birth canal causing juvenile laryngeal papillomatosis (HPV 6 and HPV 11) after birth.

Anogenital warts. http://www.patient.co.uk/health/Anogenital-Warts.htm

21. **A True.** Recurrent bacteriuria is diagnosed when there is >100,000 bacteria per mL on a mid-stream urine specimen. Following one episode, about 15% will have a recurrent bacteriuria during their pregnancy and require a second course of antibiotics. Regular urine cultures should be done in such women to ensure eradication of the causative organism.

    B True.

    C True.

    D False.

    E False.

    Ampicillin, amoxicillin and cephalosporins are considered safe for use during pregnancy. Trimethoprim should be avoided in the first trimester due to its antifolate action.

    Nitrofurantoin can be used but bear in mind the risk of haemolytic anaemia in women with glucose 6 phosphate dehydrogenase deficiency.

    Nelson-Piercy C. Handbook of Obstetric Medicine (4th edn). London: Informa Healthcare, 2010.

22. **A True.**

    B True. Metoclopramide is a dopamine antagonist and bromocriptine is a dopamine agonist, therefore there is antagonistic action.

    C True. Rifampicin induces liver enzymes and therefore reduces the efficacy of COCP. The other liver enzyme-inducing drugs which reduce the efficacy of COCP include griseofulvin, carbamazepine, primidone and phenobarbital.

    D True. They reduce the gut flora and enterohepatic circulation and therefore reduce the efficacy of COCP. One should advise the use of additional contraception during the first 7 days when women are taking broad spectrum antibiotics while using COCP for contraception.

    E True. Both are antifolate drugs and therefore increase the effect of each other.

    Guillebaud J. Your Questions Answered: Contraception (4th edn). Edinburgh: Churchill Livingstone, 2004.

Chapter 6

Early pregnancy

1. **With regards to recurrent miscarriage:**
   A   It is defined as three or more consecutive miscarriages after 24 weeks of gestation
   B   It is unexplained with regards to aetiology in nearly 80% of women attending recurrent miscarriage clinics
   C   Robertsonian translocation is the most frequent chromosomal abnormality found in women with recurrent miscarriage
   D   There is a definite association with arcuate uterus and recurrent miscarriage
   E   Women with syphilis have a very high incidence of recurrent early miscarriage

2. **With regards to miscarriage:**
   A   Sporadic miscarriage occurs in approximately 25% of all clinically recognised pregnancies
   B   The incidence of sporadic miscarriage increases with increasing paternal age
   C   Most early miscarriages are due to chromosomal abnormalities
   D   Miscarriage is defined as loss of intrauterine pregnancy after 28 weeks of gestation
   E   In endemic areas, malaria in non-immune women has been associated with recurrent miscarriage

3. **With regards to methotrexate in the treatment of ectopic pregnancy:**
   A   It is highly effective in treating ectopic pregnancy because proliferating trophoblastic tissue is very sensitive to the action of this drug
   B   Single dose regimens are as effective as multiple dose regimens with fewer side effects
   C   There is an increase in the rate of miscarriage following treatment with methotrexate for ectopic pregnancy
   D   It can be used to treat patients with persistent trophoblastic disease following salpingotomy
   E   It can be safely used in women with hepatic dysfunction

4. **With regards to gestational trophoblastic disease (GTD):**
   A   In a partial mole, the fertilisation of a diploid oocyte occurs by two haploid sperms
   B   In a complete mole, the fertilisation of an empty oocyte occurs by one sperm which duplicates its genetic material
   C   The risk of developing GTD is highest in women with blood group 'A'

   D   The risk of malignant change is higher with complete mole compared with partial mole

   E   The risk of recurrent molar pregnancy is around 1%

5.   **With regards to miscarriage:**

   A   Anti-D immunoglobulin should be given when spontaneous miscarriage occurs at 5 weeks of pregnancy

   B   Threatened miscarriage is defined as any bleeding from the genital tract before 24 completed weeks of pregnancy in the context of opened internal cervical os and viable pregnancy

   C   Incomplete miscarriage is defined as the passage of some products of conception from the uterus

   D   Complete miscarriage is defined as the passage of all products of conception from the uterus

   E   Early fetal demise and missed miscarriage are interchangeable terms

Answers

1. **A False.** Recurrent miscarriage is defined as three or more consecutive miscarriages before 24 completed weeks of gestation.

   B False. It is unexplained miscarriage in around 50% of women attending recurrent miscarriage clinics.

   C False. Balanced reciprocal translocation is the most often identified chromosomal abnormality in couples with recurrent miscarriage.

   D False. The association of uterine anomalies with recurrent miscarriage is unclear.

   E False. Syphilis is a recognised cause of recurrent late second trimester miscarriage and stillbirth. It is a rare cause of recurrent miscarriage in developed countries.

   Robertsonian translocation

   This involves two acrocentric chromosomes that fuse near the centromere region with loss of the short arms, and this results in a human karyotype of 45 chromosomes (two chromosomes have fused together). Generally it has no effect on the phenotype (as these genes are common to all chromosomes and are present in variable numbers). The most common translocation is between chromosomes 13 and 14 which is seen in 1 in 1000 newborns. Carriers of this translocation have a normal phenotype. However, there is increased risk of unbalanced gametes leading to miscarriage or abnormal offspring (translocations involving chromosome 21 have a higher risk of having a child with Down syndrome due to non-disjunction during gametogenesis). The risk is 10% if the mother is a carrier and 1% if the father is a carrier.

   Buckett W and Regan L. Chapter 23: Sporadic and recurrent miscarriage. In: Shaw RW, Luesley D, Monga A (eds). Gynaecology (4th edn). Edinburgh: Churchill Livingstone, 2011.
   Royal College of Obstetricians and Gynaecologists. Recurrent miscarriage, investigation and treatment of couples (guideline 17). London: RCOG Press, 2011.

2. **A False.** It is around 15% (range 10–15%).

   B False. The incidence of miscarriage increases with increasing maternal age.

   C True. Peri-implantation loss is seen in 50–70%, post-implantation and biochemical pregnancy loss is seen in around 30% and clinically recognised pregnancy loss is seen in 10–15%.

   D False. In the UK, miscarriage is defined as the loss of an intrauterine pregnancy before 24 completed weeks of gestation. The WHO defines this as expulsion of the fetus or embryo with a fetal weight of 500 g or less before 22 completed weeks of pregnancy.

   E True.

   Buckett W and Regan L. Chapter 23: Sporadic and recurrent miscarriage. In: Shaw RW, Luesley D, Monga A (eds). Gynaecology (4th edn). Edinburgh: Churchill Livingstone, 2011.

3. **A True.** The indications include small (<3.5 cm) unruptured ectopic pregnancy in an asymptomatic, haemodynamically stable woman and persistent trophoblastic disease.

B True. The success rate after a single dose is up to 94%. When resolution is not attained with a single dose, a second dose may be administered which increases the success rate to almost 98%.

C False. There is no increase in either rate of miscarriage or congenital anomalies following treatment with methotrexate for ectopic pregnancy. However, women should be advised to avoid pregnancy for 3 months and use a reliable form of contraception (methotrexate is an antifolate).

D True. The risk of persistent trophoblastic disease with salpingotomy is 4–8%. Follow-up after the operation should be done with serial beta human chorionic gonadotropin (hCG). There will be a rise in the beta hCG in women with persistent trophoblastic disease. This is one of the indications for the use of methotrexate in gynaecology.

E False. Methotrexate is hepatotoxic and nephrotoxic. It can cause myelosuppression leading to neutropenia and thrombocytopenia. Therefore, baseline blood tests in the form of full blood count, liver function tests and renal function tests should be done before initiating treatment with this drug. The patient should be reliable and compliant in order to monitor during therapy with repeat blood tests and symptom review in an early pregnancy assessment unit.

The other side effects include nausea, vomiting, gastritis, diarrhoea, stomatitis, conjunctivitis, photosensitivity and abdominal pain (seen in 7% of women following methotrexate therapy for ectopic pregnancy).

Anti-D immunoglobulin should be given for rhesus (RHD)-negative women.

Royal College of Obstetricians and Gynaecologists. Green-top Guideline No. 21. Management of tubal pregnancy. London: RCOG Press, 2004.
Lipscomb GH, Stovall TG, Ling FW. Nonsurgical treatment of ectopic pregnancy. N Eng J Med 2000; 343:1325–1329.

4.   **A False.** A haploid oocyte is fertilised by two haploid sperm.

B True. There is no genetic material in an oocyte in these circumstances.

C False.

D True. The risk of malignancy with a complete mole is around 15% and a partial mole is <1%.

E True. The risk of recurrence is 1 in 80 and more than 98% will not have a molar pregnancy in subsequent pregnancies. However, if a molar pregnancy recurs, 68–80% of them will be of the same histological type.

Royal College of Obstetricians and Gynaecologists. Green-top Guideline No. 38. The management of gestational trophoblastic disease. London: RCOG Press, 2010.

5.   **A False.**

B False. Threatened miscarriage is defined as any bleeding from the genital tract before 24 completed weeks of pregnancy in the context of closed internal cervical os and viable pregnancy. Opened internal cervical os and intact products of conception are seen in inevitable miscarriage.

C True. Bleeding usually continues following incomplete miscarriage.

D True. Bleeding usually stops following complete miscarriage.

E True. The words delayed miscarriage and silent miscarriage were used previously. Ultrasound scan usually confirms a non-viable pregnancy with intact intrauterine sac or the absence of a fetus and/or yolk sac with intact intrauterine sac.

Royal College of Obstetricians and Gynaecologists. Green-top Guideline No. 25. The management of early pregnancy loss. London: RCOG Press, 2006.

Chapter 7

Fetal medicine

1. **With regards to the soft marker echogenic bowel on ultrasound scan:**
   - A It is associated with cardiac abnormality in fetus
   - B It is associated with bowel obstruction in the baby
   - C It is associated with Huntington's disease
   - D It is associated with intrauterine fetal death
   - E It is associated with cystic fibrosis

2. **With regards to anencephaly:**
   - A It can be diagnosed as early as 11 weeks of gestation by ultrasound scan
   - B The characteristic feature in the first trimester is the absence of calvaria or vault of skull
   - C The cerebral hemispheres are in direct contact with amniotic fluid
   - D It is associated with post-dated pregnancy
   - E It is a non-lethal anomaly of the fetus

3. **With regards to spina bifida (SB):**
   - A It is diagnosed reliably during the dating scan in the first trimester
   - B It is associated with Arnold–Chiari malformations
   - C A banana sign is seen with encephalocele but not with Arnold–Chiari malformation
   - D A lemon sign is seen with Arnold–Chiari malformation
   - E The incidence has decreased with the recommended intake of folic acid during the first trimester of pregnancy

4. **With regards to ventriculomegaly in the fetus:**
   - A It is detected in 10% of pregnancies
   - B It is diagnosed when the anterior ventricle is >20 mm
   - C It may be associated with intraventricular haemorrhage
   - D It may be associated with infection
   - E It may be associated with chromosomal abnormalities

5. **Dandy–Walker syndrome:**
   - A Is associated with the presence of a posterior fossa cyst which is not continuous with the fourth ventricle
   - B Is associated with the absence of the cerebellar vermis situated below the fourth ventricle
   - C Is not associated with chromosomal abnormalities such as aneuploidy
   - D Is associated with hydrocephalus
   - E Can be inherited as an autosomal dominant condition

6. **With regards to congenital cytomegalovirus (CMV) infection:**

    A   It is the most common cause of congenital viral infection
    B   Only primary infection is transmitted to the fetus but not secondary infection
    C   Ninety per cent of the fetuses are affected when the mother suffers primary infection
    D   It is said to be the leading cause of cardiac defects in childhood
    E   Ninety per cent of the infants with congenital infection do not exhibit any symptoms

7. **Toxoplasma infection:**

    A   Is acquired by ingestion of tissue cysts in undercooked meat
    B   Is acquired by ingestion of infectious oocysts excreted by cats
    C   Can infect the fetus in all trimesters
    D   Can cause ventriculomegaly
    E   Can cause microcephaly

8. **With regards to CMV infection during pregnancy:**

    A   There is a 2% risk of fetal transmission of infection with recurrent maternal infection
    B   The incidence of primary maternal infection during pregnancy is around 10%
    C   It infects 40% of fetuses if maternal infection occurs in the first and second trimesters
    D   It infects all fetuses when maternal infection occurs in the third trimester
    E   With recurrent maternal infection, the vertical transmission rate is >50%

9. **With regards to parvovirus infection and pregnancy:**

    A   It has a predilection towards erythroid precursors
    B   The incubation period is 10–21 days
    C   In adults, the infection is frequently subclinical
    D   Children may present with fifth disease
    E   It can cause immune hydrops in the fetus

10. **With regards to rubella infection and pregnancy:**

    A   The incubation period is 14–21 days
    B   It occurs in 1–2% of women of reproductive age
    C   The earlier the infection during pregnancy, the higher the risk of fetal damage
    D   The risk of fetal infection and damage is highest in the third trimester
    E   Termination of pregnancy should be considered if maternal infection occurs in the first trimester

11. **With regards to varicella infection and pregnancy:**

    A   The highest risk to the fetus is when the maternal infection occurs after 20 weeks of gestation
    B   The incubation period is 6–10 days
    C   The fetus is not affected if the maternal infection occurs in second trimester
    D   The risk to the fetus before 20 weeks is 10%
    E   The period of infectivity is 7 days before to 7 days after the appearance of rash

12. **With regards to hepatitis B infection during pregnancy:**
    A The woman is considered infectious in the presence of anti-e antibodies
    B The highest risk to the fetus is during childbirth
    C Breast feeding is absolutely contraindicated if the mother is positive for surface antigen
    D The risk of fetal infection is highest if the mother has 'e' antigen and antigen from the core of the virus
    E The risk to the fetus is almost 90% in the presence of 'e' antigen and absence of anti-e antibody

13. **The following can be associated with trisomy 18:**
    A Exomphalos
    B Rocker bottom feet
    C Micrognathia
    D Echogenic bowel
    E Low set ears

14. **With regards to Turner syndrome:**
    A A mosaic pattern is seen in 50% of cases
    B The gonads are usually dysgenetic
    C The presence of the X chromosome is associated with gonadoblastoma
    D Carriers of X-linked recessive disorder are asymptomatic
    E Occasionally X:autosome translocation is seen

15. **The following are features of Turner syndrome:**
    A Cubitus valgus
    B Large testis
    C Protruding tongue
    D Tall stature
    E Early menarche

16. **With regards to trisomy 21:**
    A The incidence is 1 in 100 at the age of 40 years
    B The incidence is 1 in 350 at the age of 35 years
    C Overall 100% are due to non-dysjunction
    D The incidence decreases with increasing paternal age
    E There is increased risk of cardiac abnormalities

17. **Potter syndrome:**
    A Is associated with polyhydramnios
    B Is associated with bilateral renal agenesis
    C Is associated with cystic lung disease
    D Is associated with long limbs
    E Is associated with pulmonary hyperplasia

18. **The following syndromes are correctly matched:**
    A 47XXY – Klinefelter syndrome

B   45XO/XY – Turner mosaic
C   45XO/XX – Turner mosaic
D   Trisomy 18 – Down syndrome
E   Trisomy 13 – Cri du chat syndrome

19. **Increased nuchal translucency (NT) in the fetus is associated with:**
    A   Cardiac abnormalities
    B   Abdominal wall defects
    C   Renal abnormalities
    D   Diaphragmatic hernia
    E   Down syndrome

20. **Maternal illnesses which increase the risk of fetal malformations are:**
    A   Phenylketonuria
    B   Alcohol abuse
    C   Gestational diabetes
    D   Epilepsy
    E   Pregnancy-induced hypertension

21. **With regards to congenital adrenal hyperplasia (CAH):**
    A   It can cause virilisation
    B   It is caused due to decreased adrenocorticotropic hormone production
    C   The most common enzyme deficiency is 21-hydroxylase
    D   It can present with female pseudohermaphroditism
    E   It can present with ambiguous genitalia at birth

22. **With regards to fetal invasive testing:**
    A   Amniocentesis is usually done at 14 weeks
    B   Chorionic villus sampling (CVS) may cause limb defects when undertaken
         after 11 weeks
    C   The risk of miscarriage with CVS is 0.5%
    D   Placental mosaicism is more common with amniocentesis compared to CVS
    E   Amniotic fluid can leak following amniocentesis

23. **Maternal serum alpha fetoprotein (MSAFP):**
    A   Is synthesized in the maternal gastrointestinal tract
    B   Is raised in women carrying a fetus with anencephaly
    C   Is raised in women carrying a fetus with Down syndrome
    D   Reaches a peak at around 32 weeks of gestation in maternal serum in normal
         pregnancy and then falls gradually
    E   Is raised in maternal serum if the fetus is diagnosed with exomphalos

24. **With regards to pregnancy-associated plasma protein A (PAPP-A):**
    A   It is a glycolipid that can be detected in the maternal serum in early pregnancy
    B   It can be detected in the maternal serum at 4 weeks of gestation
    C   It is decreased in maternal serum if carrying a fetus with trisomy 13
    D   It is raised in maternal serum if carrying a fetus with trisomy 18

E   It is detected in maternal serum throughout pregnancy

25. **With regards to cardiac echogenic foci or golf ball sign:**
    A   It is defined as hyperechogenicity located on the ventricular walls
    B   It resolves spontaneously in most cases
    C   It is a soft marker for chromosomal abnormalities
    D   It is associated with trisomy 21 in 1 in 500 cases if it is an isolated finding
    E   It is associated with congenital multiple arterial thrombus in the fetus

26. **Hyperechogenic bowel is associated with an increased risk of:**
    A   Meconium ileus
    B   Fetal death
    C   Fetal growth restriction
    D   Sickle cell disease
    E   Parvovirus infection

27. **With regards to raised nuchal translucency (NT):**
    A   There is increased risk of transposition of aorta in the fetus
    B   There is increased risk of ventricular septal defect
    C   The risk of Klinefelter's syndrome is 8%
    D   There is increased risk of other genetic syndromes even in the presence of a normal karyotype
    E   There is increased risk of perinatal mortality and fetal loss

28. **Congenital rubella is associated with:**
    A   Pulmonary valvular stenosis
    B   Pulmonary artery stenosis
    C   Microphthalmia
    D   Bilateral and progressive sensorineural deafness
    E   Bilateral cataracts in the newborn

29. **With regards to parvovirus infection and pregnancy:**
    A   It is caused by RNA virus with double stranded genome
    B   If the maternal infection occurs during pregnancy, fetal infection occurs in 90% of cases
    C   It can cause transient maternal aplastic crisis
    D   The fetal loss rate is 10% if maternal infection occurs in the second trimester
    E   The fetal infection is an indication for termination in the third trimester of pregnancy

30. **With regards to maternal infection with hepatitis B virus:**
    A   It is caused by single stranded RNA virus
    B   It is transmitted to the fetus by transplacental transfer in 90% of cases
    C   It is transmitted to the fetus during delivery in 10% of cases
    D   It causes fetal congenital abnormalities
    E   Without vaccination of the newborn, 90% of babies with vertically acquired infection become chronic carriers

31. **With regards to Robertsonian or unbalanced translocation:**
    A   It most commonly involves translocation between chromosomes 13 and 14 t (13; 14)
    B   There is a 20% risk of having a child born with Down syndrome if the mother is a carrier of translocation between chromosomes 14 and 21 t (14; 21)
    C   There is a 5% risk of having a child born with Down syndrome if the father is a carrier of translocation between chromosomes 14 and 21 t (14; 21)
    D   All children would have Down syndrome if their parents are carriers of translocation of chromosomes 21 and 21 t (21; 21)
    E   Breaks are usually near the centromere in acrocentric chromosomes

32. **The following are associated with low MSAFP:**
    A   Maternal diabetes
    B   Trisomy 21
    C   Trisomy 18
    D   Trisomy 13
    E   Body mass index (BMI) >40

33. **The following conditions can be diagnosed by preimplantation genetic diagnosis:**
    A   Congenital adrenal hyperplasia
    B   Fragile X syndrome
    C   Beta thalassaemia
    D   Cystic fibrosis
    E   Charcot Marie–Tooth syndrome

34. **The causes of immune hydrops include:**
    A   Anti-Kell antibodies
    B   Anti-Duffy antibodies
    C   IgM antibodies to parvovirus B19
    D   IgG antibodies to cytomegalovirus
    E   Anti-Ro antibodies

35. **With regards to congenital diaphragmatic hernia:**
    A   It is not associated with other structural anomalies
    B   Right-sided hernias are more common than left-sided hernias
    C   Almost 50% have an abnormal karyotype
    D   Less than 50% are detected antenatally
    E   It may be associated with polyhydramnios

36. **Oesophageal atresia:**
    A   Is usually associated with tracheo-oesophageal fistula
    B   Is associated with polyhydramnios
    C   Is associated with chromosomal abnormalities
    D   Is not associated with other structural abnormalities
    E   Is associated with pre-term labour

Answers

1. A False.

    B True.

    C False.

    D True.

    E True.

    A fetal bowel is defined as hyperechogenic if it appears similar to or more echogenic than the surrounding bone in the same machine settings. It is associated with:

    - cytomegalovirus infection
    - cystic fibrosis
    - meconium ileus
    - aneuploidy (Down syndrome)
    - intra-amniotic bleeding
    - fetal growth restriction
    - intrauterine fetal death

    Therefore it is important to screen the parents for cystic fibrosis and if they are found to be carriers, it is advisable to undertake amniocentesis for DNA mutation analysis to detect whether the fetus is affected (the same sample can be used for karyotyping to diagnose aneuploidy). Maternal serum for cytomegalovirus (CMV) IgM titres should be performed to exclude infection. If the fetus is affected, a termination of pregnancy can be offered. However, if the woman wants to continue with the pregnancy, she should be supported and serial fetal growths scans should be arranged as hyperechogenic bowel can be associated with fetal growth restriction.

    James D, Steer PJ, Weiner CP, Gonik B, Crowther C, Robson S (eds). High Risk Pregnancy: Management Options (4th edn). St Louis: Saunders, 2011.

2. A True. Incidence of anencephaly is 1 in 1000 births.

    B True. It occurs when the head end of the neural tube fails to close.

    C True.

    D True. Affects more girls than it does boys.

    E False. The risk of recurrence is 4%.

    Anencephaly (lethal anomaly) is the absence of the skull vault and cerebral cortex. It is always an open defect with no skin covering the affected area and as a result maternal serum alpha fetoprotein is exceptionally high. Thus the sensitivity of measuring maternal serum alpha fetoprotein is practically 100%. Currently, this condition is diagnosed as early as the dating scan (11–14 weeks of gestation). It is described to be abnormal not to visualise the bony structures of the skull after 14 weeks of gestation.

James D, Steer PJ, Weiner CP, Gonik B, Crowther C, Robson S (eds). High Risk Pregnancy: Management Options (4th edn). St Louis: Saunders, 2011.
Magowan B. Churchill's Pocketbook of Obstetrics and Gynaecology (3rd edn). Edinburgh: Churchill Livingstone, 2005.

3. **A True.** A neural tube defect (NTD) is a congenital malformation which occurs between 20 and 28 days after conception.

    B True.

    C False.

    D True.

    E True.

    Terminology

    - anencephaly: absent cranial vault and cerebral cortex

    Spina bifida (SB)

    - meningocele: dura and arachnoid matter bulge through the defect (no skin in open neural tube defect [NTD] and closed skin in closed NTD)
    - myelomeningocele: the spinal cord canal is exposed
    - encephalocele: defect in the cranial vault leads to protrusion of the dura matter with or without brain tissue; alpha fetoprotein is normal in 95% of cases as they are closed defects
    - an isolated lesion of meningocele carries a good prognosis; association with microcephaly (caused by brain herniation) carries a very poor prognosis

    Embryology

    Following conception, a neural groove appears at 20 days, almost closed at 23 days and fully closed at 28 days. Inadequate closure of the neural tube at the cephalic end leads to anencephaly (40%) or encephalocele (5%) while incomplete closure at the lower end would lead to SB (55%).

    Aetiology

    SB is a defect of the spinal vertebra. The aetiology is multifactorial with both genetic and environmental associations. It can be associated with chromosomal abnormalities such as aneuploidy. In view of its multifactorial nature, the risk is variable and is dependent on race, sex and geographic location. The other factors which may predispose women to have NTD babies include women with diabetes, those taking antiepileptic medications during pregnancy or large doses of vitamin A, women who have an affected child or siblings or if she herself has been affected by this condition.

    Markers of SB

    MSAFP starts to rise at 10 weeks of gestation and peaks around 31 weeks of gestation before falling at term. Conventionally, NTDs were suspected in the fetuses of women with raised maternal serum alpha fetoprotein in mid-pregnancy, especially open NTDs (SB and anencephaly make up to 90% of NTDs). If the level of serum alpha fetoprotein is above the 95th centile (equivalent to two multiples of median [MOM] for that gestation), a detailed ultrasound is indicated as the risk of NTD is 2%.

With advances in the fetal medicine technology, SB is diagnosed as early as the dating scan. Normally the spine narrows caudally when viewed longitudinally. With a defect in the vertebra, the posterior ossification centres are more widely spaced than those in vertebrae above and below the defect and there is loss of skin continuity. When viewed transversely, SB appears as a splaying of the posterior ossification centres producing a U-shaped vertebra. During the third trimester, the absence of laminae and spinous process will support the diagnosis of SB.

Associations

SB can be associated with hydrocephalus (poor prognostic factor) in about 90% of cases and with Arnold–Chiari malformations in 90–95% of cases. In the latter condition, the cerebellum, fourth ventricle and medulla are displaced caudally. Two characteristic signs (99% sensitivity) on sonography include lemon-shaped skull (scalloping of the frontal bones due to caudal displacement of cranial content) and banana-shaped cerebellum (flattened cerebellar hemisphere with obliteration of the cisterna magna). The cerebellum can be totally absent. The caudal displacement of the above structures can obstruct the flow of cerebrospinal fluid leading to hydrocephalus.

Prognosis

The prognosis for SB depends on several factors which include the length of lesion, the spinal level of lesion and if the neural tissue is present in the meningeal sac. The severity can be reflected in symptoms such as lower extremity paralysis, incontinence of faeces and urine and low intelligent quotient (IQ). The treatments include early closure of the defect, ventriculoperitoneal shunting, surgical treatment of incontinence of faeces and urine, dietary management and support.

Recurrence

There is a definite risk of recurrence if the woman has had an affected child with SB in the past. In the UK, the risk of recurrence after an affected pregnancy is 3–4% which can be reduced to 1% by folic acid supplementation. If two or more siblings are affected the risk of recurrence increases to 10% and if the parent is affected the risk is 4%. Women with a previous affected child should be advised to take 5 mg folic acid starting before conception and continuing through the first trimester.

James D, Steer PJ, Weiner CP, Gonik B, Crowther C, Robson S (eds). High Risk Pregnancy: Management Options (4th edn). St Louis: Saunders, 2011.
Magowan B. Churchill's Pocketbook of Obstetrics and Gynaecology (3rd edn). Edinburgh: Churchill Livingstone, 2005.

4. A False.

 B False.

 C True.

 D True.

 E True.

Ventriculomegaly is seen in 1% of pregnancies. It is an ultrasound scan finding and is diagnosed when the lateral ventricular atrium size is >10 mm (the size of the head is generally normal). The obstruction is usually at the aqueduct of Sylvius or at the foraminae of Luschka and Magendi. If it is an isolated finding, the prognosis is better, but association with other factors may carry a poor prognosis. The risk of recurrence for isolated hydrocephalus is around 1 in 30; for sex-linked aqueduct stenosis it is 1 in 4.

Ventriculomegaly can be associated with SB (30%), hydrocephalus and Dandy–Walker malformation. Holoprosencephaly and agenesis of the corpus callosum are rare forms of ventriculomegaly. The former is associated with single cerebral ventricle with absent cavum septum pellucidum (associated with trisomy 13) and the latter is associated with absent cavum septum pellucidum, third ventricle dilatation and separation of anterior horns of the lateral ventricle. Agenesis of corpus callosum can be an isolated finding or associated with other anomalies in 80% of cases (hydrocephalus, Arnold–Chiari malformations, Dandy–Walker syndrome and holoprosencephaly). The prognosis with both forms of ventriculomegaly is poor.

James D, Steer PJ, Weiner CP, Gonik B, Crowther C, Robson S (eds). High Risk Pregnancy: Management Options (4th edn). St Louis: Saunders, 2011.
Magowan B. Churchill's Pocketbook of Obstetrics and Gynaecology (3rd edn). Edinburgh: Churchill Livingstone, 2005.

5. A False.

    B True.

    C False.

    D True.

    E False.

Dandy–Walker syndrome is associated with partial or complete absence of the cerebellar vermis and the presence of a posterior fossa cyst in continuation with the fourth ventricle. It may be caused by atresia of the foramina of Luschka and Magendie and hypoplasia of the cerebellum. On ultrasound, the posterior fossa cyst appears as an anechoic area in the posterior fossa and the cerebellar vermis (bright echogenic structure in the midline) below the fourth ventricle is absent or defective. Hydrocephalus (usually involves all four ventricles) develops sooner or later. The prognosis is poor and termination of pregnancy should be offered to women following thorough counselling.

It has been associated with chromosomal abnormalities such as aneuploidy and is also said to occur increasingly in families with a history of polycystic kidney disease and a previous affected child with cranial abnormality. It can also be inherited as an autosomal recessive condition.

James D, Steer PJ, Weiner CP, Gonik B, Crowther C, Robson S (eds). High Risk Pregnancy: Management Options (4th edn). St Louis: Saunders, 2011.
Magowan B. Churchill's Pocketbook of Obstetrics and Gynaecology (3rd edn). Edinburgh: Churchill Livingstone, 2005.

6. A True.

    B False.

C **False.**

D **False.**

E **True.**

CMV is common during pregnancy with a seroconversion rate of 2.5%. Forty per cent of the fetal transmission is mainly following primary CMV infection in the mother and 1–2% is after secondary infection. Ninety per cent of these infants with congenital infection do not exhibit any symptoms but 10% will have fetal defects at birth and are at risk of developing long-term neurological sequelae. It is the leading cause of deafness in children.

James D, Steer PJ, Weiner CP, Gonik B, Crowther C, Robson S (eds). High Risk Pregnancy: Management Options (4th edn). St Louis: Saunders, 2011.
Magowan B. Churchill's Pocketbook of Obstetrics and Gynaecology (3rd edn). Edinburgh: Churchill Livingstone, 2005.

7. A **True.**

B **True.**

C **True.**

D **True.**

E **True.**

Toxoplasma gondii

Toxoplasma gondii is an obligate intracellular parasite responsible for causing toxoplasmosis. The life cycle of this parasite shows three forms: trophozoite, tissue cyst and oocyst. In the cat intestine, the organism becomes sexually mature and produces oocysts. These are excreted in the stool and can remain infectious for up to 1 year or more. Ingestion of either oocysts or tissue cysts will lead to invasion of the human or host intestinal epithelium. Subsequently trophozoites enter the lymphatics and infect the musculoskeletal system and nervous system where trophozoites develop into tissue cysts.

Mother

Ingestion of cat litter or undercooked meat (pork and beef) causes human infection. The incidence of maternal infection during pregnancy is 1 in 2000 pregnancies. Primary infection is often asymptomatic or women may suffer mild symptoms such as malaise, fever and lymphadenopathy (which involves the posterior cervical chain) that are usually unnoticeable. Immunosuppression facilitates development of severe disease and can cause chorioretinitis and encephalitis.

Fetus

Maternal infection can affect the fetus in all trimesters but the severity of fetal damage is higher in the first and second trimesters than in the third trimester. Following primary maternal infection during pregnancy, fetal transmission is 25% in the first trimester (75% severely affected), 50% in the second trimester (55% severely affected) and 65% after 28 weeks or the third trimester (<5% severely affected).

The fetal sequelae include hydrocephalus, microcephaly, intracerebral calcification, cataract, chorioretinitis and ventriculomegaly. The newborn child may have learning disabilities, seizures, spasticity, chorioretinitis and blindness. It may also be associated with hepatosplenomegaly, anaemia, rash, blindness and neonatal jaundice (70% are born without damage, 10% with ocular manifestations and 20% with severe sequelae).

Diagnosis

The diagnosis of acute infection is made by paired serological samples from the mother (four-fold rise in IgG titres, elevated IgM titres or concurrent high IgG and IgM titres). The other methods described for diagnosis include culture of the parasite in laboratory rodents or biopsy of enlarged lymph nodes.

Management

The best strategy is prevention of primary infections by taking hygienic precautions.

The mother should be managed symptomatically as the disease is usually mild. For the fetus, she should be referred to a fetal medicine specialist unit. One should consider invasive testing (amniocentesis) for polymerase chain reaction (PCR) detection of *T. gondii* genome in amniotic fluid. In the presence of a negative amniocentesis, one should still arrange serial ultrasound scans for fetal follow-up. Fetal infection should be assumed or suspected if the amniocentesis is positive. Drug therapy with spiramycin (3 g/day) should be initiated and continued throughout pregnancy (fetal infection is reduced by 60% but there is no evidence that it reduces severity). It has been found to be safe for the baby as well as mother. In addition, pyrimethamine and sulfadiazine with folic acid supplementation may be of benefit. A termination of pregnancy should be offered if the mother had a primary infection before 20 weeks of gestation. If the ultrasound shows no abnormalities, the risk of congenital toxoplasmosis is low.

The neonatal team should be involved sooner rather than later.

James D, Steer PJ, Weiner CP, Gonik B, Crowther C, Robson S (eds). High Risk Pregnancy: Management Options (4th edn). St Louis: Saunders, 2011.
Magowan B. Churchill's Pocketbook of Obstetrics and Gynaecology (3rd edn). Edinburgh: Churchill Livingstone, 2005.

8. **A** True.

    B False.

    C True.

    D False.

    E False.

CMV, presentation and complications

CMV is a DNA virus and belongs to the herpes family. An adult with primary infection can present with flu-like illness and malaise but usually recovers with a benign course. The differential diagnosis is infectious mononucleosis caused by Epstein–Barr virus. The complications include interstitial pneumonitis, meningoencephalitis, thrombocytopaenia, haemolytic anaemia and Guillain–Barré syndrome (rare). The virus can be shed in the urine for a long time and can be isolated from urine culture. Reactivation and reinfection are not uncommon with latent CMV infections.

Routes of transmission

CMV can be transmitted through breast milk, urine, saliva, genital secretions, perinatal transmission to fetus, organ donation, transfused blood and bone marrow.

Fetal transmission

CMV is the commonest cause of fetal and perinatal infection in the UK. Although 40% of pregnant women are susceptible, the incidence of maternal infection during pregnancy is 0.5–2%. Women are generally asymptomatic and most of them might have had an infection in the past (50–60%). The earlier the fetus is infected, the greater the damage. During the first and second trimesters, maternal infection can infect 40% of fetuses but can affect (clinically symptomatic) 10% of them (90% are asymptomatic). The risk of vertical transmission with recurrent maternal infection is 1–2%.

Fetal sequelae

- ocular: chorioretinitis, microphthalmia, cataract, blindness and optic atrophy
- auditory: sensorineural deafness (most common cause of deafness and developmental delay)
- hepatic: hepatosplenomegaly, jaundice
- haematological: thrombocytopaenic purpura
- neurological: microcephaly, neuro developmental delay, cerebral palsy, learning difficulties and seizures

Diagnosis

Diagnosis is usually made by paired serological samples (enzyme-linked immunosorbent assay [ELISA] or radioimmunoassay) from the mother (IgM is detected as early as 2 weeks following infection and remains in the blood for 4 months while IgG is detected at 2–3 weeks and remains for a lifetime). However, women with reactivation of latent infection do not show either an increase or reappearance of IgM antibodies in immunocompetent individuals. This may help to differentiate between the two.

Fetal infection can be based on the detection of CMV from the amniotic fluid and blood serology. A diagnosis of congenital CMV infection can be made, if the virus is found in an infant's urine, saliva, blood or other body tissues 2–3 weeks after birth.

Counselling

Women should be thoroughly counselled about the risk of damage to the fetus during pregnancy and consider invasive procedures to establish the risk to the fetus (if affected one should consider termination of pregnancy).

Serial ultrasound scans should be arranged to detect abnormalities such as microcephaly, cerebral atrophy, intracerebral calcification, lecucomalacia, fetal growth restriction and echogenic bowel. Women should also be informed that a normal scan does not guarantee a normal baby and all infected fetuses may not be affected.

James D, Steer PJ, Weiner CP, Gonik B, Crowther C, Robson S (eds). High Risk Pregnancy: Management Options (4th edn). St Louis: Saunders, 2011.
Magowan B. Churchill's Pocketbook of Obstetrics and Gynaecology (3rd edn). Edinburgh: Churchill Livingstone, 2005.

9. A True.

 B False.

 C True.

 D True.

 E False.

Human parvovirus B19

The infection is caused by human parvovirus B19, which is a DNA virus in the family Parvoviridae. The incubation period is 4–14 days. Women are infectious 3–10 days post exposure or until a rash appears. Maternal infection is often subclinical but symptomatic women may have a rash (erythema infectiosum), fever and arthralgia (which affects 80% of adults and 10% of children). In children it can cause mild infection (e.g. slapped cheek or fifth disease).

Fetal infection and sequelae

Infection can occur in 15% of fetuses before 15 weeks, in 25% between 15 to 20 weeks and in 70% at term. The fetal sequelae include miscarriage, severe anaemia, non-immune hydrops, cardiac failure and intrauterine death. The risk of fetal loss is approximately 10% if the mother is positive for IgM and most occur 4–6 weeks from the onset of maternal symptoms or infection. Non-immune hydrops occurs in 3% of fetuses, with a fatality rate of 50%. Spontaneous resolution occurs in one in three cases. It is noted that there are no long-term sequelae following resolution of infection.

Diagnosis in the mother

Diagnosis is made by taking paired maternal serum samples and also by using polymerase chain reaction (PCR) parvovirus genome. The absence of both IgM and IgG antibodies suggests no previous infection but the person is susceptible to infection. The presence of only parvovirus B19 IgG indicates previous infection at least 4 months ago while the presence of only parvovirus B19 IgM indicates recent infection, within the last 7 days. When both parvovirus B19 IgM and IgG antibodies are present, it indicates recent infection between 7 days and 4 months ago. IgM is identified as early as 7–10 days and remains for 4 weeks whereas IgG is identified at 2 weeks and stays for a lifetime. The mother should be treated symptomatically.

Diagnosis and follow-up of the baby

Amniotic fluid or cord blood sampling can be used to detect parvovirus DNA (using the most sensitive assay) or IgM antibody (sometimes serology may be negative until late after delivery). Termination of pregnancy should be discussed if infection occurs in early pregnancy. In late pregnancy, confirmation of fetal infection by invasive procedures should be considered.

One should arrange weekly serial ultrasound scans after 4 weeks of maternal exposure or infection in order to identify signs of hydrops (ascites, pericardial effusion) early.

Currently, peak systolic velocity (PSV) in the middle cerebral artery has been used to identify fetal anaemia. If PSV is high, cord blood sampling (1% fetal loss) and *in utero* blood transfusion (mature erythrocytes are not susceptible to parvovirus infection) has been shown to benefit and promote resolution of fetal hydrops. The finding of anaemia in the presence of reticulocytosis indicates that the fetus may already have started recovering and therefore may not need a blood transfusion as hydrops usually resolves spontaneously. Fetal growth scans should be arranged following recovery of the hydrops. Delivery is indicated if the pregnancy is advanced.

James D, Steer PJ, Weiner CP, Gonik B, Crowther C, Robson S (eds). High Risk Pregnancy: Management Options (4th edn). St Louis: Saunders, 2011.
Magowan B. Churchill's Pocketbook of Obstetrics and Gynaecology (3rd edn). Edinburgh: Churchill Livingstone, 2005.

10. A **True.**

  B **True.**

  C **True.**

  D **False.**

  E **True.**

Rubella or German measles

Rubella (or third disease) is a single-stranded RNA virus which belongs to the togavirus family. It is acquired via exposure to respiratory droplets and women are usually asymptomatic. Fifty to seventy five per cent of infected individuals are symptomatic and develop a rash after an incubation period of 14–21 days. The rash spreads from the face to the trunk and lastly to the extremities and lasts for 3 days. The period of infectivity is 7 days before to 7 days after the appearance of the rash. Severe but rare complications include encephalitis, arthritis and bleeding diathesis.

Fetal transmission

The fetus can be affected by vertical transmission. The earlier the maternal infection occurs, the greater the fetal infection and damage (**Table 7.1**).

Table 7.1 Maternal rubella infection and risks to the fetus		
Gestation (weeks)	**Fetal infection (%)**	**Fetal affection or damage (%)**
4–12*	>80	>80
12–16†	55	20–25
>16‡	45	Very low risk

There is <5% risk to the fetus with reinfection

*It is reasonable to consider termination of pregnancy. If the woman does not opt for termination, she should be supported and offered fetal surveillance, e.g. serial ultrasound scan and fetal echocardiogram.

†Prenatal diagnosis

‡Negligible risk

Fetal sequelae

The classic triad of congenital rubella syndrome includes eye, ear and heart abnormalities, along with other manifestations:

- **ocular:** cataract, glaucoma, microphthalmia and retinopathy
- **cardiac:** patent ductus arteriosus, pulmonary arterial stenosis and pulmonary valvular stenosis
- **auditory:** sensorineural deafness which is bilateral and progressive
- **central nervous system:** mental retardation, microcephaly, meningoencephalitis and behavioural disorders
- **lung:** interstitial pneumonitis
- **hepatic:** hepatitis, hepatosplenomegaly and jaundice
- **haematological:** haemolytic anaemia and thrombocytopenic purpura
- **endocrine:** diabetes, thyroid dysfunction and growth hormone deficiency
- **skin:** blueberry muffin spots and chronic rubelliform rash

Serologic testing of the mother is the primary mode of diagnosis. Seroconversion in paired samples is indicative of infection (IgG immunoglobulin is positive for life). Ninety-seven per cent of women in the UK are immune to rubella. If the mother is not immune to rubella (IgG immunoglobulin <10 IU/mL), postnatal vaccination is recommended (avoid pregnancy for 1 month following vaccination).

Rubella vaccine is routinely given to children in the UK as part of the measles, mumps and rubella (MMR) vaccine. The first dose is usually given at around 13 months and a second dose at the age of 3–5 years. If the second dose is delayed for any reason, it can still be given at a later age.

James D, Steer PJ, Weiner CP, Gonik B, Crowther C, Robson S (eds). High Risk Pregnancy: Management Options (4th edn). St Louis: Saunders, 2011.
Magowan B. Churchill's Pocketbook of Obstetrics and Gynaecology (3rd edn). Edinburgh: Churchill Livingstone, 2005.

11. **A** False.

    B False.

    C False.

    D False.

    E False.

Varicella zoster virus

Varicella zoster virus (VZV) is a DNA virus and belongs to the herpes family. It causes a childhood exanthematous disease known as chickenpox.

Clinical presentation

Clinical symptoms develop 10–20 days following exposure to infection (the incubation period is 14–21 days). The disease can be severe in pregnant women. Symptoms include malaise, fever and rash (maculopapules which vesiculate and finally crust over). At first, the rash develops on the face and scalp before spreading to the trunk. The contagious period (or the period of infectivity) is 1–2 days, prior to the onset of the rash, to 6 days after the rash disappears, or until all the ruptured vesicles have crusted over. The virus can remain dormant in the body for a long time and may surface in the form of shingles or zoster (painful pruritic vesicles along the course of cutaneous nerve in the dermatomal pattern) in immunosuppressed individuals.

Fetal transmission of infection

The fetus is at risk in all trimesters but the highest risk is when maternal infection occurs before 20 weeks of gestation (25% fetal transmission of infection with a 2% risk of embryopathy). The risk is negligible thereafter but can still occur. There is a 20% risk of neonatal varicella syndrome if the maternal symptoms start 5 days before delivery to 2 days after delivery, as not enough time is available for antibody formation and transfer to the fetus. After 20 weeks, if the fetus acquires VZV *in utero*, they can develop zoster (2% risk) in the first 2 years of life following birth. Reactivation of maternal infection (shingles) poses little risk to the fetus (embryopathy) in the absence of viraemia. However, the risk exists if a non-immune mother comes into contact with a person with shingles.

Fetal sequelae

- hypoplasia or aplasia of limbs
- scarring of skin
- psychomotor retardation
- deafness and eye abnormalities
- cerebral cortical atrophy
- chorioretinal scarring
- childhood zoster
- convulsions
- microcephaly
- muscle atrophy
- limb paralysis

Diagnosis and follow-up of mother and fetus

The clinical manifestation is obvious and usually aids diagnosis. In case of doubt, serological testing for IgM and IgG antibodies may be necessary. The presence of varicella IgM or a four-fold rise in varicella IgG is proof of recent infection. A viral culture using vesicle fluid or Tzanck smear preparations can be used for diagnosis.

Fetal blood for serology or viral DNA detection from amniotic fluid can be performed but may not always be positive. Laboratory tests are not always useful in predicting the severity of disease in a newborn baby. Fetal infection can be diagnosed by ultrasonographic detection of fetal abnormalities (all sonographic abnormalities manifest before 20 weeks of gestation). If the initial scan is normal, a repeat scan 5 weeks later should be performed after maternal infection to detect late sequelae.

Management of women exposed to chickenpox during pregnancy

Most women (>90%) in the UK are immune to VZV infection. Pregnant women exposed to people with chickenpox should have a serology test to detect VZV IgG. If this is positive, they are diagnosed as immune and should be reassured. If they are not immune, they are at high risk of developing chickenpox infection and should be administered VZV immunoglobulin (125 U/10 kg) intramuscularly. Despite all these measures if the pregnant woman develops chickenpox, she should be closely observed to identify severe illness and disseminated disease. Women should be asked to report if they develop respiratory or neurological symptoms and a spreading haemorrhagic rash. The mortality rate with varicella pneumonia is 10%.

Royal College of Obstetricians and Gynaecologists. Green-top Guideline No. 13. Chicken pox in pregnancy. London: RCOG Press, 2007.
James D, Steer PJ, Weiner CP, Gonik B, Crowther C, Robson S (eds). High Risk Pregnancy: Management Options (4th edn). St Louis: Saunders, 2011.
Magowan B. Churchill's Pocketbook of Obstetrics and Gynaecology (3rd edn). Edinburgh: Churchill Livingstone, 2005.

12. A False.

   B True.

   C False.

   D True.

   E True.

Hepatitis B virus

Hepatitis B virus (HBV) is a DNA virus and belongs to the Hepadnaviridae family. The virus has a predilection to hepatocytes and therefore mainly causes hepatitis. The incubation period is 2–6 months.

Symptoms

Most acute infections in adults (two thirds) are subclinical and mild, and consequently usually go unnoticed. The presentation in symptomatic patients includes malaise, nausea, vomiting, right upper quadrant pain and mild diarrhoea. About 50% of HBV-infected individuals do not develop jaundice. Generally 90% of acute infections resolve completely within 6 months while 10% become chronic carriers (positive for hepatitis B surface antigen). The latter (chronic carrier state) predisposes to the following conditions: chronic active hepatitis, chronic persistent hepatitis, cirrhosis, hepatocellular carcinoma, fulminant hepatitis, hepatic failure and death.

Infectivity

Serological testing for various antibodies and antigen is important to determine infectivity:

- HBsAg (surface antigen): antigen presence indicates infectivity while antibody to surface antigen indicates immunologic response and cure
- HBeAg and core antigen: the presence of hepatitis 'e' antigen and antigen from the core of virus indicates high infectivity
- anti-HBe (antibody against 'e' antigen): indicates less infectivity

Prevalence

HBV is the most common blood-borne viral infection in the world with a prevalence of 0.5–1% in pregnant women in the UK (this number is greater in Asian women).

Fetus

The modes of transmission include blood-borne, sexual intercourse, splashing of the blood and body fluids into open wounds or mucous membranes, and perinatal transmission to the fetus. Vertical transmission depends on the degree of maternal infectivity status, e.g. the presence of 'e' antigen indicates high infectivity and continuous viral replication.

The reverse is true for the chronic carrier state in newborns. The chronic carrier rate is 85–90% in babies if mother is positive for 'e' antigen versus 31% if the mother is negative for 'e' antigen. Passive (within 12 hours of birth) and active immunoprophylaxis (within 7 days of birth) with hepatitis B immunoglobulin (at birth) and hepatitis B vaccine (at birth, 1 month and 6 months) is 95% effective in reducing the risk of HBV transmission but is less effective in hepatitis 'e' antigen (HBeAg)-positive mothers.

Prevention

Prevention of HBV infection through vaccination is still, therefore, the best strategy for decreasing the incidence of hepatitis B-associated morbidity.

Screening

All pregnant women should be routinely screened for HBsAg at booking as only 50% of carriers are identified with risk assessment during pregnancy. Women arriving without prior antenatal care (unbooked) or unscreened women presenting for delivery should be screened, with results made available within 24 hours.

James D, Steer PJ, Weiner CP, Gonik B, Crowther C, Robson S (eds). High Risk Pregnancy: Management Options (4th edn). St Louis: Saunders, 2011.
Magowan B. Churchill's Pocketbook of Obstetrics and Gynaecology (3rd edn). Edinburgh: Churchill Livingstone, 2005.

13. **A True.**

   B True.

   C True.

   D True.

   E False.

Aneuploidy

Most chromosomal abnormalities are due to aneuploidy. These are mainly numerical abnormalities caused by loss or gain of one, two or even the whole set of chromosomes. Non-dysjunction is the most common cause with a high occurrence in women with increased maternal age. The prevalence of these conditions is higher during pregnancy than at birth.

Trisomy 18 or Edwards syndrome

Ninety-five per cent of fetuses with trisomy 18 spontaneously miscarry. The morphological and sonographic features include rocker bottom feet, clenched fist, increased nuchal translucency, congenital heart abnormalities (ventricular septal defect, atrial septal defect and patent ductus arteriosus), omphalocele, oesophageal atresia, choroid plexus cyst, deformed ears, overlapping fingers, early onset fetal growth restriction and low serum screening markers (low maternal serum alpha fetoprotein, oestriol and beta human chorionic gonadotropin [βhCG]) in the second trimester.

Trisomy 21 or Down syndrome

Features include congenital heart defects, duodenal atresia, congenital heart defect (atrioventricular septal defect), hypotonia, small ears, upward and outward slanting of the palpebral fissures, epicanthic folds, single transverse palmar crease, Brushfield spots on iris and flat nape of the neck. Life expectancy is 50–55 years.

Children with Down syndrome are at a higher risk of developing thyroid disorders (hypothyroidism), gastro-oesophageal reflux disease, Hirschsprung disease, severe mental retardatation, infertility, early onset Alzheimer disease, leukemia and epilepsy.

Trisomy 13 or Patau syndrome

It is a lethal abnormality and almost all fetuses miscarry. Features include microphthalmia, cleft lip and palate, clenched fist, holoprosencephaly, cardiac defects, single palmar crease and polydactyly.

James D, Steer PJ, Weiner CP, Gonik B, Crowther C, Robson S (eds). High Risk Pregnancy: Management Options (4th edn). St Louis: Saunders, 2011.
Magowan B. Churchill's Pocketbook of Obstetrics and Gynaecology (3rd edn). Edinburgh: Churchill Livingstone, 2005.

14. A **False.** Mosaics account for approximately 15%; monosomy X accounts for 60% of cases.

B **True.**

C **False.** The presence of the Y chromosome is associated with a risk of gonadoblastoma

D **False.** This is a rare situation.

E **True.** This leads to the deletion of Xp.

Turner syndrome

The incidence is 1 in 3000 live births. The occurrence is usually sporadic with incidence increasing with increasing paternal age and decreasing with increasing maternal age. Pure XO abnormality is seen in 60% of cases; mosaics (usually XO/XX) are seen in approximately 15% and the rest are due to deletions, rings or isochromosomes of Xq or Xp.

Turner syndrome is one of the most common chromosomal causes of primary infertility. Spontaneous menarche occurs in 10% of women and fertile women are usually Turner mosaic. Women should be informed about increased incidence of fetal loss during pregnancy and premature ovarian failure.

Fetus and risk

Turner syndrome is associated with cystic hygroma, hydropic changes and cardiac abnormalities in the fetus. Following birth, the features include short stature, cubitus valgus, coarctation of aorta, atrial septal defect and streak gonads.

At conception, the frequency of this condition is approximately 1% and the majority of these pregnancies will end in miscarriage (98%). It accounts for 20–30% of all abnormal karyotypes detected at spontaneous miscarriage. Ultrasound appearance of nuchal oedema or cystic hygroma (around 68% of cystic hygromas are associated with fetal aneuploidy, of which 74% is associated with Turner syndrome) in a female fetus should raise the suspicion of Turner syndrome. Occasionally, the condition can be diagnosed at birth but mostly it is undiagnosed until investigated for short stature in childhood (absence of growth spurt) or infertility in adults. There is no significant increase in recurrence risk in offspring.

Management includes use of growth-promoting agents in childhood and the replacement of female sex hormones for the development of secondary sexual characters.

Connor JM. Medical Genetics for MRCOG and Beyond. London: RCOG Press, 2005.
James D, Steer PJ, Weiner CP, Gonik B, Crowther C, Robson S (eds). High Risk Pregnancy: Management Options (4th edn). St Louis: Saunders, 2011.
Magowan B. Churchill's Pocketbook of Obstetrics and Gynaecology (3rd edn). Edinburgh: Churchill Livingstone, 2005.

15. A **True.**

   B **False.**

   C **False.**

   D **False.**

   E **False.**

The features of Turner syndrome include:

- broad chest with widely spaced nipples
- coarctation of aorta
- cubitus valgus
- deep-set nails
- generally normal intelligence
- Hashimoto's thyroiditis
- hypoplasia of nails
- horseshoe kidney
- low-set ears
- swollen hands and feet or peripheral lymphoedema
- short fourth metacarpal
- short stature
- systemic hypertension
- webbed neck
- wide carrying angle

Prenatal features during pregnancy include nuchal oedema and hydrops. There is also an increased risk of intrauterine fetal death.

Connor JM. Medical Genetics for MRCOG and Beyond. London: RCOG Press, 2005.
James D, Steer PJ, Weiner CP, Gonik B, Crowther C, Robson S (eds). High Risk Pregnancy: Management Options (4th edn). St Louis: Saunders, 2011.
Magowan B. Churchill's Pocketbook of Obstetrics and Gynaecology (3rd edn). Edinburgh: Churchill Livingstone, 2005.

16. A **True.**

    B **True.**

    C **False.**

    D **False.**

    E **True.**

    Trisomy 21

    The overall incidence is 1 in 600 live births. The incidence increases with increasing maternal age. It is associated with learning disabilities, congenital heart disease (ventricular septal defect, atrial septal defect primum, patent ductus arteriosus, atrioventricular canal defects and Fallot tetralogy), congenital cataract, thyroid disease, atresia of the gastrointestinal tract, leukaemia and early dementia. The risk of recurrence at birth is 1%.

    Ninety-five per cent of cases of Down syndrome are due to non-dysjunction at the first meiotic division (extra chromosome 21 of maternal origin in 90% of the cases), 4% are due to translocations involving chromosome 21 and 1% are due to mosaicism. The clinical features of Down syndrome due to translocations are similar to those due to trisomy 21.

    James D, Steer PJ, Weiner CP, Gonik B, Crowther C, Robson S (eds). High Risk Pregnancy: Management Options (4th edn). St Louis: Saunders, 2011.
    Magowan B. Churchill's Pocketbook of Obstetrics and Gynaecology (3rd edn). Edinburgh: Churchill Livingstone, 2005.

17. A **False.**

    B **True.**

    C **False.**

    D **False.**

    E **False.**

    Potter syndrome

    Potter syndrome is rare, with a reported incidence of 1 in 10,000. In this condition bilateral renal agenesis is associated with severe oligohydramnios and as a result leads to pulmonary hypoplasia and limb deformities. It carries a poor prognosis and is lethal.

    Any cause leading to reduced amniotic fluid beginning in mid trimester (e.g. rupture of membranes) can lead to such abnormalities and the prognosis is poor.

Fetal diagnosis can be difficult due to reduced amniotic fluid. Adrenal glands can be mistaken for kidneys and Doppler studies may show the absence of renal arteries. Scanning for a few hours can identify the absence of the bladder. The risk of recurrence is 3%.

Magowan B. Churchill's Pocketbook of Obstetrics and Gynaecology (3rd edn). Edinburgh: Churchill Livingstone, 2005.

18. A **True.**

 B **True.**

 C **True.**

 D **False.**

 E **False.**

- trisomy 21 – Down syndrome
- trisomy 18 – Edwards syndrome
- trisomy 13 – Patau syndrome
- deletion of chromosome 5p – Cri du chat syndrome

James D, Steer PJ, Weiner CP, Gonik B, Crowther C, Robson S (eds). High Risk Pregnancy: Management Options (4th edn). St Louis: Saunders, 2011.
Magowan B. Churchill's Pocketbook of Obstetrics and Gynaecology (3rd edn). Edinburgh: Churchill Livingstone, 2005.

19. A **True.**

 B **True.**

 C **True.**

 D **True.**

 E **True.**

NT is used for first trimester screening for Down syndrome along with serum screening beta human chorionic gonadotrophin (βhCG) and PAPP-A. It is performed between 11 and 14 weeks. Raised NT (>3 mm) is also associated with structural defects in 4% of cases including diaphragmatic hernia, cardiac or renal abnormalities and abdominal wall defects. If the risk is higher, women should be offered invasive testing in the form of CVS in early pregnancy and amniocentesis after 15 weeks of gestation. Women should be informed about the risk of miscarriage with these procedures.

Magowan B. Churchill's Pocketbook of Obstetrics and Gynaecology (3rd edn). Edinburgh: Churchill Livingstone, 2005.

20. A **True.** If untreated, phenylketonuria can cause damage to the fetus (25% risk) leading to microcephaly, congenital heart defects and learning disabilities.

 B **True.** This leads to fetal alcohol syndrome.

 C **False.** Type 1 diabetes mellitus (i.e. insulin-dependent diabetes mellitus) increases the risk of congenital malformations by 5–15%. These include neural tube defects, congenital heart defects and sacral agenesis. Strict diabetic control and folic acid supplementation (5 mg) is recommended before conception and during pregnancy to minimise the risks.

D **True.** There is a 2–3-fold increase in congenital malformations (orofacial, cardiac and neural tube defects) during pregnancy. Also, the child may develop epilepsy later in life (the risk is 4–5% if either parent has epilepsy and 15–20% if both parents have epilepsy). If there is an affected sibling, the risk increases to 10%. Various antiepileptic drugs increase the risk of fetal abnormalities. These include sodium valproate (up 10%, especially neural tube defects), phenytoin (4–5%), carbamazepine (neural rube defects) and lamotrigine (2–3%).

E **False.** It is associated with fetal growth restriction and intrauterine death.

Connor JM. Medical Genetics for MRCOG and Beyond. London: RCOG Press, 2005.
Magowan B. Churchill's Pocketbook of Obstetrics and Gynaecology (3rd edn). Edinburgh: Churchill Livingstone, 2005.
Nelson-Piercy C. Handbook of Obstetric Medicine (4th edn). London: Informa Healthcare, 2010.

21. **A** **True.**

B **False.** It is due to increased ACTH production.

C **True.**

D **True.**

E **True.**

Steroid hormones are derived from the cyclopentanophenanthrene nucleus:

- cholesterol contains 27 carbon atoms
- pregnane derivatives contain 21 carbon atoms (progesterone and corticosteroids)
- androstane derivatives contain 19 carbon atoms (androgens)
- estrane derivatives contain 18 carbon atoms (oestrogens)

The normal structure and biosynthesis of adrenocortical hormones are:

- ACTH stimulates glucocorticoid production
- the adrenal cortex secretes primarily C21 and C19 steroids
- C21 steroids are classified as mineralocorticoids and glucocorticoids; all C21 steroids have both effects
- mineralocorticoids predominantly effect Na^+ and K^+ excretion (aldosterone, deoxycorticosterone [has 3% mineralocorticoid activity of aldosterone])
- glucocorticoids predominantly have an effect on glucose and protein metabolism (cortisone and corticosterone)
- C19 steroids, androgens, DHEA and androstenedione
- most oestrogens that are not formed in the ovary are derived from androstenedione in circulation

Congenital adrenal hyperplasia (CAH)

- is the most common cause of female pseudohermaphroditism
- is an autosomal recessive disorder
- is caused by enzyme deficiency in the biosynthesis of cortisol in the adrenal gland

- adrenal hyperplasia is a result of increased ACTH production which in turn is a result of cortisol deficiency
- deficiency of the enzyme to produce glucocorticoids will lead to a default pathway producing excess androgens and therefore its consequences
- 21 hydroxylase deficiency is the most common enzyme deficiency (occurs in 90–95% of cases) and is an autosomal recessive disorder. The gene for 21 hydroxylase is on the short arm of chromosome 6. This results in an increase in progesterone and 17 alpha-hydroxyprogesterone and their subsequent conversion to androstenedione and testosterone
- 11-beta hydroxylase deficiency is the second most common enzyme deficiency (5–8%). It leads to an increase in 11-deoxycorticosterone, resulting in sodium retention and hypertension
- both of the above enzyme deficiencies cause virilisation because of increased androgen production
- the characteristic pattern that develops is adrenogenital syndrome (baldness, receding hairline, hirsutism, small breasts, male escutcheon, enlarged clitoris, fused labioscrotal folds and heavy arms and legs)
- 3-beta–hydroxysteroid dehydrogenase deficiency is a rare form of CAH. It causes salt-losing adrenal hyperplasia and mild virilisation

Presentations

- female pseudohermaphroditism – requires plastic surgery to feminise the genitalia and is usually advised before 18 months of age
- salt-losing form of congenital virilising form – requires correction of electrolyte imbalance
- hypertensive form of congenital virilising form – requires glucocorticoid replacement therapy

Investigations

- karyotyping
- pelvic ultrasound
- 17-alpha-hydroxyprogesterone
- 24-hour urinary 17 ketosteroids

Treatment

Long-term glucocorticoid replacement therapy is indicated in all virilising congenital forms of CAH (it replaces the glucocorticoid deficit and inhibits ACTH secretion, thus decreasing the abnormal secretion of androgens and other steroids). Psychological support for both the parents and the growing child is important.

Balen A. Chapter 14: Disorders of puberty. In: Shaw RW, Luesley D, Monga A (eds). Gynaecology (4th edn). Edinburgh: Churchill Livingstone, 2011.
Khan R. Chapter 12: Principles and new developments in molecular biology. In: Shaw RW, Luesley D, Monga A (eds). Gynaecology (4th edn). Edinburgh: Churchill Livingstone, 2011.

22. **A False.** Amniocentesis should be performed after 15 weeks of gestation because early amniocentesis (<14 weeks of gestation) is associated with a higher rate of fetal loss and increased incidence of neonatal talipes and respiratory morbidity compared with other procedures.

B False. CVS is usually done from 11 weeks to 14 weeks of gestation. Limb defects are common when performed before 10 weeks of gestation and hence CVS should not be performed before 10 completed weeks of gestation.

C False. The risk of miscarriage with amniocentesis is 1% and with CVS is 1–2%.

D False. There is risk of culture failure and placental mosaicism with CVS. Placental mosaicism is more common with CVS.

E True. There is also risk of infection with both amniocentesis and CVS.

Royal College of Obstetricians and Gynaecologists. Green-top Guideline No. 8. Amniocentesis and chorionic villus biopsy. London: RCOG Press, 2010.
Royal College of Obstetricians and Gynaecologists. Patient information. Amniocentesis: what you need to know. London: RCOG, 2006.
Royal College of Obstetricians and Gynaecologists. Patient information. Chorionic villus biopsy: what you need to know. London: RCOG, 2006.

23. **A False.** It is synthesised by fetal yolk sac, liver and gastrointestinal tract.

    B True.

    C False. MSAFP is reduced in trisomy 21 but can be raised in fetal conditions including neural tube defects, anencephaly, exomphalos, congenital nephrosis, trisomy 13 and Turner syndrome. It is also raised in obstetric conditions which include antepartum haemorrhage, fetal growth restriction, perinatal death and threatened miscarriage

    D True. After delivery MSAFP decreases rapidly with a half-life of 5 days.

    E True.

MSAFP is above normal in multiple gestation, placental abruption, neural tube defects (SB and anencephaly) and abdominal wall defects. One should also consider any error in the date of gestation. Rarely, it can be raised due to endodermal sinus tumour in pregnant women or in the fetus.

MSAFP is decreased in Down syndrome (trisomy 21) and Edwards syndrome (trisomy 18).

Physiological herniation of gut

Physiological herniation of the abdominal contents into the base of the umbilical cord is normal up to 13 weeks of gestation.

Exomphalos

It is an extraembryonic hernia due to the arrest of ventral medial migration of the dermatomyotomes. The incidence is between 1 in 2500 and 1 in 5000 pregnancies and is associated with other abnormalities in 60–80% of cases. It may be associated with polyhydramnios, fetal growth restriction and chromosomal abnormality in one in six fetuses.

- Ultrasound findings: an extra-abdominal mass is detected into which the umbilical cord is inserted rather than to the anterior abdominal wall (a sac or membrane is seen around the contents with the cord inserting into it).

- Biochemical markers: AFP is raised in both omphalocele and gastroschisis during the second trimester.

Amniotic fluid sample

It reveals a faint acetylcholinesterase band and a dense pseudocholinesterase band (opposite pattern to neural tube defects).

Role of prenatal diagnosis

A detailed ultrasound examination by a fetal medicine specialist is required to rule out other malformations and fetal karyotyping is indicated to exclude chromosomal abnormalities.

Labour and delivery

Delivery should be undertaken in a tertiary care centre with neonatal and surgical teams on board in order to optimise the preoperative care and life after delivery. Caesarean section is indicated only for obstetric reasons.

Down syndrome

Serum screening reveals decreased levels of AFP, oestriol, PAPP-A and increased levels of inhibin A and βhCG.

James D, Steer PJ, Weiner CP, Gonik B, Crowther C, Robson S (eds). High Risk Pregnancy: Management Options (4th edn). St Louis: Saunders, 2011.
McGill Nelson S, Grudzinskas JG. Chapter 10: Hormones, their actions and measurements in gynaecological practice. In: Shaw RW, Luesley D, Monga A (eds). Gynaecology (4th edn). Edinburgh: Churchill Livingstone, 2011.

24. **A False.** It is a glycoprotein which is used in the combined screening test in the first trimester.

  B False. It can be detected in maternal serum at 6–8 weeks of gestation.

  C True. PAPP-A levels are decreased in fetal chromosomal abnormalities (trisomy 21, trisomy 13 and trisomy 18).

  D False.

  E True. Its concentration gradually rises throughout pregnancy.

  Low PAPP-A at serum screening for Down syndrome is associated with increased risk of pre-eclampsia and fetal growth restriction during pregnancy. Therefore it is important to watch for raised blood pressure and arrange regular growth scans.

McGill Nelson S, Grudzinskas JG. Chapter 10: Hormones, their actions and measurements in gynaecological practice. In: Shaw RW, Luesley D, Monga A (eds). Gynaecology (4th edn). Edinburgh: Churchill Livingstone, 2011.

25. **A False.** It is defined as hyperechogenicity, believed to be located in the chordate tendineae, not attached to the ventricular walls and moving together with the atrioventricular walls.

  B True.

  C True.

D True. The risk of trisomy is lower than the procedure-related loss and the risk of trisomy in women over 35 years of age. Therefore, invasive testing is not advisable in women who are below 35 years of age (considered low risk) with an isolated finding of cardiac echogenic focus.

E False.

Abdalla MGK and Beattie B. Ultrasound screening for chromosomal abnormalities in the second trimester. Personal assessment in continuing education. Reviews, questions and answers. Volume 3. London: RCOG Press, 2003: 70–72.

26. **A True.**

    B True. The increased risk is almost 23%.

    C True. It is associated with intrauterine fetal growth restriction (IUGR) in 8% of cases. Therefore surveillance by ultrasound (serial growth scans) should be arranged in such cases.

    D False. Sickle cell disease in the fetus can be associated with non-immune hydrops.

    E False. Parvovirus infection is associated with non-immune hydrops.

Echogenic bowel is defined as echogenicity of the fetal bowel similar to or greater than that of the surrounding bone regardless of the shape of the echogenic mass. It is also associated with trisomy 21, cystic fibrosis and CMV infection. The investigations include serum IgM for CMV, amniotic fluid for CMV polymerase chain reaction, chromosomal analysis for aneuploidy and testing for the cystic fibrosis gene.

Abdalla MGK and Beattie B. Ultrasound screening for chromosomal abnormalities in the second trimester. Personal assessment in continuing education. Reviews, questions and answers. Volume 3. London: RCOG Press, 2003: 70–72.

27. **A False.**

    B True. There is an increased risk of congenital heart disease.

    C False. It increases the risk of Turner syndrome in 8% of cases.

    D True. It is associated with Noonan syndrome and Robert syndrome.

    E True.

NT should be described as simple or septated as the risk of aneuploidy is very high in the presence of septation.

Abdalla MGK and Beattie B.Ultrasound screening for chromosomal abnormalities in the second trimester. Personal assessment in continuing education. Reviews, questions and answers. Volume 3. London: RCOG Press, 2003: 70–72.

28. **A True.**

    B True.

    C True.

    D True.

    E True.

Congenital rubella causes a triad (called triad of Gregg) of abnormalities affecting the eyes, ears and the heart:

- **eyes:** bilateral cataract, retinopathy (salt and pepper appearance of funduscopy), microphthalmia and glaucoma
- **ears:** mainly sensorineural deafness. It is rare if the maternal infection occurs after 16 weeks of pregnancy
- **heart:** common abnormalities are patent ductus arteriosus, pulmonary artery stenosis and pulmonary valvular stenosis while rare abnormalities are ventricular septal defect, atrial septal defect and coarctation of the aorta.

James D, Steer PJ, Weiner CP, Gonik B, Crowther C, Robson S (eds). High Risk Pregnancy: Management Options (4th edn). St Louis: Saunders, 2011.

29. **A False.** It is a DNA virus with single stranded DNA genome. Parvovirus B19 is the only pathogenic parvoviridae that causes infection in humans. The infection is transmitted by respiratory droplets and has an incubation period of 4–14 days. A rash (usually facial) appears after the viraemia is resolved. Therefore patients with a rash are no longer infectious.

B False. The vertical transmission rate is 30%.

C True. Parvovirus B19 can cause transient aplastic crisis in women with sickle cell disease and other hereditary anaemias including thalassaemia, spherocytosis, pyruvate kinase deficiency and autoimmune haemolytic anaemia. Aplastic crisis is also the fetal pathology.

D True. Fetal complications may occur over 4–6 weeks following maternal symptoms or infection when maternal IgM may be undetectable. Of these 34% are self-limiting but 3% develop non-immune hydrops (which accounts for 10–20% of non-immune hydrops), severe fetal anaemia and cardiac failure. Therefore ultrasound examination should be arranged in the next 4–6 weeks to check for any fetal signs of anaemia (middle cerebral artery, peak systolic velocity). Fetal reticulocytosis (>20%) is a good prognostic factor (but requires fetal blood sampling which is an invasive procedure) and usually suggests that fetal haemoglobin has probably reached its nadir and spontaneous recovery may occur soon. Following resolution, it does not cause any late sequelae.

E False. Fetal infection is not an indication for termination of pregnancy as 33% resolve spontaneously. Termination of pregnancy should be considered if infection occurs during early pregnancy.

James D, Steer PJ, Weiner CP, Gonik B, Crowther C, Robson S (eds). High Risk Pregnancy: Management Options (4th edn). St Louis: Saunders, 2011.
Magowan B. Churchill's Pocketbook of Obstetrics and Gynaecology (3rd edn). Edinburgh: Churchill Livingstone, 2005.

30. **A False.** It is caused by DNA virus.

B False. Transplacental transfer to fetus occurs in only 5% of cases.

C False. Vertical transmission to the fetus during childbirth occurs in 90% of cases.

D False. It does not cause congenital abnormalities.

E True. In adults 90% resolve within 6 months and only 10% develop chronic carrier state.

James D, Steer PJ, Weiner CP, Gonik B, Crowther C, Robson S (eds). High Risk Pregnancy: Management Options (4th edn). St Louis: Saunders, 2011.
Magowan B. Churchill's Pocketbook of Obstetrics and Gynaecology (3rd edn). Edinburgh: Churchill Livingstone, 2005.

31. **A True.** The second most common translocation is between chromosomes 14 and 21 t (14; 21).

    B False. The risk of having a baby born with Down syndrome is 10–15% if the mother is a carrier of translocation between chromosomes 14 and 21 t (14; 21).

    C False. The risk of having a baby born with Down syndrome is 1% if the father is a carrier of translocation between chromosomes 14 and 21 t (14; 21).

    D True. Translocations involving chromosome 21 give rise to familial Down syndrome.

    E True.

    Chromosomal translocation is the transfer of genetic material between two chromosomes, which usually happens during meiosis.

    - **Balanced translocation:** the exchange occurs between chromosomes distal to the breakpoint. In this condition the individuals are normal as no genetic material is lost and there is no risk of abnormality if it is inherited as balanced translocation.
    - **Unbalanced or Robertsonian translocation:** breaks occur near the centromere in two acrocentric chromosomes. The individual may be healthy but there is risk of loss or duplication of the genetic material during cell division.

    Risk for Down syndrome

    - absence of translocation = age-related risk plus 0.34% at term
    - presence of translocation
    - mother carrier t (14; 21) = 10–15%
    - father carrier t (14; 21) = 1%
    - mother or father t (21; 21) = 100%

    Connor JM. Medical Genetics for MRCOG and Beyond. London: RCOG Press, 2005.

32. **A True.** It is also associated with wrong dates.

    B True.

    C True.

    D False.

    E True.

    Factors that cause raised MSAFP include:

    - placental and umbilical cord tumours
    - Afro-Caribbean origin
    - anencephaly

- congenital nephrosis
- cystic adenomatoid malformation of the lung
- exomphalos
- fetal growth restriction
- fetomaternal haemorrhage
- multiple pregnancies
- obstructive uropathy
- maternal liver disease
- neural tube defects
- sacrococcygeal teratoma
- smoking
- wrong dates

High MSAFP is associated with an increased risk of fetal growth restriction, intrauterine death and pre-eclampsia.

Trisomy 21 is associated with low MSAFP and unconjugated oestriol and high serum βhCG.

Trisomy 18 is associated with low MSAFP, unconjugated oestriol and serum βhCG.

Trisomy 13 is associated with normal alpha fetoprotein and low βhCG

Connor JM. Medical Genetics for MRCOG and Beyond. London: RCOG Press, 2005.
James D, Steer PJ, Weiner CP, Gonik B, Crowther C, Robson S (eds). High Risk Pregnancy: Management Options (4th edn). St Louis: Saunders, 2011.

33. A True.

  B True.

  C True.

  D True.

  E True.

The other conditions which can be diagnosed by preimplantation diagnosis include:

- Duchenne muscular dystrophy
- familial adenomatous polyposis coli
- Marfan syndrome
- retinitis pigmentosum
- spinal muscular atrophy
- Tay–Sachs disease
- osteogenesis imperfect

The following cells are used for preimplantation diagnosis:

- polar body from oocyte
- blastomeres from cleavage stage embryos – most commonly used method
- trophectoderm cells from blastocysts

Connor JM. Medical Genetics for MRCOG and Beyond. London: RCOG Press, 2005.

34. A **True.** They also include anti-D rhesus antibodies.

   B **True.**

   C **False.**

   D **False.**

   E **False.**

   The causes of non-immune hydrops include:

   - idiopathic
   - infections (parvovirus B19, toxoplasmosis, cytomegalovirus, syphilis)
   - fetal causes of anaemia (alpha thalassaemia, glucose-6-phosphate dehydrogenase deficiency, chronic fetomaternal haemorrhage, twin-to-twin transfusion)
   - cardiac (arrhythmias, myocarditis, premature closure of ductus arteriosus, congenital heart block)
   - pulmonary (diaphragmatic hernia, congenital pulmonary adenomatoid malformation)
   - renal (bladder neck obstruction)
   - placental (chorioangioma)
   - chromosomal (trisomies, Turner syndrome, triploidy)

   The maternal risks with fetal hydrops include increased risk of pre-eclampsia, placental abruption, polyhydramnios, dystocia, caesarean section and postpartum haemorrhage.

   James D, Steer PJ, Weiner CP, Gonik B, Crowther C, Robson S (eds). High Risk Pregnancy: Management Options (4th edn). St Louis: Saunders, 2011.
   Magowan B. Churchill's Pocketbook of Obstetrics and Gynaecology (3rd edn). Edinburgh: Churchill Livingstone, 2005.

35. A **False.** It is associated with other structural anomalies.

   B **False.** Left-sided hernias are more common.

   C **False.** Only 10–20% are associated with an abnormal karyotype.

   D **True.** The newborn baby manifests with cyanosis (needing oxygen and intubation), barrel shaped chest and dextrocardia.

   E **True.**

   Diaphragmatic hernia is herniation of the abdominal contents or organs into the thoracic cavity. This may lead to the underdevelopment of lungs and pulmonary hypoplasia, which is often lethal. The reported incidence in live births is 1 in 3500. The most common site of herniation is through the posterolateral defect (foramen of Bochdalek) in the pleuroperitoneal canal. Also, left-sided hernias are more common than right-sided hernias. Even in the best hands small hernias can be missed on ultrasound and only less than 50% are diagnosed antenatally. The possible diagnostic signs on ultrasound include migration of the stomach into the chest and its abscence in the abdominal cavity, abnormal location of the heart in the thorax and presence of the bowel or stomach at the level of the heart. Antenatally the condition can present with polyhydramnios.

In almost 50% of cases, there are other associated abnormalities (VSD, tetralogy of Fallot, gastrointestinal and skeletal). It can be associated with syndromes which include Beckwith–Wiedemann syndrome, Pierre Robin syndrome, Fryns syndrome and chromosomal abnormalities (10–20%) such as trisomy 13, trisomy 18 and deletion of 9p-syndrome (hence the karyotype is indicated). Termination of pregnancy can be offered in the presence of other associated abnormalities or an abnormal karyotype.

The most common presentation after birth is cyanosis and decreased oxygen saturation which warrants intubation and ventilation of the newborn baby. It is also a common cause of dextrocardia in a newborn baby.

James D, Steer PJ, Weiner CP, Gonik B, Crowther C, Robson S (eds). High Risk Pregnancy: Management Options (4th edn). St Louis: Saunders, 2011.

36. **A True.** The diagnosis of oesophageal atresia can be made when the stomach is not visualised after 20 weeks of pregnancy on an ultrasound. It is associated with tracheoesophageal fistula in 87% of cases.

    B True.

    C True. It is associated with an abnormal karyotype in 10% of cases.

    D False. It is associated with other structural abnormalities. An isolated finding with no associated structural anomalies and a normal karyotype has good prognosis. One should aim for planned vaginal delivery and avoid neonatal feeding at birth (pass nasogastric tube and get chest X-ray done).

    E True. Pre-term labour or polyhydramnios is the usual presentation during the antenatal period.

    Oesophageal atresia can be isolated and most often associated with tracheoesophageal fistula (this is explained by their common origin of oesophagus and trachea from diverticulum in primitive pharynx and failure to separate between 3 and 5 weeks). The most common abnormality is oesophageal atresia with distal tracheoesophageal fistula (87%) whereas isolated tracheoesophageal fistula and isolated oesophageal atresia account for 4% and 8% of cases, respectively.

    Absence of stomach bubble on ultrasound scans from 20 weeks onwards should raise a strong suspicion of oesophageal atresia (differentials: oesophageal atresia, congenital diaphragmatic hernia and impaired fetal swallowing). It can also be associated with other abnormalities such as VACTERAL (vertebral, anal, cardiac [atrial septal defect and ventricular septal defect], renal, limb, abnormal location of ears and malformation of mandible and temporal bones) and aneuploidy in 10% of cases (hence karyotyping is indicated). Antenatally the condition can present with polyhydramnios and pre-term labour.

    Isolated abnormalities without any other associated abnormalities carry a good prognosis with a survival rate of almost 100%.

James D, Steer PJ, Weiner CP, Gonik B, Crowther C, Robson S (eds). High Risk Pregnancy: Management Options (4th edn). St Louis: Saunders, 2011.

Chapter 8

Gynaecological oncology

1. **With regards to familial breast/ovarian cancer:**
   A   It is inherited as an autosomal dominant trait
   B   It can be due to mutations in the BRCA1 gene on the short arm of chromosome 17
   C   The lifetime risk of breast cancer is 99% if a woman carries the BRCA1 mutation
   D   The lifetime risk of ovarian cancer is 10% if a woman carries the BRCA1 mutation
   E   Men with the mutant gene usually develop cancer

2. **With regards to the staging of endometrial cancer:**
   A   Stage Ia: Endometrial adenocarcinoma confined to the uterus but involving less than half of the myometrium
   B   Stage II: Endometrial adenocarcinoma involving more than half of the myometrium and cervical stroma
   C   Stage IVa: Endometrial adenocarcinoma invading bladder mucosa
   D   Stage IVb: Endometrial adenocarcinoma involving inguinal lymph nodes
   E   Stage IIIC2: Endometrial adenocarcinoma involving more than half of the myometrium and involvement of pelvic nodes

3. **The following are true with regards to epithelial ovarian cancer:**
   A   Peak incidence is at 50–70 years
   B   Late presentation
   C   Vague symptoms
   D   Most are advanced stage at diagnosis
   E   Overall 5-year survival is around 30%

4. **The following are correctly matched:**
   A   Dermoid cyst – Immature teratoma
   B   Germ cell tumour – Endodermal sinus tumour
   C   Diethylstilboestrol – Vaginal squamous cell carcinoma in offspring
   D   Aniline dyes – Uterine carcinoma
   E   HPV 18 – Adenocarcinoma of cervix

5. **The following tumour markers are correctly matched:**
   A   Seminomas – alpha fetoprotein (AFP)
   B   Endodermal sinus tumour – AFP
   C   Choriocarcinoma – beta human chorionic gonadotrophin (hCG)
   D   Granulose cell tumour – inhibin
   E   Dysgerminoma – lactate dehydrogenase

6. **Serum testosterone levels are increased in the following conditions:**
    A   Late onset congenital adrenal hyperplasia (CAH)
    B   Polycystic ovary syndrome
    C   Granulosa cell tumour
    D   Brenner tumour
    E   Theca cell tumour

7. **With regards to cervical glandular intraepithelial neoplasia:**
    A   It usually presents with intermenstrual bleeding
    B   The majority of lesions are within 1 cm adjacent to the squamocolumnar junction
    C   It has definite well-defined identified patterns for colposcopic diagnosis
    D   It is associated with human papilloma virus 18
    E   It is associated with skip lesions higher up in the endocervical canal

8. **Atypical endometrial hyperplasia is associated with:**
    A   Coexistent endometrial carcinoma
    B   Coexistent ovarian tumour
    C   Coexistent cervical carcinoma
    D   Progression to uterine sarcoma
    E   Abnormal uterine bleeding

9. **With regards to premalignant lesions of the genital tract:**
    A   One third of untreated women with cervical intraepithelial neoplasia (CIN) III will progress to cancer in 5 years
    B   CIN I progresses to CIN III or worse in 26% of women within 2 years
    C   Glandular lesions of the cervix can coexist with squamous lesions
    D   Glandular abnormality on cervical smear may be associated with fallopian tube cancer
    E   Glandular abnormality on cervical smear may be associated with endometrial cancer

10. **With regards to treatment methods for cervical intraepithelial neoplasia (CIN):**
    A   Invasive disease needs to be excluded before choosing any destructive methods
    B   The use of cryotherapy does not require general anaesthesia
    C   Electrodiathermy requires general anaesthesia
    D   Knife cone biopsy can be performed under local anaesthesia
    E   Cold coagulation uses a temperature of –20°C

11. **With regards to vulval intraepithelial neoplasia (VIN):**
    A   Most women present with an ulcer on the vulva
    B   VIN is usually a unifocal disease
    C   It can be associated with cervical intraepithelial neoplasia (CIN)
    D   The natural history is well-known
    E   Malignant change is more common in women who are immunosuppressed

Answers

1. **A True.** The lifetime risk of ovarian cancer is 1 in 50–100 women.

    B False. It can be due to mutations in the BRCA1 gene (35–50%) on the long arm of chromosome 17.

    C False. The lifetime risk of breast cancer is 80% if a woman carries the BRCA1 mutation.

    D False. The lifetime risk of ovarian cancer is 60% if a woman carries the BRCA1 mutation.

    E False. Men with the mutant gene usually do not develop cancer but transmit the gene to approximately 50% of their offspring.

    Connor JM. Medical Genetics for MRCOG and Beyond. London: RCOG Press, 2005.
    Tobias ES and Connor JM. Medical Genetics for the MRCOG and Beyond (2nd edn). London: RCOG Press, in press.

2. **A True.**

    B True.

    C True.

    D True.

    E False.

    The new International Federation of Gynecology and Obstetrics (FIGO) staging (2009) for endometrial cancer is as follows:

    - **IA:** Tumour confined to the uterus, or less than half the myometrium invaded
    - **IB:** Tumour confined to the uterus, more than half the myometrium invaded
    - **II:** Cervical stromal invasion, but not beyond the uterus
    - **IIIA:** Tumour invades serosa or adnexa
    - **IIIB:** Vaginal and/or parametrial involvement
    - **IIIC1:** Pelvic node involvement
    - **IIIC2:** Para-aortic involvement
    - **IVA:** Tumour invasion bladder and/or bowel mucosa
    - **IVB:** Distant metastases including abdominal metastases and/or inguinal lymph nodes

    Endocervical glandular involvement is no longer considered stage II.

    Positive peritoneal cytology does not alter the surgico-pathological FIGO stage.

    Holland C. Endometrial cancer. Obstet Gynaecol Reprod Med 2010; 20:347–352.

3. **A True.**

    B True.

    C True.

    D True.

    E True.

Risk factors for ovarian cancer:

- nulliparity
- ovulation induction
- familial
- age: epithelial cell tumours are common in old age and germ cell tumours in young age (less than 20% of ovarian cancers occur before the age of 45 years)

Protective factors for ovarian cancer:
- long-term use of combined oral contraceptive pills (COCP)
- pregnancy
- breastfeeding

The risk of malignancy is high with the following:

- age >45 years
- bilateral tumours
- solid areas and irregular growth on surface of ovaries or ovarian cyst
- multilocular cyst

Risk of malignancy index (RMI):

- ultrasound score: 1 point for each of the features: multilocular, solid, bilateral, metastasis, ascites
- U = 0 (no points), U = 1 (1 point) and U = 3 (2 – 5 points)
- menopausal status: M = 1 if premenopausal and M = 3 if postmenopausal

Protocol for triaging women:

- risk/low = RMI <25 = <3% risk of cancer
- risk/moderate = RMI 25–250 = risk of cancer is 20%
- risk/high = RMI >250 = risk of cancer is 75%

Familial breast and ovarian cancer

Inherited genes play an important role in the development of breast, ovarian and colorectal cancers (**Table 8.1**).

The lifetime risk of developing breast cancer in the UK is 1 in 12 while ovarian cancer is 1 in 80. The incidence of breast cancer goes up to 300 per 100,000 in women aged

Table 8.1 Genes associated with breast, ovarian and colorectal cancers

Inherited genes	Cancers
ATM, BRCA1, BRCA2, CHEK2, RAD51, DIRAS3, and ERBB2	Breast
BRCA1 and BRCA2	Ovarian
MSH2 and MSH6, both on chromosome 2 and MLH1, on chromosome 3	Colorectal

over 85 years compared to fewer than 10 per 100,000 in women who are under the age of 30 years. This can occur in either sporadic or hereditary forms. Of the hereditary forms, up to 10% are known to be inherited as dominant genes before the age of 35 years, while only 1% have such inheritance over the age of 80 years.

About 1 in 800 women in the general population may have the BRCA1 mutation and somewhat less than this may have the BRCA2 mutation, which varies further with ethnic populations and geographical location (e.g. about 1 in 50 Ashkenazi Jews carry these mutations).

The presence of BRCA1 or BRCA2 equally increases the risk of developing breast cancer by 40–85% during a woman's lifetime depending on the population. The risk of ovarian cancer is higher with BRCA1 compared to BRCA2 (**Table 8.2**).

Genetics: family history

- Risk: Relative risk 1.1 for mother, 3.8 for sister and 6 for daughter.
- If there is one affected primary relative aged <50 years, the lifetime risk is 5%.
- If there are two affected primary relatives aged <50 years, the lifetime risk is 25%.
- Five to ten per cent of ovarian cancers are hereditary (e.g. BRCA1 and HNPCC).

BRCA1 and BRCA2 mutation

- Overall these mutations account for 3% of ovarian tumour cases (5% aged <40 years).
- They are associated with a 10–50% lifetime risk of developing ovarian tumour.
- Mutation occurs in 80% of families with breast or ovarian cancer.

Risk reduction measures for women who carry BRCA1 or BRCA2 mutations

Breast cancer

- self-breast examination
- early screening with mammogram
- prophylactic mastectomy does not eliminate the risk of cancer

Ovarian cancer

- yearly screening with transvaginal scan and Ca 125
- COCP use is associated with risk reduction of ovarian cancer by 40%. This is a good option in women who have not completed their family yet. The protecting effect lasts up to at least 10 years after stopping the pill
- prophylactic oophorectomy once the family is complete (this does not prevent primary peritoneal cancers)

Table 8.2 BRCA1 and BRCA2 lifetime risk

Lifetime risk	BRCA1	BRCA2
Breast cancer	60–80%	30–60%
Ovarian cancer	30–60%	20–30%

Royal College of Obstetricians and Gynaecologists. Green-top Guideline No. 34. Ovarian cysts in postmenopausal women. London: RCOG Press, 2003.

Morrison PJ, Hodgson SV, Haites NE (eds). Familial Breast and Ovarian Cancer, Genetics, Screening and Management. Cambridge: Cambridge University Press, 2002.

Shafi MI, Luesley DM, Jordan JA. Handbook of Gynaecological Oncology. Edinburgh: Churchill Livingstone, 2001.

4. A **False.** A dermoid cyst is a mature teratoma.

   B **True.**

   C **False.**

   D **False.** It is bladder carcinoma.

   E **True.**

   Tumours and tissues of origin are shown in **Table 8.3**.

   Viruses and cancer are shown in **Table 8.4**.

   Chemicals and cancer are shown in **Table 8.5**.

Table 8.3 Tumours and tissues of origin

Tissue of origin	Benign	Malignant
Germ cells	Mature teratoma	Immature teratoma
Placenta tissue	Hydatidiform mole	Choriocarcinoma
Neuroectoderm	Naevus	Malignant melanoma
Glands or ducts	Adenoma	Adenocarcinoma
Squamous cells	Papilloma	Squamous cell carcinoma
Smooth muscle	Leiomyoma	Leiomyosarcoma

Table 8.4 Viruses and cancer

Virus	Cancer
Human papillomavirus 16, 18	Cervical cancer
Human T-cell lymphotropic virus-1	T-cell lymphoma/leukaemia
Hepatitis B	Hepatocellular carcinoma
Epstein–Barr virus	Nasopharyngeal carcinoma, Burkitt lymphoma

Table 8.5 Chemicals and cancer

Carcinogen	Cancer
Aflatoxin B1	Liver cancer
Asbestos	Mesothelioma
Diethylstilboestrol	Vaginal clear cell carcinoma in offspring
Alkylating agents (especially melphalan)	Leukaemia
Aniline dyes	Bladder cancer

Shafi MI, Luesley DM, Jordan JA. Handbook of Gynaecological Oncology. Edinburgh: Churchill Livingstone, 2001.

Sanusi FA, Carter P, Barton DPJ. Non-Epithelial Ovarian Cancers. Personal assessment in continuing education. Reviews, questions and answers. Volume 3. London: RCOG Press, 2003.

5. A **True.**

B **True.**

C **True.**

D **True.**

E **True.**

The following parameters are used for making a tumour diagnosis:

*   clinical symptoms
*   clinical signs
*   imaging
*   tumour markers
*   morphology and histopathology
*   molecular

A tumour marker is a biochemical marker which may indicate the presence of a tumour. It can support in making a diagnosis and can also be used for screening purposes, localisation of the primary tumour, and response to therapy or relapse of a tumour. Examples of tumour markers are shown in **Table 8.6**.

Ovarian cancer is the fourth most common cause of cancer death but sixth most common cancer. Two thirds of them are diagnosed at FIGO stage III and IV (advanced disease) and hence the poor prognosis. Obviously women diagnosed in the early stages carry a better prognosis and good survival rate (89% and 67% for stages I and II, respectively). This does not apply to clear cell carcinoma.

CA 125 is raised in approximately 80% of all women with epithelial ovarian cancer but only 50% of patients with FIGO stage I disease. However, one should remember

Table 8.6 Examples of tumour markers

Tumour markers (oncofetal proteins)	Cancer
Carcinoembryonic antigen	Colonic, stomach and pancreatic. It is also raised in mucinous ovarian tumours
Alpha fetoprotein	Endodermal sinus tumour, embryonal carcinoma, seminomas and hepatocellular carcinoma

Tumour markers (hormones)	Cancer
Catecholamines and vanillylmandelic acid	Phaeochromocytoma
Calcitonin	Medullary carcinoma of thyroid
Human chorionic gonadotrophin (hCG)	Gestational trophoblastic tumours, choriocarcinomas and embryonal carcinoma (3% of dysgerminomas produce beta hCG)
5-hydroxytryptamine (5-HT)	Carcinoid tumour

Tumour markers (enzymes and proteins)	Cancer
CA 15.3	Breast carcinoma
CA 19.9	Colonic and pancreatic carcinoma
CA 125	Ovarian carcinoma (epithelial and primary peritoneal carcinoma)
Lactate dehydrogenase	Dysgerminomas

that CA 125 has low specificity in women <45 years of age as it can be elevated in several benign conditions which include endometriosis, pelvic inflammatory disease, adenomyosis, fibroids, lymphoma, during menstruation, ovarian hyperstimulation syndrome and pregnancy.

Shafi MI, Luesley DM, Jordan JA. Handbook of Gynaecological Oncology. Edinburgh: Churchill Livingstone, 2001.
Sanusi FA, Carter P, Barton DPJ. Non-Epithelial Ovarian Cancers. Personal assessment in continuing education. Reviews, questions and answers. Volume 3. London: RCOG Press, 2003.
Kumar B and Davies-Humphreys J. Tumour Markers and Ovarian Cancer Screening. Personal assessment in continuing education. Reviews, questions and answers. Volume 3. London: RCOG Press, 2003.

6. **A True.** High levels of 17 hydroxyprogesterone confirm the diagnosis of CAH. Once diagnosed, the treatment is administration of dexamethasone for life.

    B True.

    C False. Oestrogen and inhibin levels are increased in women with granulosa cell tumour.

    D False.

    E True.

    The serum testosterone levels are normally <2 nmol/L. It can be raised in ovarian or adrenal conditions. Ovarian conditions causing raised serum testosterone levels include theca cell tumours, arrhenoblastoma, gynandroblastoma (levels >5 nmol/L), ovarian hyperthecosis and polycystic ovary syndrome (levels >3 nmol/L). Adrenal conditions causing raised serum testosterone levels include Cushing syndrome (levels >4 nmol/L) and adrenal tumours (if levels are >7 nmol/L suspect an androgen-secreting tumour).

    Sanusi FA, Carter P, Barton DPJ. Non-Epithelial Ovarian Cancers. Personal assessment in continuing education. Reviews, questions and answers. Volume 3. London: RCOG Press, 2003.
    Critchley HOD, Horne A, Munro K. Chapter 16: Amenorrhoea and oligomenorrhoea, and hypothalamic–pituitary dysfunction. In: Shaw RW, Luesley D, Monga A (eds). Gynaecology (4th edn). Edinburgh: Churchill Livingstone, 2011.
    James D, Steer PJ, Weiner CP, Gonik B, Crowther C, Robson S (eds). High Risk Pregnancy: Management Options (4th edn). St Louis: Saunders, 2011.
    Magowan B. Churchill's Pocketbook of Obstetrics and Gynaecology (3rd edn). Edinburgh: Churchill Livingstone, 2005.

7. **A False.** It is usually asymptomatic. Glandular lesions are either an incidental finding on cervical smear or diagnosed associated with squamous lesions.

    B True.

    C False. There are no definitive identified patterns for CGIN unlike squamous intraepithelial lesions.

    D True.

    E True. It therefore poses difficulty in diagnosis, treatment and follow-up.

    Personal assessment in continuing education. Reviews, questions and answers. Volume 3. London: RCOG Press, 2003.
    NHS Cervical Screening Programme. Colposcopy and Programme Management. Guidelines for the NHS Cervical Screening Programme (2nd edn). Publication No 20. NHSCSP, 2010. http://www.bsccp.org.uk/docs/public/pdf/nhscsp20.pdf
    Wuntakal R and Hollingworth T. Chapter 3: Management of abnormal Pap smears. In: Cervical Cancer: Contemporary Management. [Rajaram S, Maheswari A, Chitrathara (eds)]. New Delhi: Jaypee Brothers Medical Publishers, 2011.

8. **A True.**

    B True.

    C False.

    D False. It is a premalignant condition and progresses to endometrial cancer.

E True.

Women with endometrial hyperplasia can present with postmenopausal bleeding, abnormal vaginal bleeding and/or infertility problems in premenopausal women. Endometrial hyperplasia is classified as simple hyperplasia with or without atypia and complex hyperplasia with or without atypia.

The risk of progression to endometrial cancer with various types of hyperplasia is as follows:

- simple hyperplasia without atypia (around 1%)
- complex hyperplasia without atypia (3%)
- simple hyperplasia with atypia (8%)
- complex hyperplasia with atypia (29%)

The treatment depends on age, fertility wishes and type of hyperplasia. The main aim of treatment is identification and removal of the excessive source of oestrogen. Women who wish to preserve fertility and have hyperplasia without atypia can be treated with high dose oral progesterone or levonorgestrel IUS to be followed by hysteroscopy and endometrial biopsy 3 months later. Women with atypical hyperplasia should have a hysterectomy and bilateral salpingo-oophorectomy because of the increased risk of coexistent endometrial carcinoma (25–50% of the cases).

Moss E, Redman CW, Ganeshan R. Chapter 38: Premalignant diseases of the genital tract. In: Shaw RW, Luesley D, Monga A (eds). Gynaecology (4th edn). Edinburgh: Churchill Livingstone, 2011.
Fritz MA and Speroff L. Clinical Gynaecologic Endocrinology and Infertility (8th edn). Philadelphia: Lippincott Williams and Wilkins, 2011.

9. **A False.** One third of untreated women with CIN III will progress to cancer in 20 years.

   B True.

   C True. Cervical glandular neoplasia is associated with CIN in almost 50% of cases.

   D True.

   E True. In light of this association, women with cervical glandular neoplasia should be investigated further (with transvaginal pelvic scan and hysteroscopy and endometrial biopsy), especially when they present with abnormal vaginal bleeding and have a negative colposcopy on examination.

Moss E, Redman CW, Ganeshan R. Chapter 38: Premalignant diseases of the genital tract. In: Shaw RW, Luesley D, Monga A (eds). Gynaecology (4th edn). Edinburgh: Churchill Livingstone, 2011.
NHS Cervical Screening Programme. Colposcopy and Programme Management. Guidelines for the NHS Cervical Screening Programme (2nd edn). Publication No 20. NHSCSP, 2010. http://www.bsccp.org.uk/docs/public/pdf/nhscsp20.pdf
Wuntakal R and Hollingworth T. Chapter 3: Management of abnormal Pap smears. In: Cervical Cancer: Contemporary Management. [Rajaram S, Maheswari A, Chitrathara (eds)]. New Delhi: Jaypee Brothers Medical Publishers, 2011.

10. **A True.** The use of destructive methods depends on the exclusion of invasive disease by colposcopy and tissue diagnosis.

   B True. Cryotherapy has the highest treatment failure.

C **True.** Electrodiathermy destroys tissue up to a depth of 10 mm.

D **False.** Knife cone biopsy is done under general anaesthesia. The excision method, large loop excision of transformation zone (LLETZ), is the most commonly used method for treatment of CIN in the UK. The majority of these are done in a colposcopy clinic under local anaesthesia (according to the British Society for Colposcopy & Cervical Pathology [BSCCP] guideline, 80% of LLETZ should be done under local anaesthesia) and the rest under general anaesthesia for indications such as patient's request, anxiety and a large lesion with a large transformation zone.

E **False.** Cold coagulation uses a temperature of 100–120°C and destroys tissue up to a depth of 4 mm. General anaesthesia is not required.

NHS Cervical Screening Programme. Colposcopy and Programme Management. Guidelines for the NHS Cervical Screening Programme (2nd edn). Publication No 20. NHSCSP, 2010. http://www.bsccp.org.uk/docs/public/pdf/nhscsp20.pdf

11. A **False.** Most women present with pruritus vulvae.

B **False.** Vulval intraepithelial neoplasia (VIN) is usually a multifocal disease.

C **True.** It is called field phenomenon. CIN can be associated with vaginal intraepithelial neoplasia (VAIN) or VIN in the genital tract and anal intraepithelial neoplasia (AIN).

D **False.** The natural history is not well-known. However, the malignant potential is much lower compared to CIN.

E **True.** Malignant change is also common in older women.

Nunns D and Scott IV. Ulcers and Erosions of the Vulva. Personal assessment in continuing education. Reviews, questions and answers. Volume 3. London: RCOG Press, 2003.

Chapter 9

Management of labour and delivery

1. **With regards to caesarean section:**

   A The incidence of postoperative morbidity is increased following classical caesarean section compared to lower segment caesarean section (LSCS)

   B The risk of peripartum hysterectomy is quoted to be 1 in 500 with first caesarean section

   C Dissection of the bladder is always required while performing classical caesarean section

   D A subsequent trial of labour is allowed for women with previous classical caesarean section

   E The risk of uterine rupture with vaginal birth after caesarean (VBAC) is less than 1% in women with one previous LSCS

2. **With regards to shoulder dystocia:**

   A Fifty per cent of cases occur in babies weighing less than 4 kg

   B It occurs due to obstruction at the pelvic outlet

   C It resolves with simple manoeuvres (like McRoberts and suprapubic pressure) in more than 90% of cases

   D It is increased in women who receive pethidine for pain relief in labour

   E It is definitely a preventable condition

3. **The following information should be given to women choosing epidural analgesia:**

   A It is associated with prolonged second stage of labour

   B It is always associated with long-term backache

   C Its effectiveness is less than parenteral opioids

   D Epidural solutions containing opioids can cross the placenta and cause respiratory distress in the baby

   E It is associated with longer first stage of labour

4. **The following are indications to switch to continuous electronic fetal monitoring (EFM) from intermittent auscultation in low-risk women:**

   A Maternal pyrexia of 37.1°C on two occasions 2 hours apart

   B Oxytocin use for augmentation of labour

   C Maternal pyrexia of 38°C on two occasions

   D Abnormal fetal heart rate (FHR) detected on intermittent auscultation

   E The woman's request

5. **Concerning interventions to reduce perineal trauma during childbirth:**
   A   Perineal massage should be routinely performed in the second stage of labour
   B   Episiotomy should be carried out for vaginal births
   C   Episiotomy should be performed to assist instrumental deliveries if necessary
   D   Unless fetal compromise is suspected, tested effective analgesia should be offered before undertaking episiotomy
   E   Episiotomy should be routinely offered to women with previous history of third- and fourth-degree tear

6. **The third stage of labour is said to be:**
   A   Actively managed if the cord is clamped and cut early
   B   Actively managed if the placenta is delivered by maternal effort
   C   Actively managed in the absence of use of oxytocin
   D   Actively managed if clamping of the cord is withheld until the pulsations cease
   E   Prolonged if the placenta is not delivered 30 minutes after the birth of the baby with physiological management

7. **With regards to perineal trauma:**
   A   Injury to the skin is classified as a first-degree tear
   B   injury to the anal sphincter <50% thickness and anal mucosa is classified as 3B (third-degree tear)
   C   Injury to the perineal muscles but not the perineal skin is classified as a first-degree tear
   D   Injury to the perineal muscles but not the anal sphincter is classified as a second-degree tear
   E   Injury to the perineal muscles and both external and internal sphincter is classified as 3B (third-degree tear)

8. **With regards to prelabour spontaneous rupture of membranes (SROM) at term:**
   A   Speculum examination should always be done irrespective of the history
   B   Digital examination should be done to check cervical dilatation in the absence of contractions
   C   Women should be informed that 90% will go into spontaneous labour within 24 hours
   D   Women should be informed that there is a 1% risk of serious neonatal infection
   E   Lower vaginal swabs should be routinely done in women with SROM

9. **With regards to FHR trace on cardiotocograph (CTG):**
   A   It is said to be suspicious if two or more features are classified as non-reassuring
   B   It is said to be suspicious if there is reduced variability for more than 40 minutes and three accelerations in the last 30 minutes
   C   It is said to be suspicious if there is reduced variability for more than 90 minutes with baseline FHR of 165 bpm
   D   It is said to be pathological if it shows recurrent late deceleration down to 60 bpm with slow recovery for 35 minutes
   E   It is said to be suspicious if the CTG shows recurrent atypical variable decelerations for more than 30 minutes

10. **With regards to Sheehan syndrome:**
    A   The first sign may be failure of lactation in the puerperium
    B   The onset may be late with loss of axillary and pubic hair and atrophic vaginal changes
    C   It can present with hypothyroidism
    D   It can present with oligomenorrhoea or amenorrhoea
    E   Hormonal therapy may be used to achieve pregnancy in these women

11. **With regards to magnesium sulphate ($MgSO_4$) therapy for treatment of eclampsia:**
    A $MgSO_4$ can be administered by the intramuscular route
    B $MgSO_4$ is known to be significantly more effective than phenytoin or diazepam in prevention of recurrent seizures
    C $MgSO_4$ is a cerebral vasodilator
    D $MgSO_4$ has uterine muscle relaxing properties
    E   The CTG show features of reduced variability following intravenous $MgSO_4$ administration

12. **With regards to $MgSO_4$ toxicity when used for treating eclampsia:**
    A   Reduced patellar reflexes usually precede respiratory depression
    B $MgSO_4$ can cause both oliguria and anuria
    C $MgSO_4$ can cause respiratory depression at serum levels 2–4 mmol/L
    D   Calcium carbonate can be used to reverse respiratory depression caused by $MgSO_4$ administration
    E $MgSO_4$ crosses the placenta and causes fetal sedation

13. **Vaginal colonisation by group B streptococcus (GBS) during pregnancy:**
    A   Is caused by *Streptococcus agalactiae*
    B   Is caused by an obligate anaerobic gram-positive bacillus
    C   Is an indication for antenatal treatment to eradicate colonisation
    D   Is an indication for intrapartum antibiotic prophylaxis
    E   Is an indication for postpartum antibiotic prophylaxis in asymptomatic women

14. **The following are recommended by the National Institute for Health and Clinical Excellence (NICE) with regards to first stage of normal labour:**
    A   Once labour is established, the partogram should be initiated
    B   Check FHR after a contraction every 30 minutes
    C   Document frequency of contractions every 30 minutes
    D   Check vitals, including pulse and temperature, every 4 hours
    E   Check blood pressure every hour

15. **Acute uterine inversion:**
    A   Can occur following vaginal delivery
    B   Can occur following caesarean section
    C   Can occur following manual removal of placenta
    D   Can occur following active management of the third stage of labour
    E   Can occur following physiological management of the third stage of labour

16. With regards to acute uterine inversion:

   A   Women can present with massive haemorrhage

   B   Women can present with shock

   C   Women can present with neurogenic shock

   D   Women can present with sudden collapse

   E   Women can present with severe abdominal pain

Answers

1. **A True.**

    B False. See **Table 9.1** for UK Obstetric Surveillance System (UKOSS) figures for risk of peripartum hysterectomy.

    C False. Dissection of the bladder is not required with a classical caesarean section.

    D False. Trial of labour is contraindicated in women with a previous classical caesarean section due to increased risk of uterine rupture.

    E True. See **Table 9.2** for UKOSS figures for women undergoing vaginal birth after caesarean after one lower segment caesarean section (LSCS).

Table 9.1 UKOSS figures for risk of peripartum hysterectomy

Risk groups	Relative risk of hysterectomy
First vaginal delivery	1 in 30,000
First caesarean section	1 in 1700
One previous caesarean section	1 in 1300
Two or more caesarean sections	1 in 220

Table 9.2 UKOSS figures for risk of uterine rupture

Risk groups	Relative risk of uterine rupture
No prostaglandin or oxytocin	1.0
Oxytocin only	3.0
Prostaglandin only	2.9
Both prostaglandin and oxytocin	4.1

Royal College of Obstetricians and Gynaecologists. Green-top Guideline No. 45. Birth after Previous Caesarean Section. London: RCOG Press, 2007.

2. **A True.**

    B False. The problem is at the pelvic inlet.

    C False. The reported success rate is up to 90%.

    D False. Analgesia (parenteral or epidural) does not have an effect on the incidence of shoulder dystocia.

Table 9.3 Absolute risk of uterine rupture

Risk groups	Absolute risk of uterine rupture
Previous one LSCS	22–74 in 10,000
Previous inverted 'T' or 'J' incision	190 in 10,000
Previous low vertical incision	200 in 10,000
Previous high vertical incision	200–900 in 10,000

E False. Shoulder dystocia is not preventable but can be anticipated in women with fetal macrosomia. However, 50% occur with normal weight babies.

Shoulder dystocia is defined as a failure to deliver the shoulders after delivery of the head. The incidence is 0.5–2% of all vaginal deliveries.

It is associated with maternal obesity, diabetes (which increases the risk of shoulder dystocia by more than 70%), fetal macrosomia, previous shoulder dystocia (12% recurrence in future pregnancies), prolonged labour (labour progresses normally in 70% of women) and difficult instrumental delivery.

There is no evidence to support induction of labour in women with fetal macrosomia as this has not been shown to reduce either shoulder dystocia or caesarean section rate.

Elective caesarean section is not recommended for women with fetal macrosomia on scan as this has not shown to decrease operative delivery, shoulder dystocia or birth trauma. However, this rule does not apply to diabetic women. It is reasonable to do a planned caesarean section in diabetic women with estimated birth weight >4500 g.

Fetal complications include birth trauma, brachial plexus injury (due to excessive neck traction) and fractured clavicle or humerus, while the maternal complications include genital tract trauma and postpartum haemorrhage.

Neill AMC and Thornton S. Shoulder Dystocia. Personal assessment in continuing education. Reviews, questions and answers. Volume 3. London: RCOG Press, 2003:55–57
Royal College of Obstetricians and Gynaecologists. Green-top Guideline No. 42. Shoulder Dystocia. London: RCOG Press, 2005
Royal College of Obstetricians and Gynaecologists. Green-top Guideline No. 45. Birth after Previous Caesarean Section. London: RCOG Press, 2007.
American College of Obstetricians and Gynecologists. www.acog.org/publications.cfm

3. **A True.** It is associated with an increased chance of instrumental delivery.

    B False. It is not associated with long-term backache.

    C False. Epidural is more effective than opioids.

    D True.

E False. It is not associated with a longer first stage of labour or an increased risk of caesarean section.

The National Centre for Health and Clinical Excellence (NICE) recommendations for care of women with regional analgesia:

- Intravenous access prior to commencing regional analgesia.
- Preloading with fluids need not be administered routinely before establishing low-dose epidural analgesia.
- While establishing regional analgesia or administration of further boluses, blood pressure should be measured every 5 minutes for 15 minutes.
- The anaesthetist should be called for review if the woman is not pain-free 30 minutes after each administration of local anaesthetic/opioid solution.
- Sensory block assessment should be done hourly.
- Women should be encouraged to move and adopt upright positions with which they are comfortable.
- Effective regional analgesia should be continued till the completion of the third stage of labour and any necessary procedure.
- Maternal pushing can be delayed for at least 1 hour after full dilatation unless the woman has the urge to push or the head is on the perineum.
- Regardless of parity, delivery should be accomplished within 4 hours of full dilatation.
- Oxytocin use should not be routine in the second stage of labour for women with regional analgesia.
- Continuous EFM is recommended for at least 30 minutes during establishment of regional analgesia and after administration of each further bolus of 10 mL or more of low dose solutions.

National Institute for Health and Clinical Excellence. Intrapartum care. Care of healthy women and their babies during childbirth (CG55). NICE, 2008.

4. **A False.**

    B True.

    C True.

    D True. FHR <110 bpm or >160 bpm or any decelerations.

    E True.

    The other indications include significant meconium staining of liquor, fresh vaginal bleeding and maternal pyrexia of 37.5°C on two occasions, 2 hours apart.

    National Institute for Health and Clinical Excellence. Intrapartum care. Care of healthy women and their babies during childbirth (CG55). NICE, 2008.

5. **A False.** Perineal massage should not be performed routinely in the second stage of labour.

    B False. A routine episiotomy should not be carried out during spontaneous vaginal birth.

    C True. If there is a need, episiotomy should be performed.

D True.

E False. Episiotomy should not be routinely offered to women with previous history of third- and fourth-degree perineal tear.

Other recommendations by NICE regarding perineal trauma during labour:

- The recommended technique is a mediolateral episiotomy originating at the vaginal fourchette and usually directed to the right side.
- The risk of repeated severe perineal trauma is not increased in a subsequent birth in women with a previous history of severe perineal trauma, compared with women having their first baby.
- Women with infibulated genital mutilation need to be informed about the difficulty in performing any vaginal procedures, the need for an anterior episiotomy and possible defibulation during labour.

National Institute for Health and Clinical Excellence. Intrapartum care. Care of healthy women and their babies during childbirth (CG55). NICE, 2008.

6. **A True.** Active management includes the use of intramuscular oxytocin (10 IU) followed by early clamping and cutting of the cord and controlled cord traction (CCT). Physiological management is just opposite.

B False. It is said to be actively managed if the placenta is delivered by CCT.

C False. It is said to be actively managed with routine use of uterotonic drugs.

D False.

E False. It is diagnosed to be prolonged if the placenta is not delivered 30 minutes after the birth of the baby with active management and 60 minutes with physiological management.

National Institute for Health and Clinical Excellence. Intrapartum care. Care of healthy women and their babies during childbirth (CG55). NICE, 2008.

7. **A True.**

B False. It is a fourth-degree tear as anal mucosa is involved.

C False. Involvement of perineal muscles is a second-degree tear.

D True.

E False. It is 3C according to the third-degree classification.

A systematic assessment of the perineum includes visual inspection of the perineum to assess the extent and structures involved and rectal examination to assess anal sphincter or mucosal involvement.

Classification of perineal tears caused by either tearing or episiotomy:

- **first degree:** injury to the skin only
- **second degree:** injury to the perineal muscles but not the anal sphincter
- **third degree:** injury to the perineum involving the anal sphincter complex
- **3a:** less than 50% of the external anal sphincter thickness torn
- **3b:** more than 50% of the external anal sphincter thickness torn
- **3c:** internal anal sphincter torn

- **fourth degree:** injury to the perineum involving the anal sphincter complex (external and internal anal sphincter) and the anal epithelium

National Institute for Health and Clinical Excellence. Intrapartum care. Care of healthy women and their babies during childbirth (CG55). NICE, 2008.

8.   A **False.** One may avoid speculum examinations in women with a strong history and upon visualisation of leaking fluid at vulva and the wet pad.

B **False.** There is a risk of introducing an infection and it is better avoided in the absence of strong contractions. A speculum examination should give some idea about the cervical status.

C **False.** Sixty per cent will go into labour within 24 hours of spontaneous rupture of membranes (SROM).

D **True.**

E **False.** In the absence of suspected signs of infection, vaginal swabs and tests for C-reactive protein should not be routinely performed.

Counselling women with SROM at term:

- The pros and cons of expectant management versus immediate induction of labour should be discussed with the patient and an informed choice made by the patient.
- Expectant management for 24 hours after SROM is reasonable in the absence of an infection or fetal compromise.
- Induction of labour should be offered 24 hours after SROM.
- Women should be advised to take their temperature every 4 hours at home.
- Bathing and showering are not associated with an increase in infection.
- Sexual intercourse may be associated with an increase in infection.
- Women should report any reduction in fetal movement.
- Antibiotics are not routinely advised in the absence of infection, while definitely indicated in the presence of infection, even before 24 hours have elapsed.

National Institute for Health and Clinical Excellence. Intrapartum care. Care of healthy women and their babies during childbirth (CG55). NICE, 2008.

9.   A **False.** One non-reassuring feature is said to be suspicious, while two or more non-reassuring features is said to be pathological.

B **False.** Reduced variability in the presence of repeated acceleration is said to be normal CTG.

C **False.** Reduced variability for more than 90 minutes is a pathological CTG, while >40 minutes and <90 minutes is said to be suspicious.

D **True.** Late deceleration is an abnormal feature of the trace and is said to be pathological CTG.

E **False.** Recurrent atypical variable deceleration is an abnormal feature and the CTG is said to be pathological.

National Institute for Health and Clinical Excellence. Intrapartum care. Care of healthy women and their babies during childbirth (CG55). NICE, 2008.

10. **A True.**

  B True.

  C True. It can be diagnosed with a finding of low or normal thyroid-stimulating hormone in concurrence with low serum (secondary hypothyroidism) thyroxine levels. Similarly, low cortisol levels which fail to increase with stress and which are associated with low serum adrenocorticotropic hormone levels support the diagnosis of adrenocortical deficiency.

  D True.

  E True.

  Sheehan syndrome is a result of avascular necrosis of the pituitary gland. This is caused by severe and long-lasting hypotension due to a major obstetric haemorrhage on the pituitary gland, which is usually enlarged during pregnancy (especially the anterior pituitary, as it increases 2- to 3-fold in late pregnancy). It is associated with lactation failure, symptoms and signs of hypothyroidism, adrenocortical insufficiency and amenorrhoea.

  The pituitory gland is supplied by an end artery with no collateral supply.

  Critchley HOD, Horne A, Munro K. Chapter 16: Amenorrhoea and oligomenorrhoea, and hypothalamic–pituitary dysfunction. In: Shaw RW, Luesley D, Monga A (eds). Gynaecology (4th edn). Edinburgh: Churchill Livingstone, 2011.
  James D, Steer PJ, Weiner CP, Gonik B, Crowther C, Robson S (eds). High Risk Pregnancy: Management Options (4th edn). St Louis: Saunders, 2011.

11. **A True.**

  B True.

  C True.

  D True.

  E True.

  Magnesium sulphate:

  - Conventionally, diazepam and phenytoin were preferred and used in the UK for treating eclampsia.
  - Today, $MgSO_4$ is the anticonvulsant of choice for the treatment of eclampsia and for seizure prophylaxis in women with severe pre-eclampsia (it reduces the risk by half).
  - Its mechanism of action includes cerebral vasodilatation, increased production of endothelial prostacyclin (a vasodilator), reduced neuronal damage associated with ischaemia, protecting endothelial injury from free radicals and suppression of electroencephalogram activity and neuronal burst responses.
  - Toxicity is easy to detect and treat. It can be monitored clinically by checking the patellar reflex (forearm reflex in women with epidural), respiratory rate, oxygen saturation and urine output.
  - It is mainly excreted by the kidney and therefore increases the risk of renal toxicity leading to oliguria or anuria.

- MgSO$_4$ causes a decline in the available calcium which leads to impaired muscle strength and cardiac arrest.
- It easily crosses the placenta and fetal serum levels equilibrate with maternal levels. It does not result in maternal or fetal sedation.
- The antidote for treating its toxicity is intravenous calcium gluconate (10 mL of 10% solution).
- Its use is associated with reduced maternal morbidity and mortality.

Duley L. Magnesium sulphate regimens for women with eclampsia: messages from the Collaborative Eclampsia Trial. BJOG 1996; 103:103–105.
Robson SC. Magnesium sulphate: the time of reckoning. BJOG1996; 103:99–102.

12. **A True.** Loss of patellar reflex is the first sign of MgSO$_4$ toxicity.

   B True.

   C False. The normal required therapeutic range is 2–4 mmol/L.

   D True.

   E False. Calcium gluconate is used to reverse MgSO$_4$ toxicity.

Duley L. Magnesium sulphate regimens for women with eclampsia: messages from the Collaborative Eclampsia Trial. BJOG 1996; 103:103–105.
Robson SC. Magnesium sulphate: the time of reckoning. BJOG1996; 103:99–102.

13. **A True.**

   B False. It is caused by facultative anaerobic gram-positive cocci.

   C False. Antenatal treatment to eradicate maternal vaginal colonisation is not effective. The evidence regarding screening and treating women during the antenatal period is not strong. Based on current evidence, at least 600–700 women will be treated to prevent one case of early onset GBS disease (7000 women will need to be treated and 24,000 women screened to prevent one neonatal death).

   D True. The indications for intrapartum antibiotic prophylaxis include (a) GBS carriage in women who are either positive on their vaginal swab or their mid-stream urine sample and (b) women with a previous baby affected by early onset GBS. Therefore screening is not effective or cost-effective.

   E False. Antibiotic prophylaxis should be stopped after delivery if the mother is asymptomatic (postpartum endometritis with GBS should be treated with broad spectrum antibiotics).

Intrapartum antibiotic prophylaxis includes:

- intravenous penicillin G: 3 g immediately after the onset of labour, followed by 1.5 g every 4 hours until delivery, or:
- intravenous clindamycin (in women allergic to penicillin) 900 mg every 8 hours until delivery

Intrapartum antibiotics prophylaxis are offered to all women to prevent early onset GBS disease if the following risk factors are present:

- previous baby affected by GBS
- pre-term labour

- GBS bacteriuria detected during the current pregnancy
- prolonged rupture of membranes (>18 hours)
- fever in labour

Royal College of Obstetricians and Gynaecologists. Green-top Guideline No. 36. Prevention of early onset neonatal group B streptococcal disease. London: RCOG Press, 2003.

14. **A** **True.** A 4-hour action line should be used.

    B **False.** Every 15 minutes, check FHR after a contraction.

    C **True.**

    D **False.** Every 4 hours, blood pressure and temperature should be recorded and vaginal examination offered.

    E **False.** Check pulse every hour.

    Delay in the first stage of labour should be considered if there is :

    - less than a 2 cm cervical dilatation over 4 hours in nulliparous women
    - less than a 2 cm cervical dilatation over 4 hours or a slowing in the progress of labour for second and subsequent labours

    In the second stage of labour:

    - check fetal heart rate after a contraction every 5 minutes
    - check blood pressure, pulse and offer a vaginal examination every hour
    - check temperature every 4 hours
    - document the frequency of contractions every 30 minutes
    - regularly check the frequency of bladder emptying

    A delay in the second stage of labour should be considered if:

    - the active second stage is >2 hours in nulliparous woman
    - the active second stage is >1 hour in parous woman

    National Institute for Health and Clinical Excellence. Intrapartum care. Care of healthy women and their babies during childbirth (CG55). NICE, 2008.

15. **A** **True.**

    B **True.**

    C **True.**

    D **True.**

    E **True.**

    Uterine inversion is rare in the UK (reported incidence: 1 in 28,000) but is associated with an increase in morbidity and mortality of 15%. It has been known since time immemorial; Hippocrates mentioned inversion in 430–370 BC. Inversion of the uterus is defined as the inversion of the fundus into the uterine cavity 'the turning inside out of the uterus'. The inversion can be acute or chronic. The most common cause of this condition is inappropriate management of the third stage of labour but it can also occur following a caesarean section and the reported incidence by Baskett is 1 in 2000. Diagnosis is based on clinical signs and symptoms.

Reported associations for uterine inversion include the following:

- idiopathic
- spontaneous 40–50%
- excessive cord traction or a short umbilical cord
- credé (fundal) pressure
- placenta accreta, increta or percreta
- fundal implantation of the placenta
- chronic endometritis
- fetal macrosomia
- trial of vaginal birth following caesarean delivery
- myometrial weakness or uterine sacculation
- precipitate labour
- acute tocolysis with nitroglycerine or other potent tocolytic drugs, including magnesium sulfate

Classification

- acute: when it occurs immediately after delivery to <24 hours (contraction ring may or may not form)
- sub-acute: more than 24 hours and <4 weeks after delivery (contraction ring is present)
- chronic: when it occurs after 4 weeks of delivery

Degrees of inversion

- first degree: the inverted fundus extends to the level of the cervical os
- second degree: the inverted uterine fundus extends through the cervical os but not to the introitus
- third degree: the fundus extends to the introitus
- fourth degree: the inverted uterus extends below the introitus with associated vaginal inversion

Management

- identify
- call for help
- resuscitate
- manual replacement
- hydrostatic methods for uterine replacement
- surgery for uterine replacement.

Bhalla R, Wuntakal R, Odejinmi F, Khan RU. Acute inversion of the uterus. The Obstetrician and Gynaecologist 2009; 11:13–18.
Mehra U and Ostapowicz F. Acute puerperal inversion of the uterus in a primipara. Obstet Gynecol 1976; 47:S30–S32.
Calder AA. Emergencies in operative obstetrics. Baillieres Best Pract Res Clin Obstet Gynaecol 2000; 14:43–55.
Baskett TF. Acute uterine inversion: a review of 40 cases. J Obstet Gynaecol Can 2002; 24:953–956.

16. **A True.**

    B True.

C True.

D True.

E True.

The most common presentation is haemorrhage (seen in 94% of cases) and the next common is shock (seen in 39% of cases). The shock is generally out of proportion to blood loss. If this is the finding, a high index of suspicion is necessary and the diagnosis is confirmed by bimanual examination. The management is treatment for shock and manual repositioning of the uterus to reduce morbidity and mortality.

The other signs and symptoms include sudden severe abdominal pain in the third stage of labour, a lump in the vagina, a large polypoidal mass coming out of the vagina with or without the placenta attached to it, an absence of uterine fundus on abdominal palpation and abdominal tenderness.

The differential diagnosis includes:

- lump protruding through the vagina: utero-vaginal prolapse, large fibroid polyp protruding through the cervix, rare vaginal tumours, a foreign body in the vagina
- postpartum collapse: uterine atony, genital tract lacerations, coagulopathy, retained placenta without inversion.

Bhalla R, Wuntakal R, Odejinmi F, Khan RU. Acute inversion of the uterus. The Obstetrician and Gynaecologist 2009; 11:13–18.

Platt LD and Druzin ML. Acute puerperal inversion of the uterus. Am J Obstet Gynecol 1981; 141:187–189.

Chamberlain G, Steer PJ. Turnbull's Obstetrics (3rd edn). Edinburgh: Churchill Livingstone, 2002: 622–623.

Tank PD, Mayadeo NM, Nandanwar YS. Pregnancy outcome after operative correction of puerperal uterine inversion. Arch Gynecol Obstet 2004; 269:214–216.

Watson P, Besch N, Bowes WA Jr. Management of acute and subacute puerperal inversion of the uterus. Obstet Gynecol 1980; 55:12–16.

Vijayaraghavan R and Sujatha Y. Acute postpartum uterine inversion with haemorrhagic shock: laparoscopic reduction: a new method of management? BJOG 2006; 113:1100–1102.

Chapter 10

Menopause

1. **Hormone replacement therapy (HRT):**
   A   Increases the risk of colon cancer
   B   Increases the risk of a brain tumour
   C   Increases the risk of stroke
   D   Increases the risk of coronary heart disease
   E   Increases the risk of venous thromboembolism (VTE)

2. **Hormone replacement therapy (HRT) is indicated:**
   A   To prevent Alzheimer disease
   B   To treat overactive bladder
   C   To treat psychosis in postmenopausal women
   D   To treat severe vasomotor symptoms in postmenopausal women
   E   To treat vulval dystrophic disorders

3. **Lichen sclerosus is associated with:**
   A   Type 1 diabetes mellitus
   B   Vaginal cancer
   C   Alopecia areata
   D   Primary biliary cirrhosis
   E   Labial adhesions

4. **With regards to premature ovarian failure:**
   A   It is associated with osteoporosis
   B   One of the most common chromosomal causes is trisomy 13
   C   The classic picture is raised steroid hormones with decreased follicle-stimulating hormone (FSH)
   D   It can occur in women with galactosaemia
   E   Women diagnosed with this condition require only cyclical oestrogen therapy as progesterone is produced peripherally

5. **With regards to VTE:**
   A   Oral oestrogen HRT increases the risk of VTE three-fold in the first year of use
   B   Raloxifene is associated with a three-fold increase in risk of VTE in the first year of use
   C   Progestogen only pill used for contraception significantly increases the risk of VTE

  D The risk of postoperative deep venous thrombosis (DVT) following major surgery is roughly doubled in women taking a combined oral contraceptive pill (COCP)

  E The risk of VTE is 40 in 100,000 in postmenopausal women who do not use HRT

6. **HRT:**

  A Decreases the risk of breast cancer

  B Increases the risk of osteoporotic fractures

  C Increases the risk of thrombosis

  D Increases the risk of stroke

  E Reduces the risk of colorectal cancer

Answers

1. A False.

   B False.

   C True.

   D True.

   E True.

   Hormone replacement therapy (HRT)

   HRT increases the risk of breast cancer (especially with the use of combined oestrogen and progesterone HRT), endometrial cancer and venous thromboembolism.

   The risk of endometrial cancer increases with the use of unopposed oestrogen replacement therapy and this risk persists for 5 years or more after discontinuation of unopposed oestrogen therapy.

   Women with a uterus *in situ* should use combined oestrogen and progestogen for HRT, while women without a uterus (who have already had a hysterectomy) should use oestrogen only HRT.

   HRT can be used as a short-term therapy for the relief of severe menopausal symptoms (hot flushes and night sweats). The symptoms can improve within 1 month of starting the HRT.

   It also decreases the risk of osteoporosis significantly including fractures. Bone gain is expected in the first 16–24 months of starting HRT but thereafter bone mineral density tends to remain steady or plateau.

   In view of the above risks, women should be counselled appropriately before prescribing HRT and it has to be an informed choice.

   Rees M. Chapter: 28: The menopause. In: Shaw RW, Luesley D, Monga A (eds). Gynaecology (4th edn). Edinburgh: Churchill Livingstone, 2011.
   Beral V; Million Women Study Collaborators. Breast cancer and hormone-replacement therapy in the Million Women Study. Lancet 2003; 362:419–427.

2. A **False.** Epidemiological studies suggest that oestrogen may prevent or delay the onset of Alzheimer disease or that the age of onset is later in women who have taken oestrogen before. However, HRT did not slow the progression of Alzheimer disease or improve cognitive function in women with the disease already established.

   B **False.** HRT may be helpful in women with recurrent urinary tract infections during menopause but the right dose and duration of therapy are not known. It is also used to treat vaginal dryness but the response to therapy may take as long as 1 year.

   C **False.** HRT may have psychological benefits following the initiation of therapy.

   D **True.** It is the only indication for HRT. Women with severe vasomotor symptoms (hot flushes and night sweats) can be given HRT along with adequate counselling to improve the quality of life.

E **False.** HRT is beneficial in managing genital atrophy.

Rees M. Chapter: 28: The menopause. In: Shaw RW, Luesley D, Monga A (eds). Gynaecology (4th edn). Edinburgh: Churchill Livingstone, 2011.

3.   A **True.** Lichen sclerosus is more common in older age groups (it usually presents with vulval pruritus) but it can occur at any age. It is associated with autoimmune diseases in less than 10% of cases. The more common ones are vitiligo and alopecia areata but it is also associated with insulin-dependent diabetes mellitus, bullous pemphigoid, thyroid disorders and systemic lupus erythematosus (SLE). The local steroid clobetasol 0.05% (Dermovate) is used for treating symptomatic women.

B **False.** Lichen sclerosus is a premalignant condition. The risk of developing cancer is up to 4–5% and therefore long-term follow-up is recommended for such women.

C **True.**

D **True.**

E **True.** It may cause clitoral or labial adhesions.

Shaw RW, Luesley D, Monga A (eds). Gynaecology (4th edn). Edinburgh: Churchill Livingstone, 2011.

4.   A **True.** This is due to oestrogen deficiency.

B **False.** One of the most common chromosomal causes is Turner syndrome.

C **False.** The classic picture is amenorrhoea and raised gonadotrophin levels (both FSH and LH) in women <40 years of age.

D **True.** It is also associated with autoimmune diseases.

E **False.** Women diagnosed with this condition require both cyclical oestrogen and progestogen replacement (progestogen is required to protect the endometrium).

Critchley HOD, Horne A, Munro K. Chapter 16: Amenorrhoea and oligomenorrhoea, and hypothalamic–pituitary dysfunction. In: Shaw RW, Luesley D, Monga A (eds). Gynaecology (4th edn). Edinburgh: Churchill Livingstone, 2011.
Rees M. Chapter: 28: The menopause. In: Shaw RW, Luesley D, Monga A (eds). Gynaecology (4th edn). Edinburgh: Churchill Livingstone, 2011.

5.   A **True.**

B **True.** Raloxifene is a selective oestrogen receptor modulator and equally increases the risk of VTE when compared to oral oestrogen.

C **False.** There is no evidence that low dose progestogens (used for contraception) increase the risk of VTE.

D **True.** The suggestion was to stop COCP 4–6 weeks prior to major surgery in view of increased risk of VTE in postoperative women. However, this has to be balanced with the risk of unwanted pregnancy, the need for subsequent termination and the effect of surgery and anaesthesia on the fetus.

E **False.** The risk of VTE in women who use HRT is quoted to be 30 in 100,000 women per year while it is 10 in 100,000 women per year for non-users.

Letsky E, Murphy MF, Ramsay JE, Walker I. Venous Thromboembolism in Obstetrics and Gynaecology. London: RCOG Press, 2005.

6. **A** False.

B False.

C True.

D True.

E True.

Breast cancer and HRT in the Million Women Study (**Table 10.1**):

- current users of HRT were more likely to develop breast cancer than those who had never used HRT
- current users of HRT were more likely to die of breast cancer than those who had never used HRT
- past users of HRT were not at increased risk of breast cancer
- the incidence of breast cancer increased for current users of oestrogen only, oestrogen plus progesterone and tibolone
- the association with breast cancer was significantly greater for oestrogen plus progesterone preparations than for other types of HRT
- in current users of HRT, the risk of breast cancer increased with increasing duration of use

Table 10.1 Breast cancer risk for HRT users		
Duration of HRT use	**Breast cancer risk over 20 years from the of age 50–70 years**	**Extra breast cancers in HRT users**
Never	45 in 1000	–
5 years	47 in 1000	2 in 1000
10 years	51 in 1000	6 in 1000
15 years	57 in 1000	12 in 1000

Rees M. Chapter: 28: The menopause. In: Shaw RW, Luesley D, Monga A (eds). Gynaecology (4th edn). Edinburgh: Churchill Livingstone, 2011.
Beral V; Million Women Study Collaborators. Breast cancer and hormone-replacement therapy in the Million Women Study. Lancet 2003; 362:419–427.
Collaborative Group on Hormonal Factors in Breast Cancer. Breast cancer and hormone replacement therapy: collaborative reanalysis of data from 51 epidemiological studies of 52 705 women with breast cancer and 108 411 women without breast cancer. Lancet 1997; 350:1047–1059.

Chapter 11

Puerperium

1. **Haemolytic disease of the newborn (erythroblastosis fetalis):**
    A   Is characterised by the presence of erythroblasts in the cord blood
    B   Is associated with a positive direct Coombs test in the cord blood
    C   Is characterised by the presence of jaundice at birth
    D   Is associated with a prolonged prothrombin time
    E   Is associated with persistence of the placental syncytiotrophoblast

2. **With regards to fetal circulation before birth:**
    A   Blood returning through the umbilical vein from placenta is well oxygenated
    B   The ductus venosus connects the umbilical vein to the inferior vena cava
    C   The ductus arteriosus connects the pulmonary trunk to the aorta
    D   Most of the blood which enters the right atrium is directed through the foramen ovale into the left atrium
    E   Most of the blood which enters the right ventricle is pumped into the pulmonary trunk to the lungs for reoxygenation

3. **With regards to infant mortality:**
    A   Perinatal death is defined as sum of stillbirths and neonatal deaths within the first 28 days of life
    B   The infant mortality rate: number of deaths per year, babies aged less than 1 year in 1000 live births, including neonatal deaths
    C   Early neonatal death: death of a live born infant at less than 7 completed days from the time of birth
    D   Neonatal death: death rate between days 0 and 28 of life in 1000 live births
    E   In England and Wales, stillbirth is defined as the death of a fetus after the 24th week of gestation with no sign of life at birth

4. **Cephalohaematoma:**
    A   Is swelling above the periosteum of skull bones
    B   Usually crosses the suture lines
    C   Is associated with jaundice
    D   Usually resolves within 1 week
    E   Always appears on the same day following delivery

5. **Peripartum cardiomyopathy:**
    A   Is a rare condition
    B   Carries a 10% maternal mortality
    C   Is more common in nulliparous women

D   Is associated with increased maternal age
E   Is associated with twin pregnancy

6. **With regards to neonatal thyrotoxicosis:**

A   Postnatal growth rate is decreased
B   The condition is usually self-limiting
C   A history of Graves disease in the mother is common
D   Intellectual impairment is common if timely treatment is not initiated
E   Results from Guthrie card screening will usually be uninformative

7. **With regards to early congenital syphilis in the neonate:**

A   Most infants with early congenital syphilis are asymptomatic at birth
B   Neonates with early congenital syphilis characteristically present with feeding problems
C   If early congenital syphilis is untreated, late congenital syphilis will develop
D   The symptoms for early congenital syphilis usually develop after 20 days following birth
E   Untreated maternal syphilis results in symptomatic congenital syphilis in around 50% of the neonates

8. **Regarding chlamydia infection in the newborn:**

A   It is caused by *Chlamydia trachomatis*, an obligate intracellular organism
B   The prevalence in pregnant women is 0.5%
C   Almost half of neonates born vaginally are colonised with chlamydia in the presence of maternal infection
D   Ninety per cent of exposed neonates will develop conjunctivitis in the first 1–2 weeks, in the presence of maternal infection
E   One per cent of exposed neonates may develop pneumonia in the first 8 weeks

9. **With regards to postpartum blues:**

A   About 10% of women will experience postpartum blues
B   Most women will need drug therapy
C   Women usually present in the third week following delivery
D   It is usually associated with an organic condition
E   Most women will need admission for treatment

10. **The following are risk factors for developing haemorrhagic disease of the newborn:**

A   Premature delivery
B   Maternal diabetes
C   Obstetric cholestasis during pregnancy
D   Maternal heart disease
E   Fetal sickle cell trait

11. **With regards to the repair of first- and second-degree perineal lacerations:**

A   Synthetic non-absorbable suture material should be used to repair these tears as it is associated with less pain

B   Synthetic absorbable suture material should be used to repair these tears as it is associated with the use of less analgesia

C   Synthetic non-absorbable suture material should be used to repair these tears as it is associated with less wound dehiscence

D   Continuous subcuticular sutures should be used to close the perineal skin as it is associated with less short-term pain compared with interrupted sutures

E   Interrupted suture should be used to close each layer as it is associated with less short-term pain compared to continuous non-locking sutures

12. **Regarding retained placenta in the third stage of labour:**

A   Intravenous oxytocin infusion is the recommended initial management for retained placenta

B   Oxytocin injection into the umbilical artery is the initial recommended management for retained placenta

C   Oxytocin injection into the umbilical vein is the initial recommended management for retained placenta

D   If the placenta is still retained after 30 minutes of intraumbilical oxytocin, the situation should be assessed and the woman should be offered manual removal of the placenta

E   The manual removal of the placenta should be undertaken under local anaesthesia

13. **With regards to neonatal lupus:**

A   It is mainly caused by antinuclear antibodies (ANA)

B   The most common manifestation is cutaneous lupus

C   Anti-Ro antibodies are present in more than 90% of the mothers of affected offspring

D   The incidence increases with increasing severity of maternal disease

E   It is caused by increased complement levels in the mother

Answers

1. **A True.** The initial response is reticulocytosis and when the disease becomes severe, erythroblasts are released into the fetal circulation.

    B True.

    C False. Jaundice appears after 24 hours as the bilirubin is excreted by the placenta before birth.

    D True.

    E False.

    Fifteen per cent of women in the UK are Rhesus (Rh) negative and it is recommended that all women should be screened for antibodies at the first midwife appointment during pregnancy. If anti-D prophylaxis is not administered to Rh-negative women during pregnancy, 1% of women would develop antibodies during their first pregnancy and 3–5% during subsequent pregnancies.

    If the father is homozygous for 'D' there is a 100% chance that the fetus is Rh-positive, while if he is heterozygous for 'D' there is 50% chance that the fetus will be Rh-positive. However, if the father is homozygous for 'd' then both father and the fetus will be Rh-negative and therefore Rhesus disease is said to be unlikely.

    Rhesus disease accounts for more than 95% of the haemolytic disease.

    Maternal sensitisation to fetal red blood cell antigens usually occurs at delivery but can also occur with recurrent antepartum haemorrhage, amniocentesis, external cephalic version and abdominal trauma in Rh-negative women. In 10% of cases there is no recognised cause for sensitisation.

    The first immune response in the mother is the formation of IgM antibodies (they do not cross the placenta) and therefore the first baby is usually unaffected. Subsequent antigen exposure leads to an increased response and IgG formation in the mother, which does cross the placenta and destroy the fetal red blood cells (RBC) leading to reticulocytosis, anaemia, heart failure and hydrops. If the disease is severe, erythroblasts are found in fetal circulation and therefore it is called Erythroblastosis fetalis.

    Maternal antibodies can be measured regularly in subsequent pregnancies in women with a history of Rhesus disease in her previous pregnancy. If the maternal antibody is <4 IU/mL severe haemolytic disease in the fetus is rare, while 50% of fetuses will have severe anaemia if the maternal antibody level is >15 IU/mL.

    Anti-D immunoglobulin is given to Rh-negative women following any sensitising event during pregnancy (miscarriage at >12 weeks, medical or surgical termination, ectopic pregnancy, normal delivery and antepartum haemorrhage) and prophylactically during antenatal period.

    Anti-D dose and timing

    *   if <20 weeks, 250 IU of anti-D should be given intramuscularly

- if >20 weeks, 500 IU of anti-D should be given intramuscularly
- give more anti-D if indicated by Kleihauer test; ideally this should be done for all women routinely following delivery
- it should be administered within 72 hours

Direct Coombs test to diagnose HDN

This test mainly detects fetal RBCs already bound by maternal anti-D antibodies (IgG). A sample of fetal RBCs is washed to remove any unbound antibody. When the antibodies (anti-IgG) are added, they agglutinate the fetal RBCs which are already bound by maternal antibodies.

Indirect Coombs test to diagnose HDN

This test mainly detects anti-D antibodies in the maternal serum before they attach the fetal RBCs (adding maternal serum to fetal RBCs should haemolyse them *in vitro*). The mother's serum is incubated with Rh-positive RBCs (expecting the antibodies to bind to fetal RBCs if present in the maternal serum). The cells are then washed to remove the free antibodies. Subsequently anti-IgG antibodies are added. They agglutinate the fetal RBCs which are now bound by maternal antibodies.

ABO blood group incompatibility

HDN due to ABO incompatibility is less common (fetal RBCs express less of the ABO antigens than adult RBCs) and less severe than Rhesus incompatibility. It can be caused when a mother with the blood group 'O' carries a fetus with a different blood group, e.g. types A, B or AB. The mother's serum contains natural anti-A and anti-B antibodies (IgG type) and can therefore cross the placenta resulting in the destruction of fetal RBCs.

Magowan B. Churchill's Pocketbook of Obstetrics and Gynaecology (3rd edn). Edinburgh: Churchill Livingstone, 2005.

2. A True.

B True.

C True.

D True.

E False.

Fetal circulation before birth

Three shunts which cause blood to bypass the liver and lungs are listed below.

Liver bypass:

- blood returning from the placenta in the umbilical vein is well oxygenated
- as it enters the fetus, approximately half is directed through the portal vein and through the hepatic sinusoids
- the other half of the umbilical vein blood bypasses the liver by entering the ductus venosus and passing into the inferior vena cava

Lung bypass:

Inferior vena cava

- deoxygenated blood from the lower limbs, abdomen and pelvis mixes with oxygenated umbilical vein blood and blood from hepatic sinusoids
- it then enters the right atrium. Most of it is directed through the foramen ovale by the inferior border of the septum secundum (crista dividens)
- it then enters the left atrium and mixes with a small amount of deoxygenated blood returning from the uninflated lungs
- enters the left ventricle and into the ascending aorta to supply the heart, head, neck and upper limbs

Other lung bypass:

- a small amount of oxygenated blood in the right atrium mixes with deoxygenated blood from the superior vena cava and coronary sinus
- it passes to the right ventricle and into the pulmonary trunk
- because of high pulmonary resistance, most of this blood bypasses the lungs and passes through the ductus arteriosus into the aorta
- approximately 50% of this blood supplies the abdomen, pelvis and lower limbs while 50% returns via two umbilical arteries to the placenta and is re-oxygenated

Changes at birth and later in life:

- functional closure of the umbilical arteries occurs soon after birth
- closure of the umbilical vein and the ductus venosus follows closure of the umbilical arteries
- a fall in the pulmonary vascular resistance occurs in the first few days of life
- closure of the ductus arteriosus depends on the rise in the partial pressure of oxygen (PaO_2)
- blood returning from the pulmonary veins into the left atrium causes an increase in pressure in the left atrium. The septum primum is pressed against septum secundum and the foramen ovale is functionally closed
- adult: the site of septum primum is the floor of the fossa ovalis and the former inferior edge of the septum secundum is located at the limbus fossae ovalis (anulus ovalis)

Postnatal development:

- most umbilical vessels within the infant become ligaments
- umbilical vein: ligamentum teres hepatis in the falciform ligament
- umbilical arteries distal part: medial umbilical ligaments
- umbilical arteries proximal part: persists as the superior vesical arteries

Sadler TV. Langman's Medical Embryology (11th edn). Philadelphia: Lippincott Williams and Wilkins, 2009. The RCOG online training course. www.StratOG.net

3. A False.

    B True.

    C True.

D **True.**

E **True.**

Perinatal deaths are the sum of stillbirths and early neonatal deaths and late neonatal deaths are those occurring from days 8–28 from birth.

4. A **False.** Cephalohaematoma incidence is 1%. It is swelling beneath the periosteum of the skull bones due to bleeding.

B **False.** Cephalohaematoma never crosses suture lines. On the other hand sub-galeal haematomas (may be associated with shock, anaemia and death of the baby) occur beneath the aponeurosis and cross the midline. Both are associated with ventouse delivery.

C **True.**

D **False.** Cephalohaematoma may take several weeks to resolve.

E **False.** Cephalohaematoma may not appear until the second day after birth.

Cephalohaematoma is more common with ventouse delivery than forceps delivery. One should also be cautious while assessing this condition as it can be associated with an underlying skull fracture.

Other injuries after ventouse delivery include scalp bruising, abrasion, laceration, subgaleal haematoma and intracranial haemorrhage. Retinal haemorrhage and neonatal jaundice are also common with ventouse deliveries.

James D, Steer PJ, Weiner CP, Gonik B, Crowther C, Robson S (eds). High Risk Pregnancy: Management Options (4th edn). St Louis: Saunders, 2011.

5. A **True.**

B **False.** It carries a maternal mortality rate of 25–50%.

C **False.** It is associated with high parity.

D **True.**

E **True.** It is also associated with hypertension.

Peripartum cardiomyopathy

Peripartum cardiomyopathy is a rare condition which usually presents during late pregnancy or after delivery. The most common presentation is cardiac failure. An echocardiogram will show a large dilated heart (cardiomegaly). The drugs used in its management include: frusemide, digoxin, nitrates and angiotensin-converting enzyme inhibitors. Thromboprophylaxis with heparin is very important to reduce the risk of venous thromboembolism. In women presenting during the antenatal period, delivery is indicated.

Diagnostic features

- heart failure in the last month of pregnancy or heart failure in the first 6 months after delivery

- no obvious cause identified
- no history of cardiac disease
- usually more than 30 weeks of gestation
- usually multiparous and of African descent

Complications

Cardiomyopathy during pregnancy is associated with high morbidity and mortality. Complications include cardiac arrhythmias, thromboembolism and persistent cardiac dysfunction in 45–90% of patients.

Prognosis

Long-term prognosis is reported to be good if the patient recovers (normal cardiac function at 6–12 months postpartum) fully after the first episode (mortality rate of 15%), while prognosis is poor for those with persistent ventricular dysfunction (mortality rate of around 60%). The risk of recurrence in subsequent pregnancies is high (as high as 85%).

Nelson-Piercy C. Handbook of Obstetric Medicine (4th edn). London: Informa Healthcare, 2010.
Magowan B. Churchill's Pocketbook of Obstetrics and Gynaecology (3rd edn). Edinburgh: Churchill Livingstone, 2005.
James D, Steer PJ, Weiner CP, Gonik B, Crowther C, Robson S (eds). High Risk Pregnancy: Management Options (4th edn). St Louis: Saunders, 2011.

6. A **False.**

   B **True.**

   C **True.**

   D **False.**

   E **False.**

Maternal hyperthyroidism (if untreated) is associated with an increased incidence of pre-term delivery (11–25%), stillbirth (8–15%) and a decrease in the mean infant birth weight. Fetal and neonatal thyrotoxicosis is also increased due to stimulation of the fetal thyroid gland by maternal thyroid-stimulating antibodies, crossing the placenta. Neonatal thyrotoxicosis occurs in 10% of the offspring of mothers with Graves' disease and is usually transient and self-limiting after delivery (it lasts for 2–3 months). This can also cause fetal craniosynostosis, exophthalmos, cardiac failure and hepatosplenomegaly. The severity of maternal thyroid disease does not reflect the development of fetal neonatal thyrotoxicosis (measurement of anti-TSH receptor antibodies may help to predict this condition). However, one should closely liaise with paediatricians during the prenatal and postnatal periods.

Nelson-Piercy C. Handbook of Obstetric Medicine (4th edn). London: Informa Healthcare, 2010.
James D, Steer PJ, Weiner CP, Gonik B, Crowther C, Robson S (eds). High Risk Pregnancy: Management Options (4th edn). St Louis: Saunders, 2011.

7. A **True.**

   B **False.** They usually manifest with maculopapular rash, rhinitis, jaundice, hepatosplenomegaly, chorioretinitis, lymphadenopathy and pseudoparalysis of the limbs due to osteochondritis.

C True. The features of late congenital syphilis include Hutchinson teeth, interstitial keratitis, mulberry molars, saddle nose, eighth nerve deafness, saber shins and cardiovascular lesions.

D False. Neonates usually develop signs and symptoms 10–14 days after birth.

E True. Untreated maternal primary and secondary syphilis lead to early congenital syphilis in approximately 40% of children while with late latent syphilis it is 10%.

James D, Steer PJ, Weiner CP, Gonik B, Crowther C, Robson S (eds). High Risk Pregnancy: Management Options (4th edn). St Louis: Saunders, 2011.

8. **A True.** The drug of choice for treatment during pregnancy is erythromycin for 14 days (tetracycline group of drugs are contraindicated).

   B False. The prevalence is 2–7% in pregnant women.

   C True.

   D False. Only half of exposed neonates will develop conjunctivitis in the first 1–2 weeks after birth.

   E False. Almost 10–20% of exposed neonates develop pneumonia in the first 8 weeks after birth.

Magowan B. Churchill's Pocketbook of Obstetrics and Gynaecology (3rd edn). Edinburgh: Churchill Livingstone, 2005.

9. **A False.**

   B False.

   C False.

   D False.

   E False.

Postpartum blues

Fifty to seventy per cent of women will experience postpartum blues and it usually presents in the first few days following delivery. The cause is multifactorial and affects all cultural and social groups. Symptoms may include tearfulness, lack of sleep, anxiety, headache, poor concentration, fatigue and depression. The treatment is reassurance, education and support.

Postpartum depression

This affects around 10–14% of women. Severe depression lasting more than 2 weeks after delivery is suggestive of postpartum depression. It is diagnosed when five of the following symptoms (criteria from Diagnostic and Statistical Manual of Mental Disorders, 4th edition) are present for at least 2 weeks. These include depressed mood, major changes in weight or appetite, anhedonia, fatigue, psychomotor agitation, feelings of worthlessness, decreased or lack of concentration, lack of sleep, excessive sleep and recurrent thoughts of death or suicide.

Depression can often be treated in outpatients; psychosis often needs admission. However, women with depression and suicidal tendencies need treatment with admission to a specialist mother and baby unit, psychotherapy and pharmacotherapy (selective serotonin reuptake inhibitors and tricyclics). Electroconvulsive therapy has also been used successfully to treat severe postpartum depression.

Postpartum psychosis

Postpartum psychosis is uncommon and occurs in 2 per 1000 deliveries. Women who develop postpartum psychosis will have a history of bipolar disease in 40% of cases. The condition usually presents after 2–3 days and before 3 weeks after delivery. The symptoms include mania, delusions and hallucinations (auditory commands to harm the baby). Depression is not often seen. One should also rule out organic conditions such as sepsis, electrolyte imbalance, metabolic disturbance and intoxication.

The treatment consists of admission to the mother and baby unit and antipsychotic medication (chlorpromazine or haloperidol). Antidepressants and benzodiazepines may also be necessary.

The risk of recurrence in subsequent pregnancies is between 21 and 50%.

James D, Steer PJ, Weiner CP, Gonik B, Crowther C, Robson S (eds). High Risk Pregnancy: Management Options (4th edn). St Louis: Saunders, 2011.
Magowan B. Churchill's Pocketbook of Obstetrics and Gynaecology (3rd edn). Edinburgh: Churchill Livingstone, 2005.

10. **A True.** Neonates have comparatively less vitamin K at birth (due to impaired production of coagulation factors II, VII, IX, X, C, and S by the liver) which puts them at risk of haemorrhagic complications. This is called haemorrhagic disease of the newborn, which is a rare condition with an incidence of 1 in 10,000 if vitamin K is not supplemented to newborn babies. One milligram of intramuscular vitamin K at birth is more than enough to prevent this condition.

    B False.

    C True. Women should be advised that where the prothrombin time is prolonged, the use of water-soluble vitamin K (menadiol sodium phosphate) in doses of 5–10 mg daily is indicated. Women should be advised that when prothrombin time is normal, water-soluble vitamin K (menadiol sodium phosphate) in low doses should be used only after careful counselling about the likely benefits but small theoretical risk. Postnatal vitamin K must be offered to the babies in the usual way.

    D False.

    E False.

Nelson-Piercy C. Handbook of Obstetric Medicine (4th edn). London: Informa Healthcare, 2010.
Walker SP, Permezel M, Berkovic SF. The management of pregnancy in epilepsy. BJOG 2009; 116:758–767.

11. **A False.** Synthetic absorbable suture (polyglycolic acid or polygalactin) material should be used to repair these tears as it is associated with less pain. The use of rapid absorbable sutures (polygalactin) is preferable as it is associated with less perineal pain and the need for removal of suture material.

    B True.

C **False.** Synthetic absorbable suture material should be used to repair these tears as it is associated with less wound dehiscence.

D **True.**

E **False.** Continuous non-locking sutures should be used for the closure of each layer as it is associated with less short-term pain compared with interrupted sutures.

Royal College of Obstetricians and Gynaecologists. Green-top Guideline No. 29. The management of third and fourth degree perineal tears. London: RCOG Press, 2007.

12. A **False.** Intravenous oxytocin infusion is not to be used to assist the delivery of the placenta. Intravenous access should always be secured in women with a retained placenta.

B **False.** Oxytocin injection (20 IU oxytocin diluted in 20 mL of normal saline) into the umbilical vein is the initial recommended management for retained placenta in women who are not actively bleeding and who are stable.

C **True.**

D **True.**

E **False.** Where manual removal of the placenta is necessary, it should be undertaken under effective regional anaesthesia (or general anaesthesia when necessary).

The third stage of labour (from delivery of the baby until delivery of the placenta) is said to be prolonged if not completed within 30 minutes of the birth of the baby with active management of the third stage and 60 minutes with physiological management of third stage.

National Institute for Health and Clinical Excellence. Chapter 17: Complicated labour: third stage. Intrapartum care. Care of healthy women and their babies during childbirth (CG55). NICE, 2008.

13. A **False.** It is mainly caused by the presence of anti-Ro and anti-La antibodies.

B **True.**

C **True.**

D **False.** There is no correlation between the severity of maternal disease and the incidence of neonatal lupus syndrome.

E **False.**

Systemic lupus erythematosus (SLE) is a connective tissue disease which can affect any organ in the body. The most common clinical feature is involvement of the joints causing non-erosive arthritis with tenderness and swelling. Although the exact aetiology is not known, certain factors such as genetic and environmental triggers have been associated with its occurrence.

Neonatal manifestations include cutaneous lupus and congenital heart block. The former is common while the latter is a more serious form of neonatal lupus. Anti-Ro and anti-La auto-antibodies directed against cytoplasmic ribonucleoproteins are the main culprits responsible for this. These cross the placenta and cause damage to the immune system in the fetus. Anti-Ro antibodies are present in more than 90% of mothers of affected offspring and 50–70% of mothers have anti-La antibodies.

Congenital heart block is a serious consequence of SLE disease. It is seen in 2% of babies whose mothers have either anti-Ro or anti-La antibodies. It appears *in utero* and is permanent. It is usually diagnosed later in the pregnancy and is associated with a 15–30% mortality rate. The main aetiopathogenesis is destruction of the conducting system in the heart, causing scarring. Treatment with dexamethasone may reverse milder forms of heart block but not complete heart block. Approximately 20% of affected children die in the early neonatal period and 50–60% require pacemakers in early infancy.

Nelson-Piercy C. Handbook of Obstetric Medicine (4th edn). London: Informa Healthcare, 2010.

1. **Ovarian hyperstimulation syndrome (OHSS):**
   A   Is a complication of intrauterine insemination
   B   Can cause pericardial effusion
   C   Can lead to renal failure
   D   Can cause cerebral infarction
   E   Can cause adult respiratory distress syndrome

2. **The following are autosomal recessive conditions:**
   A   Albinism
   B   Cystic fibrosis
   C   Congenital adrenal hyperplasia
   D   Galactosaemia
   E   Gaucher disease

3. **With regards to autosomal recessive inheritance:**
   A   If both parents are carriers, there is a 1 in 4 chance that the mutant gene will be transmitted to the child
   B   It is always expressed in heterozygous state
   C   Men and women have an equal chance of being affected
   D   It is more likely that affected individuals have heterozygous parents
   E   It is more common in children with parents of consanguineous marriage

4. **The following are X-linked or sex-linked recessive disorders:**
   A   Sickle cell disease
   B   Vitamin D resistant rickets
   C   Wilson disease
   D   Duchenne muscular dystrophy
   E   Hunter syndrome

5. **The following are X-linked dominant conditions:**
   A   Red/green colour blindness
   B   Turner syndrome
   C   Huntington disease
   D   Hairy ears
   E   Haemophilia

6. **The following are autosomal dominant inherited conditions:**
   A   Phenylketonuria
   B α1 antitrypsin deficiency

    C   Porphyria variegata
    D   Sickle cell disease
    E   Cri du chat syndrome

7. **A semen sample is said to be normal if:**
    A   Volume <1 mL
    B   Motility > 50%
    C   Sperm concentration 5 million/mL
    D   Liquefaction time of >120 minutes
    E   Total sperm number of > 40 million per ejaculate

8. **With regards to luteinising hormone (LH) and follicle-stimulating hormone (FSH):**
    A   LH promotes formation of androstenedione from cholesterol (in theca interna cells) which in turn is transported to granulosa cells to form oestradiol
    B   LH peaks 4 hours before ovulation
    C   LH surge occurs 4 days before ovulation
    D   FSH and LH secretion peak to the highest level during the luteal phase
    E   LH is released in pulsatile manner during proliferative phase

9. **With regards to Turner syndrome:**
    A   Women always present with secondary amenorrhoea
    B   Women have a karyotype 47XXX
    C   It is associated with cardiomyopathy
    D   The external genitalia is usually male
    E   Women are always infertile

10. **Prolactin is increased in the following situations:**
    A   Exercise
    B   Stress
    C   Nipple stimulation
    D   Sleep
    E   Pregnancy

11. **Regarding autosomal dominant disorders:**
    A   They usually affect people in each generation
    B   Men are more likely to be affected than women
    C   Men can transmit the condition only to daughters
    D   Women can transmit the condition only to sons
    E   Overall, one half of the children of an affected person will be affected

12. **The following tissues can be used for DNA analysis:**
    A   Leucocytes
    B   Cultured skin fibroblasts
    C   Buccal mucosal cells
    D   Amniotic fluid cells
    E   Chorionic villus cells

13. **Klinefelter syndrome:**
    A   Is one of the most common chromosomal causes of male fertility
    B   Is usually associated with gynaecomastia
    C   Is associated with increased risk of breast cancer in males
    D   Is associated with increased risk of diabetes
    E   Is associated with a short lifespan

14. **With regards to cystic fibrosis:**
    A   The incidence is 1 in 2500 births in the UK
    B   The affected pregnancies usually inherit one underactive cystic fibrosis transmembrane conductance regulator (CFTR) gene from one parent
    C   ΔF508 mutation is more common in northern Europe
    D   The defect is on chromosome 6
    E   ΔF508 is the single most common mutation

15. **Regarding Duchenne muscular dystrophy (DMD):**
    A   It is the most common form of muscular dystrophy in childhood
    B   The gene is located on the long arm of chromosome X
    C   Affected children show high levels of serum creatinine phosphokinase (CPK) at birth
    D   It almost always affects females
    E   The incidence at birth is 1 in 3000 females

16. **Regarding haemophilia:**
    A   Factor IX deficiency causes haemophilia A
    B   It is an autosomal recessive disorder
    C   Females should always be tested for carrier state if the father has haemophilia
    D   Chorionic villus sampling is the principle method used in early pregnancy for antenatal diagnosis
    E   Caesarean section is indicated if the fetus has haemophilia

17. **Clomiphene citrate:**
    A   Is an anti-oestrogen
    B   Decreases serum FSH levels
    C   Raises the incidence of twin pregnancy to 30%
    D   Can cause ovarian hyperstimulation
    E   May increase the risk of ovarian cancer when used for 3 months

18. **With regards to hyperprolactinaemia:**
    A   Nearly 80% of cases are due to an adenoma in the posterior pituitary
    B   Galactorrhoea occurs in almost 50% of women with hyperprolactinaemia
    C   In women with raised prolactin levels, more than 50% will have galactorrhoea
    D   It can occur in women with hypothyroidism
    E   There is increased risk of osteoporosis

19. **Premature ovarian failure:**
    A   Occurs in 10% of women

B   Is called premature when menopause occurs in women aged >40 years
C   Is associated with viral infection
D   Is associated with autoimmune disorders
E   Is most commonly due to chromosomal abnormalities

20. **Sheehan syndrome:**

A   Usually occurs following massive postpartum haemorrhage
B   Is a common cause of secondary amenorrhoea in the UK
C   May present with failure of lactation
D   May present with symptoms of hyperthyroidism
E   May present with symptoms of adrenocortical insufficiency

21. **Gonadotrophins are raised in the following conditions:**

A   Resistant ovary syndrome
B   Gonadal dysgenesis
C   Turner syndrome
D   Hyperprolactinaemia
E   Gonadotrophin receptor defect

22. **With regards to findings on semen analysis:**

A   Oligozoospermia is diagnosed only when the sperm count is <5 million per mL
B   Azoospermia should be diagnosed only after two samples have been spun and examined under oil emersion microscopy 4 weeks apart
C   A consistently low semen volume of less than 0.5 mL may be due to congenital absence of the seminal vesicles
D   The commonest cause of low volume is noted to be either spillage of sample at collection or during transport
E   A deficiency of the enzyme vesiculase may lead to prolonged liquefaction time of more than 1–2 hours

23. **With regards to azoospermia:**

A   A high serum FSH in males usually indicates obstructive cause for azoospermia
B   A low serum FSH in males is seen with non-obstructive azoospermia
C   It is common in men with Klinefelter syndrome
D   Maturation arrest is a non-obstructive cause for azoospermia
E   The cause for azoospermia may be due to sertoli cell-only syndrome

24. **The following tests can be used to assess ovulation:**

A   Basal body temperature recording
B   Mid-luteal serum progesterone level
C   Day 2 serum LH levels
D   Follicular tracking by ultrasound
E   Cervical mucus changes during the menstrual cycle

25. **Regarding twin pregnancy:**

A   The incidence of dizygotic twinning is relatively constant

B The perinatal mortality rate is five times higher in monochorionic twin pregnancies compared to dichorionic twin pregnancies
C The incidence of monozygotic twin pregnancy is increased with increased maternal age
D The incidence of cerebral palsy is increased in twin pregnancies compared to singleton pregnancy
E Twin-to-twin transfusion is more common in dichorionic twin pregnancies than those with monochorionic twin pregnancies

26. **With regards to intracytoplasmic sperm injection (ICSI):**
A There is no benefit in terms of fertilisation per retrieved oocyte or pregnancy rates between ICSI and conventional IVF for couples with normal semen
B ICSI results in higher fertilisation rates than IVF in couples with borderline semen
C In couples with poor semen, ICSI has better fertilisation outcomes than with subzonal insemination (SUZI)
D The live birth rate for ICSI per cycle is more than IVF
E The live birth rate per cycle falls to 5% or less for women aged >40 years

27. **Regarding the effect of contraception on future fertility:**
A The return of normal fertility is delayed following stopping progesterone only pill
B There is timely return of normal fertility following stopping COCP
C The return of normal fertility is not delayed following stopping depot medroxyprogesterone
D The return of normal fertility is delayed following stopping etonogestrel subdermal implant
E The return of normal fertility is delayed following removal of copper coil

28. **With regards to anti-Müllerian hormone:**
A It is a lipoprotein produced by granulose cells of primary antral follicles
B Levels vary significantly from menstrual cycle to cycle
C Levels are higher in women with polycystic ovarian syndrome (PCOS)
D It increases the sensitivity of pre-antral follicles to FSH
E Levels are higher in women with endometriosis

Answers

1. A False.

   B True.

   C True.

   D True.

   E True.

   OHSS is a complication of ovarian stimulation, especially following use of gonadotrophins for numerous follicular growths preceding assisted reproduction. Early OHSS is usually caused by excessive ovarian hyperstimulation (increased oestradiol levels, number of ovarian follicles) and late OHSS is related to pregnancy. Risk factors include thin body structure, young age, polycystic ovary syndrome (PCOS), past history of OHSS and the use of gonadotropin-releasing hormone analogues in the ovarian stimulation regime.

   The systemic symptoms and signs are a result of vasoactive substances released from enlarged ovaries. This results in increased capillary permeability, leading to a loss of protein-rich fluid into third space or serous cavities (ascites, pleural and, rarely, pericardial effusion). As a result, it causes depletion of the intravascular volume, haemoconcentration and an increased predisposition to developing thrombosis (Virchow's triad). Furthermore, it can cause renal and liver dysfunction and adult respiratory distress syndrome.

   Reported causes of death include adult respiratory distress syndrome, cerebral infarction and hepato-renal failure.

   Royal College of Obstetricians and Gynaecologists. Green-top Guideline No. 5. Management of ovarian hyperstimulation syndrome. London: RCOG Press, 2006.
   Jenkins J and Mathur R. Ovarian hyperstimulation syndrome. Personal assessment in continuing education. Reviews, questions and answers. London: RCOG Press, 2003.

2. A True.

   B True. Cystic fibrosis is an autosomal recessive condition which affects chromosome 7. It mainly affects chloride ion transport within the cells due to an inherent problem in the transmembrane regulator protein. The carrier rate for cystic fibrosis in the general population is 1 in 20 which reduces to 1 in 85 when the screening for common mutations is negative.

   C True. Congenital adrenal hyperplasia is caused by various enzyme deficiencies in the adrenal cortex resulting in excessive adrenocorticotropic hormone production. The most common type (90–95%) is due to 21 hydroxylase enzyme deficiency, for which the gene is located on the short arm of chromosome 6. The next most common abnormality is 11-beta hydroxylase deficiency (4%). Both the enzyme deficiencies cause virilisation because of an increase in androgen production. The presentation at birth is ambiguous genitalia posing problems with gender assignment. In adults, the characteristic features are development of adrenogenital syndrome (baldness, receding hairline, hirsutism, small breasts, male escutcheon, enlarged clitoris and heavy arms and legs).

D True.

E True.

Autosomal recessive inherited conditions:

- alpha-1 antitrypsin deficiency
- Fredreich ataxia
- haemoglobinopathies (e.g. thalassaemia and sickle cell disease).
- mucopolysaccharidoses (e.g. Hurler syndrome type 1)
- Niemann–Pick disease
- pentosuria
- phenylketonuria
- sickle cell disease
- spinal muscular atrophy
- thalassaemia
- Tay–Sachs disease
- Wilson disease

Connor JM. Medical Genetics for MRCOG and Beyond. London: RCOG Press, 2005.
Magowan B. Churchill's Pocketbook of Obstetrics and Gynaecology (3rd edn). Edinburgh: Churchill Livingstone, 2005.
James D, Steer PJ, Weiner CP, Gonik B, Crowther C, Robson S (eds). High Risk Pregnancy: Management Options (4th edn). St Louis: Saunders, 2011.

3. **A True.**

B False.

C True.

D True.

E True.

The prevalence of autosomal recessive inherited conditions is 2.5 in 100. They manifest only in the homozygous state. The heterozygous state represents carrier status and individuals are usually normal. When both the parents are heterozygous for the same condition, there is a 25% chance of their offspring being affected.

Features of autosomal recessive inheritance:

- rare condition
- increased risk with consanguinity (1%)
- risk of 0.3% with women without consanguineous relation
- parents are usually carriers
- twenty-five per cent recurrence risk at conception
- the rarer the autosomal recessive condition, the greater the probability that the parents of an affected homozygote are related

Connor JM. Medical Genetics for MRCOG and Beyond. London: RCOG Press, 2005.
Magowan B. Churchill's Pocketbook of Obstetrics and Gynaecology (3rd edn). Edinburgh: Churchill Livingstone, 2005.
James D, Steer PJ, Weiner CP, Gonik B, Crowther C, Robson S (eds). High Risk Pregnancy: Management Options (4th edn). St Louis: Saunders, 2011.

4. **A False.** It is an autosomal recessive disorder.

    B False. It is an X-linked dominant condition.

    C False. It is an autosomal recessive disorder.

    D True.

    E False. It is an autosomal dominant disorder.

Sex-linked recessive disease

Sex-linked recessive traits are determined by genes on the X chromosomes. Males have one X chromosome and females have two X chromosomes. The disease usually manifests in males as they have a single copy of the X chromosome. In females one copy is active and the other is inactive. It is difficult to determine if the active X chromosome is obtained from the father or the mother in an individual cell. Some women have two sets of cells, where one set are normal and the other are affected cells (mosaics). Male offspring have a 50% chance of inheriting a disease when the mother is heterozygous for an X-linked recessive disorder. On the other hand female offspring have a 50% chance of inheriting the trait but are unaffected by the disease (carrier).

X-linked recessive inherited conditions:

- Becker muscular dystrophy
- complete androgen insensitivity syndrome
- congenital aqueductal stenosis (hydrocephalus)
- Duchenne muscular dystrophy
- glucose-6-phosphate dehydrogenase (G6PD) deficiency
- haemophilia A and B
- partial colour blindness (not able to distinguish between red and green shades)

Connor JM. Medical Genetics for MRCOG and Beyond. London: RCOG Press, 2005.
Magowan B. Churchill's Pocketbook of Obstetrics and Gynaecology (3rd edn). Edinburgh: Churchill Livingstone, 2005.
James D, Steer PJ, Weiner CP, Gonik B, Crowther C, Robson S (eds). High Risk Pregnancy: Management Options (4th edn). St Louis: Saunders, 2011.

5. **A False.** It is a X-linked recessive condition.

    B False. It is a sporadic occurrence.

    C False. It is an autosomal dominant condition.

    D False. It is a Y-linked condition.

    E False. It is a X-linked recessive condition.

X-linked dominant conditions include Xg blood group and vitamin D resistant rickets.

Connor JM. Medical Genetics for MRCOG and Beyond. London: RCOG Press, 2005.

6. **A False.** It is an autosomal recessive condition.

    B False. It is an autosomal recessive condition.

    C True.

D False. Sickle cell disease is an autosomal recessive condition. It is more commonly seen in women of Afro-Caribbean origin. Testing for haemoglobinopathies is part of a booking visit during pregnancy as it helps to quantify risks to the woman depending on whether she is a sickle cell carrier (anaemia) or has sickle cell disease (miscarriage, fetal growth restriction, premature labour, thromboembolism, sickle cell crisis and pre-eclampsia).

E False. Cri du chat syndrome is due to the deletion of a portion of the short arm of chromosome 5 (characteristic features in children include mental retardation, microcephaly, atypical facial features and hypertelorism).

Autosomal dominant inheritance manifests in a heterozygous state (the affected person has one normal allele and one abnormal allele). It is vertically transmitted from one generation to the next and can vary in expression and penetrance making clinical effects on the fetus are more difficult to predict. Men and women are equally affected and each offspring of an affected person has a 50% chance of being affected. Male to male transmission can occur.

Autosomal dominant inheritance conditions:

- achondroplasia
- adult polycystic kidney
- baldness in males
- brachydactyly
- cancer susceptibility genes (BRCA1, BRCA2, HNPCC, p53)
- familial adenomatous polyposis
- Huntington disease
- haemochromatosis
- hereditary sensorimotor neuropathy
- neurofibromatosis type 1
- osteogenesis imperfecta (except type VII)
- tuberous sclerosis
- Marfan syndrome
- retinoblastoma
- hereditary spherocytosis
- von Willebrand disease
- hypokalemic periodic paralysis
- acute intermittent porphyria

Connor JM. Medical Genetics for MRCOG and Beyond. London: RCOG Press, 2005.
Magowan B. Churchill's Pocketbook of Obstetrics and Gynaecology (3rd edn). Edinburgh: Churchill Livingstone, 2005.
James D, Steer PJ, Weiner CP, Gonik B, Crowther C, Robson S (eds). High Risk Pregnancy: Management Options (4th edn). St Louis: Saunders, 2011.

7. **A False.**

   B True.

   C False

   D False.

   E True.

Normal semen analysis

Reference values:

- volume: 2 mL or more
- liquefaction time: <60 minutes
- pH: 7.2 or more
- sperm concentration: 20 million or more per mL
- total sperm number: 40 million spermatozoa per ejaculate or more
- motility: 50% or more motile or 25% or more with progressive motility (grade 'a') within 60 minutes of ejaculation
- morphology: 15% or 30% normal
- vitality: 70% or more alive
- white blood cells fewer than 1 million per mL

See **Table 12.1** for the World Health Organisation (WHO) reference values for fertile men (2009).

Table 12.1 Semen analysis: reference values

Centiles	2.5th	5th	10th
Semen volume (mL)	1.2	1.5	2
Sperm concentration (million/mL)	9	15	22
Total number (million/ejaculate)	23	39	69
Motility (%)*	34	40	45
Progressive motility (%)	28	32	39
Normal forms (%)	3	4	5.5
Vitality (%)	53	58	64

*Motility is graded as a+b (progressive) and c (non-progressive) according to the WHO 1999 classification.

Semen analysis

- If the semen analysis is normal, no further action is required.
- If the first semen analysis is abnormal, a repeat confirmatory test should be offered.
- Repeat confirmatory tests should ideally be undertaken 3 months after the initial analysis to allow time for the cycle of spermatozoa to be completed.
- A repeat test should be undertaken as soon as possible in the presence of gross spermatozoa deficiency (azoospermia or sever oligozoospermia).

The WHO definition of severe male factor infertility:

- severe abnormality of one or moderate abnormality of two or more of the three main parameters of seminal fluid analysis

Criteria used to diagnose severe abnormality:

- count <5 million/mL
- rapid progressive motility <10%
- morphology <5% normal forms

Medical management of male factor infertility

- Men with hypogonadotrophic hypogonadism should be offered gonadotrophins as these are effective in improving fertility.
- Men with idiopathic semen abnormalities should not be offered anti-oestrogenic drugs, gonadotrophins, androgens or bromocriptine as they have not been shown to be effective.
- Men should be informed that the significance of antisperm antibodies is unclear and the effectiveness of systemic corticosteroids is uncertain.
- Men with leucocytes in their semen should not be offered antibiotic treatment unless there is an identified infection as there is no evidence that this improves pregnancy rates.
- When there is severe deficit of semen quality or non-obstructive azoospermia, the man's karyotype should be established.

Surgical management of male factor infertility

- Men with obstructive azoospermia should be offered surgical correction of the epididymal blockage as it is likely to restore patency of the duct and improve fertility. Surgical correction should be considered as an alternative to surgical sperm recovery and *in vitro* fertilisation.
- Men should not be offered surgery for varicoceles as a form of fertility treatment as it does not improve pregnancy rates.

National Institute for Health and Clinical Excellence. Fertility: assessment and treatment for people with fertility problems (CG11). NICE, 2004.
World Health Organization: Infertility. http://www.who.int/reproductivehealth/publications/infertility/en/
Cooper TG, Noonan E, von Eckardstein S, Auger J, Baker HWG, Behre HM, Haugen TB, Kruger T, Wang C, Mbizvo MT, Vogelsong KM. World Health Organization reference values for human semen characteristics. Human Reproduction Update 2009; 00:1–15. http://www.who.int/reproductivehealth/topics/infertility/cooper_et_al_hru.pdf
World Health Organization reference values for human semen. http://www.who.int/reproductivehealth/publications/infertility/human_repro_upd/en/

8. A **True.**

    B **False.** LH peaks 9 hours before ovulation.

    C **False.** Between 36 and 48 hours before ovulation, oestrogen has a positive feedback effect on the anterior pituitary and therefore initiates the burst of LH secretion (LH surge) to produce ovulation.

    D **False.** During the luteal phase, secretion of FSH and LH is low because of elevated levels of oestrogen, progesterone and inhibin.

    E **True.**

    FSH and LH are secreted by the anterior pituitary. They are glycoproteins and are made up of alpha and beta subunits. The alpha subunits of LH, FSH, TSH and hCG are

Table 12.2 FSH and LH

Follicle-stimulating hormone (FSH)	Luteinising hormone (LH)
Tropic to Sertoli cells	Tropic to Leydig cells
FSH and androgens maintain gametogenesis	Stimulates the secretion of testosterone
Testosterone has no effect on FSH	Testosterone in turn has negative feedback effect and inhibits LH secretion by direct action on anterior pituitary and inhibits GnRH by direct action on the hypothalamus
Inhibin (testicular origin) inhibits FSH secretion	
Plasma FSH levels are elevated in patients with atrophy of the seminiferous tubules	

identical, and contain 92 amino acids. The beta subunits vary. FSH has a beta subunit of 118 amino acids which confers its specific biologic action. The sugar part of the hormone is composed of fucose, galactose, mannose, galactosamine, glucosamine and sialic acid.

The carbohydrate content increases their potency by slowing their metabolism.

- the half-life of FSH is 170 minutes
- the half-life of LH is 60 minutes

Hamilton M. Chapter 20: Disorders and investigation of female reproduction. In: Shaw RW, Luesley D, Monga A (eds). Gynaecology (4th edn). Edinburgh: Churchill Livingstone, 2011.
Magowan B. Churchill's Pocketbook of Obstetrics and Gynaecology (3rd edn). Edinburgh: Churchill Livingstone, 2005.

9. **A False.** Women usually present with primary amenorrhoea due to streak gonads and failure of ovarian development. Turner mosaics may present with secondary amenorrhoea.

    B False. Pure XO pattern is seen in 60% of the cases and mosaics (usually XO/XX) in approximately 15%. In the latter, the condition is not severe and women may menstruate and be able to conceive.

    C False. It is associated with coarctation of the aorta, bicuspid aortic valve, webbed neck, short stature and poorly developed secondary sexual characteristics.

    D False. Gonadal dysgenesis or Turner syndrome (XO): the gonads are rudimentary or absent, female external genitalia, short stature and no maturation at puberty.

    E False. Women can be fertile especially if Turner syndrome is due to mosaicism (45XO/46XX).

Connor JM. Medical Genetics for MRCOG and Beyond. London: RCOG Press, 2005.

Magowan B. Churchill's Pocketbook of Obstetrics and Gynaecology (3rd edn). Edinburgh: Churchill Livingstone, 2005.

10. A True.

B True. This includes psychological and surgical stress.

C True.

D True. It increases throughout sleep.

E True. It reaches peak at parturition and falls to normal, non-pregnant levels about 8 days after delivery.

Prolactin contains 199 amino acid residues and three disulphide bridges. It is structurally similar to human growth hormone and has a similar half-life (20 minutes). Its plasma levels are approximately 5 ng/mL in men and 8 ng/mL in women. Its secretion is inhibited by dopamine produced by the hypothalamus and therefore sections of the pituitary stalk increase its secretion.

Its actions during puerperium include:

- milk secretion following oestrogen and progesterone priming
- increased production of mRNA, casein and lactalbumin in the breast
- suckling increases the production of prolactin

Hyperprolactinaemia

Hyperprolactinaemia is seen in around 15–20% of women with secondary amenorrhoea. Hyperprolactinaemia should be excluded in young girls who present with primary amenorrhoea and who have normal development of the uterus and secondary sexual characteristics.

Table 12.3 Factors which increase or decrease prolactin hormone secretion

Increase prolactin secretion	Decrease prolactin secretion
Prolactinoma (40–50%)	L-Dopa: increases the formation of dopamine
Drugs (1–2%):	
· chlorpromazine (blocks dopamine receptors)	Bromocriptine and cabergoline are dopamine agonists and hence inhibit prolactin production
· metoclopramide	
· haloperidol	
· pimozide	
· cimetidine	
· reserpine	
· methyldopa	
· rauwolfia alkaloids	
· chlorpromazine	
· thioridazine	
· opiates	
· oestrogens (lactotrophs)	
End-stage renal disease (73–91%)	
Primary hypothyroidism (3–5%)	

Critchley HOD, Horne A, Munro K. Chapter 16: Amenorrhoea and oligomenorrhoea, and hypothalamic–pituitary dysfunction. In: Shaw RW, Luesley D, Monga A (eds). Gynaecology (4th edn). Edinburgh: Churchill Livingstone, 2011.

Vogiatzi M and Shaw RW. Chapter 17: Ovulation induction. In: Shaw RW, Luesley D, Monga A (eds). Gynaecology (4th edn). Edinburgh: Churchill Livingstone, 2011.

11. **A True.** Usually people are affected in each generation following a vertical pattern of inheritance.

   B False. Both men and women are equally likely to be affected.

   C False. Men can transmit the condition to sons or daughters.

   D False. Women can transmit the condition to sons or daughters.

   E True.

   Autosomal dominant inheritance

   - when only one member of an allelic pair of genes is able to express, it is called autosomal dominant inheritance
   - can be expressed in the heterozygous as well as homozygous state
   - the trait usually appears in every generation
   - fifty per cent of children would be affected irrespective of the sex of the child
   - there is a high new mutation rate

   Connor JM. Medical Genetics for MRCOG and Beyond. London: RCOG Press, 2005.
   Magowan B. Churchill's Pocketbook of Obstetrics and Gynaecology (3rd edn). Edinburgh: Churchill Livingstone, 2005.
   James D, Steer PJ, Weiner CP, Gonik B, Crowther C, Robson S (eds). High Risk Pregnancy: Management Options (4th edn). St Louis: Saunders, 2011.

12. **A True.** Lymphocytes.

   B True. Bone marrow samples can also be used.

   C True.

   D True.

   E True.

   An anticoagulated (EDTA) blood sample (10 mL) can be taken and maintained at an ambient temperature. Once DNA is extracted, it can be stored as a frozen sample for analysis in the future (years). This is particularly useful for identifying fatal inherited conditions in the family if a test is not yet available or may be required in the future long after the affected person in the family has passed away. DNA material can be extracted from paraffin blocks of stored sample but the quality of sample is not good.

   Connor JM. Medical Genetics for MRCOG and Beyond. London: RCOG Press, 2005.

13. **A True.** It is seen in 1 in 10 infertile couples.

   B True.

   C True.

D True. The risk of diabetes is 7%.

E False. The lifespan is normal.

Klinefelter syndrome is 47XXY. Its incidence increases with increasing maternal age. Affected people are tall with sparse facial hair, gynaecomastia and poor socialising skills. This condition is usually diagnosed as a result of investigation of male infertility and is the single most common cause of male hypogonadism. It is also associated with diabetes, asthma and hypothyroidism. It almost always causes azoospermia.

Lifespan and intelligence are usually within normal limits. Management will include assessment for hormone replacement and screening for future complications.

Connor JM. Medical Genetics for MRCOG and Beyond. London: RCOG Press, 2005.
Magowan B. Churchill's Pocketbook of Obstetrics and Gynaecology (3rd edn). Edinburgh: Churchill Livingstone, 2005.

14. **A True.** One in twenty-two northern Europeans is a carrier.

    B False. Cystic fibrosis is an autosomal recessive condition and is expressed in the homozygous state. The fetus must inherit one underactive CFTR gene from each parent in order to be affected (25% chance if both parents are carriers).

    For example, when two people who carry the cystic fibrosis gene have a child, there is a:
    - 1 in 4 chance that the child will have cystic fibrosis
    - 2 in 4 chance that the child will not have cystic fibrosis, but will be a carrier
    - 1 in 4 chance that the child will not have cystic fibrosis, and will not be a carrier.

    C True. This mutation is more common in northern Europe and the USA (accounting for 70–80% of cases) and is less common in Ashkenazi Jews, African Americans and southern Europeans, Afro-Caribbeans and Asians. About 1 in 25 people in the UK of Caucasian descent (white European) are carriers of the cystic fibrosis gene.

    D False. The defect is on chromosome 7. If a person is a carrier, he or she will have one copy of the normal CFTR gene and one copy of the underactive CFTR gene. If a person is affected, he or she will have two copies of the underactive CFTR gene.

    E True. Testing for mutations helps to identify nearly 90% of the CFTR gene mutations in northern European populations. For screening purposes, mouthwash samples are collected from the pregnant woman and her partner for DNA analysis. If positive, the couple can be offered prenatal diagnosis to test the fetus.

    Connor JM. Medical Genetics for MRCOG and Beyond. London: RCOG Press, 2005.
    Magowan B. Churchill's Pocketbook of Obstetrics and Gynaecology (3rd edn). Edinburgh: Churchill Livingstone, 2005.

15. **A True.**

    B False. The DMD gene is located on the short arm of chromosome X.

    C True. CPK can be raised in two thirds of carriers.

    D False. Males are always affected.

    E False. The incidence at birth is 1 in 3000 males.

DMD is a single gene disorder with the mutant gene on one X chromosome and the normal copy on the opposite X chromosome. Affected males show high serum CPK at birth and are physically normal. Later, walking may be delayed with progressive muscular weakness. Most of them will be wheelchair bound by 10–12 years and die around the age of 15–20 years due to respiratory complications.

Connor JM. Medical Genetics for MRCOG and Beyond. London: RCOG Press, 2005.
Magowan B. Churchill's Pocketbook of Obstetrics and Gynaecology (3rd edn). Edinburgh: Churchill Livingstone, 2005.

16. A **False.** There is a deficiency of factor VIII in haemophilia A and factor IX in haemophilia B.

B **False.** It is a sex-linked recessive disorder.

C **False.** Females are obligate carriers.

D **True.**

E **False.**

Vaginal delivery is safe if there are no other associated obstetric complications. Epidural anaesthesia is allowed if the factor level is more than 40 IU/dL and caesarean section may be carried out (if indicated) if the factor VIII level is more than 50 IU/dL. Ventouse delivery should be avoided due to the increased risk of cephalhaematoma or intracranial bleeding. Fetal blood sampling, application of fetal scalp electrodes or ST waveform analysis (STAN) monitoring should be avoided during labour. At birth, cord blood sampling should be sent for factor assay and intramuscular injection of vitamin K withheld until the results are available (oral vitamin K can be administered until then).

During normal pregnancy there is a marked increase in factor VIII and von Willebrand factor (VWF), especially in the third trimester. Therefore treatment with coagulation factors is rarely indicated for women who are carriers and are pregnant. If treatment is required, recombinant products should be considered as the products of choice. 1-deamino-8-D arginine vasopressin (DDAVP) (there are anecdotal reports of premature labour and hyponatraemia associated with seizures with its use during pregnancy) can be used in pregnant women with haemophilia A and von Willebrand factor deficiency to raise factor VIII and VWF levels. Its use is of no value in women with haemophilia B carrier.

Letsky E, Murphy MF, Ramsay JE, Walker I. Haemorrhagic disease and hereditary bleeding disorders. London: RCOG Press, 2005.

17. A **True**

B **False**

C **False.** It raises the incidence of twin pregnancy to 10%.

D **True.** It is rare.

E **False.**

Clomiphene citrate is an anti-oestrogen (a non-steroidal agent with structural similarity to diethylstilboestrol) used for ovulation induction (dose 25–50 mg once daily from days

3–7 of the menstrual cycle). The dose can be increased up to a maximum of 250 mg/day for 5 days. It competes with natural oestrogens in the pituitary by blocking or displacing oestrogen from oestrogen receptors and, as a result, negative feedback of oestrogen on the hypothalamo-pituitary axis is removed. This in turn results in an increase in GnRH and gonadotrophins (FSH and LH).

The side effects include hot flushes, visual disturbances, abdominal discomfort, rashes, breast tenderness and rarely ovarian hyperstimulation (these are completely reversible once the drug is stopped). There is a 10% risk of having multiple pregnancies with clomiphene citrate treatment. When clomiphene is used for more than 12 cycles, it has been linked to increased risk of ovarian cancer but this association remains uncertain.

Clomiphene citrate is used for ovulation induction in women who do not ovulate, who ovulate less, or who ovulate but did not get pregnant. It is not found to be helpful for increasing the chances of pregnancy in women who ovulate regularly but have failed to conceive after more than 1 year of unprotected intercourse. Approximately 80% of women will ovulate while using clomiphene, however only 40% of women will achieve pregnancy.

In women with clomiphene-resistant PCOS, laparoscopic ovarian drilling is recommended before gonadotrophin ovulation induction.

Tamoxifen (triphenylethylene derivative with similar structure to clomiphene citrate) is used for ovulation induction (dose 20–40 mg once daily from days 3–5 of the menstrual cycle) in women sensitive to clomiphene citrate. It is equally as effective as clomiphene citrate but with less anti-oestrogenic side effects. In the UK, it is not licensed for ovulation induction.

National Institute for Health and Clinical Excellence. Fertility: assessment and treatment for people with fertility problems (CG11). NICE, 2004.
Hughes E, Brown J, Collins JJ, Vanderkerckhove P. Clomiphene citrate for unexplained sub fertility in women. Cochrane Database Syst Rev 2000; (2):CD000057
Magowan B. Churchill's Pocketbook of Obstetrics and Gynaecology (3rd edn). Edinburgh: Churchill Livingstone, 2005.
Vogiatzi M and Shaw RW. Chapter 17: Ovulation induction. In: Shaw RW, Luesley D, Monga A (eds). Gynaecology (4th edn). Edinburgh: Churchill Livingstone, 2011.

18. **A False.** It is due to an adenoma in 40–50% of cases and actually arises from the anterior pituitary.

B True.

C False. In women with raised prolactin levels, almost 50% will have galactorrhoea and approximately 15–20% of women who present with secondary amenorrhoea will show raised serum prolactin levels.

D True. Hyperprolactinaemia is characterised by abnormally high levels of prolactin. Its levels in the body are normally regulated by dopamine. Any condition which reduces dopamine levels, disrupts the system (compression of the pituitary stalk) or increases prolactin levels (prolactinoma) will lead to hyperprolactinaemia. The physiological causes of hyperprolactinaemia include pregnancy, lactation, stress, exercise and nipple stimulation. The pathological causes of raised prolactin levels include chronic renal failure, pituitary stalk compression and drugs, which account for 1–2% of cases (phenothiazines, methyldopa, haloperidol and metoclopramide). Elevated levels are also seen in some women with PCOS (10%).

E True. Hyperprolactinaemia can also cause decreased libido.

Critchley HOD, Horne A, Munro K. Chapter 16: Amenorrhoea and oligomenorrhoea, and hypothalamic–pituitary dysfunction. In: Shaw RW, Luesley D, Monga A (eds). Gynaecology (4th edn). Edinburgh: Churchill Livingstone, 2011.
Vogiatzi M and Shaw RW. Chapter 17: Ovulation induction. In: Shaw RW, Luesley D, Monga A (eds). Gynaecology (4th edn). Edinburgh: Churchill Livingstone, 2011.

19. **A False.** It occurs in 1% of women.

    B False. It is called premature when menopause occurs in women aged <40 years.

    C True. It is associated with viral infection, e.g. mumps.

    D True. It is also associated with chemotherapy and radiotherapy.

    E False. It is most commonly idiopathic (two thirds of cases) and only rarely due to a chromosomal abnormality, e.g. Turner syndrome (45XO).

    Critchley HOD, Horne A, Munro K. Chapter 16: Amenorrhoea and oligomenorrhoea, and hypothalamic–pituitary dysfunction. In: Shaw RW, Luesley D, Monga A (eds). Gynaecology (4th edn). Edinburgh: Churchill Livingstone, 2011.

20. **A True.**

    B False. It is very rare in the UK.

    C True.

    D False. It may cause hypothyroidism.

    E True.

Sheehan syndrome is a rare complication of pregnancy and usually occurs after a massive postpartum haemorrhage. There is an enlargement of the anterior pituitary due to hyperplasia and hypertrophy of the lactotrophs during pregnancy. This occurs without a corresponding increase in blood supply. A major haemorrhage and prolonged hypotension in the peripartum period can result in ischaemia and necrosis of the affected pituitary region causing hypopituitarism.

Critchley HOD, Horne A, Munro K. Chapter 16: Amenorrhoea and oligomenorrhoea, and hypothalamic–pituitary dysfunction. In: Shaw RW, Luesley D, Monga A (eds). Gynaecology (4th edn). Edinburgh: Churchill Livingstone, 2011.

21. **A True.** It is claimed that raised gonadotrophin levels generally predict the absence of ovarian follicles. In this condition ovarian follicles are present on an ultrasound scan along with elevated gonadotrophin levels unlike premature ovarian failure or menopause where follicles are not detected on an ultrasound scan. Mutations in the FSH receptor have been described in some women.

    B True.

    C True.

    D False.

E True. Single gene mutations in the FSH-B subunit have been described with primary amenorrhoea and infertility.

Critchley HOD, Horne A, Munro K. Chapter 16: Amenorrhoea and oligomenorrhoea, and hypothalamic–pituitary dysfunction. In: Shaw RW, Luesley D, Monga A (eds). Gynaecology (4th edn). Edinburgh: Churchill Livingstone, 2011.

22. **A False.** The WHO defines oligozoospermia as having a sperm count of less than 20 million per mL.

B True. The cause is usually obstructive, either due to infection or cystic fibrosis. Therefore all men with this finding (azoospermia) should be tested for the cystic fibrosis gene as this is frequently positive. Testing the partner is suggested if the man is positive for the cystic fibrosis gene. If both are positive, the chance of having a child with cystic fibrosis is 25% with 50% being carriers and 25% being normal children.

C True. It may also be due to obstruction of the ejaculatory ducts.

D True.

E True.

Hamilton M. Chapter 20: Disorders and investigation of female reproduction. In: Shaw RW, Luesley D, Monga A (eds). Gynaecology (4th edn). Edinburgh: Churchill Livingstone, 2011.

23. **A False.** A high serum FSH indicates non-obstructive aetiology.

B False. The FSH level is normal in obstructive aetiology.

C True. There will be associated eunuchoid features and the diagnosis can be confirmed by a chromosomal analysis.

D True. A testicular biopsy should be performed to establish whether normal sperm maturation is taking place.

E True. Absence of the germinal epithelium may be congenital or acquired (via radiotherapy or chemotherapy). Sertoli cell-only syndrome can be confirmed by absence of spermatozoa on testicular biopsy.

Hamilton M. Chapter 20: Disorders and investigation of female reproduction. In: Shaw RW, Luesley D, Monga A (eds). Gynaecology (4th edn). Edinburgh: Churchill Livingstone, 2011.

24. **A True.** A rise in basal body temperature is noted during the mid-cycle (0.5–1°C) due to the thermogenic effect of progesterone.

B True. It is suggested that serum progesterone should be assessed during at least two cycles to confirm the regularity of ovulation. Serum levels of 30 nmol/mL indicate ovulation.

C False. Day 2 serum FSH and LH levels are measured during investigations into infertility. High levels indicate reduced ovarian reserve and poor results with *in vitro* fertilisation.

D True. This is useful in tracking ovarian follicles in women undergoing ovulation induction for infertility and may be used to diagnose luteinised unruptured follicle syndrome. In the UK, follicular tracking is not commonly performed. (It is recommended in the first cycle but not in subsequent stimulated cycles.)

E True. Cervical mucus levels differ between the follicular and luteal phases. Around the time of ovulation, the cervical mucus becomes thin, watery and stretchy. The latter is known as a Spinnbarkeit test. The mucus can be stretched while removing it from the cervix or in between two glass slides. It should stretch to at least 8 cm at the time of ovulation. Also the mucus can be examined under the microscope to look specifically for a ferning pattern which also is indicative of ovulatory mucus.

Basal body temperature (BBT) and Spinnbarkeit are no longer used in clinical infertility practice in the UK.

The following hormonal changes occur around the time of ovulation:

- Thirty-six to forty-eight hours before ovulation, the oestrogen feedback effect becomes positive and this initiates the burst of LH secretion (LH surge) that produces ovulation
- Ovulation occurs 9 hours following LH peak
- During the luteal phase, secretion of FSH and LH is low because of elevated levels of oestrogen, progesterone and inhibin.

Hamilton M. Chapter 20: Disorders and investigation of female reproduction. In: Shaw RW, Luesley D, Monga A (eds). Gynaecology (4th edn). Edinburgh: Churchill Livingstone, 2011.
Magowan B. Churchill's Pocketbook of Obstetrics and Gynaecology (3rd edn). Edinburgh: Churchill Livingstone, 2005.

25. A False. The incidence of monozygotic twinning is relatively constant (3 in 1000). The overall incidence of twins in the UK is 12 in 1000. The incidence increases with ovulation induction (10% with clomiphene citrate and 30% with gonadotrophins).

B True. The perinatal mortality rate is five times higher with twin pregnancies than with singleton pregnancies (due to premature delivery).

C False. The incidence of monozygotic twinning is constant (3 in 1000) and is not affected by maternal age, ethnic origin, parity and the use of assisted reproductive techniques. However, these factors do affect the incidence of dizygotic twinning.

D True. It is related to pre-term delivery and also twin-to-twin transfusion syndrome (TTTS).

E False. Vascular anastomoses only occur in monochorionic pregnancies and therefore twin-to-twin transfusion is more common in these pregnancies.

Chorionicity

The determination of chorionicity during early pregnancy is not only important for risk stratification but also has key implications for prenatal diagnosis (e.g. for monochorionic twins, testing of one amniotic sac is sufficient for Down syndrome screening) and antenatal monitoring (e.g. monochorionic twins require 2-weekly ultrasound growth monitoring compared to 4-weekly for dichorionic diamniotic twins).

Ultrasound features of dichorionic twins:

- lambda or twin peak sign
- dividing membrane >2 mm

- different sex
- two placentas
- distinct, separate sacs in first trimester

Magowan B. Churchill's Pocketbook of Obstetrics and Gynaecology (3rd edn). Edinburgh: Churchill Livingstone, 2005.

26. **A True.**

B True.

C True.

D True. The rate is 20.7% versus 14.9%.

E True. In their early 30s, the success rate is 20–25%.

Intracytoplasmic sperm injection (ICSI)

ICSI improves fertilisation rates compared with IVF alone, but once fertilisation is achieved the pregnancy rate is no better than with IVF.

Where the indication for an intracytoplasmic sperm injection is a severe deficit of semen quality or non-obstructive azoospermia, the man's karyotype should be established.

ICSI is offered to people with severe deficits in semen quality, obstructive azoospermia and non-obstructive azoospermia.

In addition, treatment by ICSI should be considered for couples with whom a previous IVF treatment cycle has resulted in a failed or very poor fertilisation.

Anderson RA and Irvine S. Chapter 21: Disorders of male reproduction. In: Shaw RW, Luesley D, Monga A (eds). Gynaecology (4th edn). Edinburgh: Churchill Livingstone, 2011.
National Institute for Health and Clinical Excellence. Fertility: assessment and treatment for people with fertility problems (CG11). NICE, 2004.
Ubaldi F, Liu J, Nagy Z, Tournaye H, Camus M, Van Steirteghem A, Devroey P. Indications for and results of intracytoplasmic sperm injection. Int J Androl 1995; 18 (Suppl. 2):88–90.

27. **A False.** Fertility is promptly resumed.

B True. Most ovulate in the first cycle and the almost all ovulate by the third cycle.

C False. The return of normal fertility is delayed (conception may be delayed from 8 to 18 months). Women who wish to conceive sooner should be warned about this effect and advised to use alternative methods.

D False. Fertility is promptly resumed.

E False. Fertility is resumed promptly following the removal of intrauterine contraceptive device or levonorgestrel IUS.

Guillebaud J. Your Questions Answered: Contraception (4th edn). Edinburgh: Churchill Livingstone, 2004.

28. **A False.**

B False.

C True.

D False.

E False.

Anti-Müllerian hormone (AMH):

- it is a growth factor hormone, which affects tissue growth and differentiation
- a glycoprotein produced by granulosa cells of the primary, pre-antral and small antral follicles (2–6 mm follicles) of the ovary
- reduces the sensitivity of pre-antral follicles to FSH
- correlates significantly with the gonadotrophin response
- there is only a small fluctuation in AMH serum levels between menstrual cycles
- serum levels are higher in women with PCOS
- AMH levels reflect the number of remaining eggs in the ovary
- AMH levels reflect the growing pool of follicles in the ovary
- low AMH means low egg numbers
- in males it continues to be secreted and reaches a mean value of 48 ng/mL in plasma in 1–2-year-old boys. Thereafter it declines towards puberty and remains at a low level throughout life
- in females the plasma levels remain low or undetectable until puberty. Thereafter they are maintained at a low level of 2 ng/mL
- it is probably involved in germ cell maturation in both sexes and control of testicular descent in males

La Marca A, Stabile G, Artenisio AC, Volpe A. Serum anti-Mullerian hormone throughout the human menstrual cycle. Hum Reprod 2006; 21:3103-3107.
La Marca A, Sighinolfi G, Radi D, Argento C, Baraldi E, Artenisio AC, Stabile G, Volpe A. Anti-Mullerian hormone (AMH) as a predictive marker in assisted reproductive technology (ART). Hum Reprod Update 2010; 16:113-130.

Chapter 13

Research, ethics, consent and risk management

1. **With reference to the Abortion Act 1967 (revised in 1991):**
   A   Abortion is legal in Northern Ireland
   B   It is readily available on request at general practitioner centres
   C   It can be done if there is substantial risk that if the child were born, it would suffer such physical and mental abnormalities as to be seriously handicapped
   D   It can be done after 24 weeks of pregnancy if the risk of continuation is greater than if the pregnancy was terminated, because of the possible physical and mental health effects to the pregnant woman
   E   It can be done if termination is necessary to prevent grave permanent injury to physical and mental health of the partner

2. **With regards to the basis of valid consent:**
   A   It rests on the principle of patient autonomy
   B   The patient should be competent
   C   The doctor should provide adequate information to a competent patient
   D   The patient should understand the information
   E   The patient should make a decision voluntarily

3. **Regarding minors (<18 years) and consent under English law:**
   A   Sixteen to seventeen year olds are presumed to have the capacity to give consent to medical procedures
   B   Children under 16 years of age are presumed not to have the capacity to consent unless a health professional's assessment declares otherwise
   C   For children aged under 13 years, the person with parental responsibility can give consent
   D   If a patient under 16 years of age refuses consent, those with parental responsibility or a court can give consent if it is in the patient's best interest
   E   If the parent refuses to give consent to the procedure that a doctor strongly believes is in the best interest of the patient, the doctor should involve the courts

4. **The following are examples where doctors may breach confidentiality to specific authorities:**
   A   Child protection
   B   Under court orders

    C   Notifiable disease

    D   Identification of donors and recipients of transplanted organs

    E   Medical conditions affecting the ability to drive

5. **Regarding the Access to Health Records Act 1990:**

    A   It gives patients the general right to see medical records

    B   It gives patients the general right to request and obtain copies of these records

    C   It applies to medical records made after 1 November 1995

    D   Doctors should provide copies of records for patients within 21 days

    E   Doctors should provide copies of records for patients within 40 days for records >40 days old

6. **The Mental Capacity Act is underpinned by five key principles:**

    A   A presumption of capacity

    B   The right for individuals to be supported in order to make their own decisions

    C   The right to make what might be seen as an unwise decision

    D   Any decision taken must be done in the individual's best interest

    E   Any decision taken should be as unrestrictive of the individual's basic rights and freedom as possible

7. **Appraisal is a process:**

    A   To give doctors feedback on their past performance

    B   To chart doctors' continuing progress

    C   To identify developmental and educational needs

    D   To criticise doctors about their current performance

    E   To highlight mistakes made in the past

8. **The following are aims of risk management:**

    A   To reduce the frequency of adverse events

    B   To promote reflective practice

    C   To reduce the chance of a claim

    D   To improve quality of life

    E   To improve one's curriculum vitae

9. **The following are true with regards to the termination of a pregnancy:**

    A   Abortion can only be offered up to a maximum of 18 weeks if the mental or physical wellbeing of the mother is likely to deteriorate if the pregnancy continues

    B   A person shall not be guilty of an offence under the law relating to abortion when a pregnancy is terminated by a registered medical practitioner and if two registered medical practitioners are of the opinion that this is the right thing to do, formed in good faith

    C   Only 50% of abortions are carried out before the 13th week of pregnancy

    D   A surgical abortion at 8 weeks of gestation can be carried out under general anaesthetic if the woman requests it

    E   Early medical abortion can be performed under general anaesthesia if the woman requests it

10. **The following statements are true with regards to induced abortions in the UK:**

    A   It is one of the most common procedures performed in gynaecology

    B   Over 98% are performed because of risk to the physical and mental health of the woman and child

    C   Both surgical and medical methods of abortion carry a risk of failure to terminate the pregnancy and hence the need for a repeat procedure

    D   There is a small risk of a uterine rupture with mid-trimester medical management

    E   There is a recognised association with subsequent placenta praevia

11. **With regards to fetal heart rate (FHR) traces:**

    A   They should be kept for a minimum of 5 years

    B   If there is concern that the baby may suffer developmental delay, FHR traces should be photocopied and stored for at least 10 years

    C   When they are stored separately from a woman's records, tracer systems should be available for all FHR traces

    D   When they are used for risk management or teaching purposes, tracer systems should be available to locate them

    E   Paired cord blood gases should be taken routinely for all deliveries

Answers

1. **A False.** It is illegal in Northern Ireland, where the 1967 Act does not apply, but it is legal in Great Britain.

    B False. Women can go to their general practitioner to be referred for an abortion at a different centre. However, is not readily available on request as two doctors have to certify that the abortion is being done within the grounds of the Abortion Act.

    C True.

    D True.

    E False. It can be done if termination is necessary to prevent grave permanent injury to the physical and mental health of the pregnant woman.

    Abortion is legal up to 24 weeks of gestation under the 1967 Abortion Act (amended by the Human Fertilisation and Embryology Act 1990). Two medical practitioners have to sign for the authorisation of an abortion. Nurses are not permitted to sign the legal forms for an abortion under the 1967 Abortion Act.

Family Planning Association. Abortion: your questions answered (information leaflet). www.fpa.org.uk
Royal College of Obstetricians and Gynaecologists. Q&A: The abortion time limit and why it should remain at 24 weeks – the O&G perspective. http://www.rcog.org.uk
National Institute for Health and Clinical Excellence. Care of women requesting inducted abortions. NICE, 2009.
O'Reilly B, Bottomley C, Rymer J. Pocket Essentials of Obstetrics and Gynaecology. London: Saunders, 2005.

2. **A True.**

    B True. There is no proxy consent for an incompetent adult in English law.

    C True.

    D True.

    E True. This is an informed choice (without coercion).

    The key words are competent patient, information given, understands information, and makes decision voluntarily.

    ### Respect for patient autonomy

    Autonomy is the capacity to think, decide and act on the basis of such thought and decision, freely and independently. Respect for patient autonomy requires that health professionals help patients to make their own decisions by providing them with all relevant information, and respecting and following those decisions even when they believe the patient's decision is wrong.

    ### Further reading

Hope T. Medical Ethics: A Very Short Introduction. Oxford: Oxford University Press, 1998.
Campbell A, Gillett G, Jones G (eds). Medical Ethics (3rd edn). Oxford: Oxford University Press, 2001.
Blackburn S. Ethics: A Very Short Introduction. Oxford: Oxford University Press, 2001.
Parker M and Hope T. Ways of thinking about ethics. Medicine 2000; 28:2–5.
Doyal. L. The moral character of clinicians or the best interests of patients? BMJ 1999; 318: 1432–1433.

3. A **True.** Capacity is the ability to make an informed choice but has no bearing on the quality of choice taken. If one has the capacity, they can give consent. The consent of anyone aged 16 years and over has the same legal status as that of an adult.

    B **True.** Children under the age of 16 years may have the capacity to consent but it should not be presumed. The principles of valid consent include: (a) capacity assessed by health professionals; (b) giving adequate information; (c) checking whether the person understands the information provided; (d) the person being able to make a decision with the information provided; and (e) the decision should be voluntary. This was originally called Gillick competence (assessing the capacity for consent in children under 16 years of age). It is now called Fraser Guidelines.

    C **True.**

    D **True.**

    E **True.**

    In England, Wales and Northern Ireland, a minor is a person under the age of 18; in Scotland, under the age of 16.

    Important points with regards to consent in English law are listed below:

    *   Patients under 18 years of age: in an emergency, if the patient or parent refuses consent and there is insufficient time to involve the courts, the doctors can act to save the child from serious harm or death.
    *   Patients between 16 and 17 years of age are presumed to have the capacity to give consent.
    *   Patients under 16 years of age are not presumed to have the capacity to consent and health professionals should assess for this before offering treatment (Fraser guidelines).
    *   Patients 18 years of age and over are adults and presumed to have the capacity to consent. An adult will lack the capacity if they cannot understand or retain the information provided.
    *   Unborn children have no rights and the duty of care of the doctor is to the mother.

    Bolam test

    A doctor is not negligent if he has acted in accordance with proper practice as accepted by a responsible body of medical personnel who specialise in that area.

    Hope T. Medical Ethics: A Very Short Introduction. Oxford: Oxford University Press, 1998.
    Campbell A, Gillett G, Jones G (eds). Medical Ethics (3rd edn). Oxford: Oxford University Press, 2001.
    Blackburn S. Ethics: A Very Short Introduction. Oxford: Oxford University Press, 2001.
    Parker M and Hope T. Ways of thinking about ethics. Medicine 2000; 28:2–5.
    Doyal L. The moral character of clinicians or the best interests of patients? BMJ 1999; 318: 1432–1433.
    General Medical Council booklets. Good medical practice regarding seeking patient consent, confidentiality and serious communicable diseases. www.gmc-uk.org

4. A **True.**

    B **True.**

    C **True.**

D True.

E True.

Situations where doctors can breach confidentiality to specific authorities:

* identification of patients undergoing *in vitro* fertility treatment with donated gametes: Human Fertilisation and Embryology Act 1990
* births: Births and Deaths Registration Act 1953
* deaths: Births and Deaths Registration Act 1953
* notifiable disease: Notifiable Disease Act 1984
* identification of doctors and recipients of transplanted organs: Human Organ Transplant Act 1989

Situations in which doctors have discretion to breach confidentiality:

* information sharing between members of the team in the interests of the patient
* a third party is at significant risk of harm (e.g. a human immunodeficiency virus [HIV]-positive patient at risk of transmitting the infection to his partner)
* a patient who is not medically fit to drive is driving

General Medical Council. Good medical practice regarding seeking patient consent, confidentiality and serious communicable diseases. www.gmc-uk.org
Hope T. Medical Ethics: A Very Short Introduction. Oxford: Oxford University Press, 1998.
Campbell A, Gillett G, Jones G (eds). Medical Ethics (3rd edn). Oxford: Oxford University Press, 2001.
Blackburn S. Ethics: A Very Short Introduction. Oxford: Oxford University Press, 2001.
Parker M and Hope T. Ways of thinking about ethics. Medicine 2000; 28:2–5.
Doyal L. The moral character of clinicians or the best interests of patients? BMJ 1999; 318: 1432–1433.
Hope T, Savulescu J, Hendrick I. Medical Ethics and Law: The Core Curriculum. Edinburgh: Churchill Livingstone, 2003.

5. **A** True.

    B True.

    C False.

    D True.

    E True.

Access to Health Records Act 1990

An application from a patient should be in writing (including children <16 years of age if they are able). A patient has the right to ask for the records to be explained to them if they are illegible. The doctor can charge a reasonable fee for providing the records and also for time spent in explaining the records.

The limitations to this Act include:

* It applies to medical records made after 1 November 1991.
* Doctors must guarantees the confidentiality of other individuals (any part of the notes which contains information given by or relating to another individual should be removed before providing copies and the patient should not be informed that such pages have been removed unless they ask).
* The doctor may refuse to provide records if he or she believes providing such records will cause serious harm to the patient's physical or mental health.

Hope T. Medical Ethics: A Very Short Introduction. Oxford: Oxford University Press, 1998.
Campbell A, Gillett G, Jones G (eds). Medical Ethics (3rd edn). Oxford: Oxford University Press, 2001.
Blackburn S. Ethics: A Very Short Introduction. Oxford: Oxford University Press, 2001.
Parker M and Hope T. Ways of thinking about ethics. Medicine 2000; 28:2–5.
Doyal L. The moral character of clinicians or the best interests of patients? BMJ 1999; 318: 1432–33.
Hope T, Savulescu J, Hendrick I. Medical Ethics and Law: The Core Curriculum. Edinburgh: Churchill Livingstone, 2003.
Beauchamp TL and Childress JF. Principles of Biomedical Ethics (4th edn). Oxford: Oxford University Press, 1994.

6. **A True.** Every adult has the right to make his or her own decisions and must be assumed to have the capacity to do so unless it is proved otherwise.

   B True. Patients must be given all appropriate help before anyone concludes that they cannot make their own decisions.

   C True. Individuals must retain the right to make what might be seen as the wrong decision.

   D True. Anything done for, or on behalf of, people without the capacity to consent must be in their best interests.

   E True. Anything done for, or on behalf of, people without the capacity to consent should be as unrestrictive of their basic rights and freedom as possible.

   The Mental Health Act 2005 provides a statutory framework to empower and protect vulnerable adults who lack the capacity to make their own decisions. It enables people to plan ahead for situations when they may lack the capacity to make decisions. It clarifies who can make decisions and how they should go about it.

   Department of Health publications. www.dh.gov.uk/en/SocialCare/Deliveringadultsocialcare/MentalCapacity/MentalCapacityActDeprivationofLibertySafeguards/index.htm

7. **A True.**

   B True.

   C True.

   D False.

   E False.

   Appraisal is a positive process and its main purpose is to improve performance and assist learning:

   - The content of an appraisal is based on the core headings set out by the General Medical Council (GMC) Good Medical Practice guidelines.
   - Standardised documentation is used so that information from various hospital services is recorded and expressed consistently.
   - It also provides a structured system for recording progress towards revalidation.
   - Appraisals have been part of contractual arrangements for consultants since April 2001 and a contractual requirement since 2002.
   - Specialist registrars' progress was assessed conventionally by RITA (Record of In Training Assessment). This is now known as ARCP (Annual Review of Competence Progression).

Revalidation assesses the standard of fitness to practise in line with the seven headings of the GMC Good Medical Practice guidelines and allows a doctor's licence to practice to be reviewed.

Appraisal and revalidation are both based on the same sources of information, but the objectives of the two processes are distinct and complementary.

The RCOG's online training course. www.StratOG.net
Appraisal. http://www.rcog.org.uk/stratog/page/introduction-appraisal

8. A True.

B True.

C True.

D False.

E False.

The components of clinical governance include:

- clinical effectiveness: education and training, clinical audit, guidelines and protocols
- continuing professional development
- clinical risk management
- formal appraisal of complaints
- information technology
- revalidation
- staff management

Risk management (RM) is defined as a process to improve the safety and quality of care through reporting, analysing and learning from adverse incidents involving patients. It is an active tool for learning and aids in problem solving (not blame). The purpose is to ensure harm to the patients, relatives and professionals is kept to a minimum in the workplace.

The aims of RM include:

- to reduce adverse events
- to reduce the chance of a claim
- to reduce the cost of a claim once made
- to improve the quality of care for patients
- to reduce harm to patients
- to promote reflective practice
- to improve future practice

The process of RM includes four key steps:

- risk identification and reporting (e.g. massive postpartum haemorrhage)
- risk analysis (determines human and other factors, analyses underlying systems, identifies risk points and determines potential improvements)
- risk control (by formulating recommendations, updating the protocols and guidelines, running drills in labour ward and debriefing the staff)
- risk funding

Royal College of Obstetricians and Gynaecologists. Clinical governance advice No. 2. Improving patient safety. Risk management for maternity and gynaecology. RCOG, 2009. http://www.rcog.org.uk/files/rcog-corp/CGA2ImprovingPatientSafety2009.pdf

9. **A False.** Termination of pregnancy is legal up to 24 weeks of gestation under the Abortion Act 1967 (revised 1991).

   B True.

   C False. Ninety per cent of abortions are carried out by the 13th week.

   D True. Local anaesthesia or conscious sedation is used for performing surgical abortion up to 15 weeks but a general anaesthesia can be provided if the woman requests it.

   E False. Early medical abortion (up to 9 weeks) can be induced with oral mifepristone, followed by vaginal or oral misoprostol depending on the local protocol.

   Family Planning Association. Abortion: your questions answered (information leaflet). www.fpa.org.uk
   National Institute for Health and Clinical Excellence. Care of women requesting inducted abortions. NICE, 2009.
   O'Reilly B, Bottomley C, Rymer J. Pocket Essentials of Obstetrics and Gynaecology. London: Saunders, 2005.

10. **A True.**

    B True.

    C True. The risk of failure to terminate is 2.3 in 1000 for surgical and between 1 and 14 in 1000 for medical abortion.

    D True. The risk of uterine rupture is 1 in 1000 for mid-trimester medical abortion.

    E False. There is no proven association of abortion and subsequent ectopic pregnancy, placenta praevia or infertility.

Ideally, women requesting an abortion should be offered an assessment appointment within 5 days or as a minimum standard, they should be offered an assessment appointment within 2 weeks of referral.

An assessment should be done pre-abortion. These include:

- a full blood count
- testing for ABO and Rhesus blood groups, with screening for red cell antibodies
- if indicated, test for other conditions such as haemoglobinopathies, HIV and hepatitis B and C

The risks of surgical abortion include:

- haemorrhage: 1 in 1000 overall. The risk increases after 13 weeks
- uterine perforation: 1–4 in 1000 for surgical abortion
- cervical trauma: 1 in 100. The risk is lower in early pregnancy
- infection post-abortion: occurs in 10% of cases (genital tract infection)
- may be associated with a small increased risk of subsequent miscarriage or pre-term delivery

Other important points to remember during practise:

- It is advised to use blunt forceps and a suction curette, not a sharp curette, while undertaking the procedure.
- Conventional suction termination should be avoided before 7 weeks of gestation because of the increased risk of failure to terminate.
- Anti-D immunoglobulin G (250 IU before 20 weeks of gestation and 500 IU thereafter) should be administered to all non-sensitised Rhesus negative women within 72 hours of an abortion, whether by surgical or medical methods.
- Cervical preparation should be routinely used for women under 18 years of age or at >10 weeks of gestation.

National Institute for Health and Clinical Excellence. Care of women requesting inducted abortions. NICE, 2009.
Royal College of Obstetricians and Gynaecologists. Consent advice No. 10. Surgical Evacuation of the Uterus for Early Pregnancy Loss. London: RCOG, 2006.
O'Reilly B, Bottomley C, Rymer J. Pocket Essentials of Obstetrics and Gynaecology. London: Saunders, 2005.

11. **A False.** FHR traces should be kept for a minimum of 25 years and stored electronically where possible.

B False. If there is concern that the baby may suffer developmental delay, FHR traces should be photocopied and stored indefinitely in case of possible adverse outcomes.

C True.

D True.

E False. Paired cord blood gases need not be taken routinely for all deliveries but need to be taken when there has been concern regarding the baby either in labour or immediately after birth.

See **Table 13.1** for fetal blood sampling classification.

Table 13.1 Interpretation of fetal blood sampling (FBS) results	
Interpretation	**FBS result (pH)**
Normal FBS result	≥ 7.25
Borderline FBS result	7.21–7.24
Abnormal FBS result	≤ 7.20

Management plans with regards to fetal blood sampling (FBS) results

- Consultant advice should be sought after one abnormal result.
- After a normal FBS result, it should be repeated in 1 hour if the FHR trace remains pathological or sooner if it deteriorates.
- After a borderline FBS result, it should be repeated 30 minutes later if the FHR trace remains pathological or sooner if it deteriorates.

- If the FBS result remains stable and there is no change in the features of the cardiotocograph (CTG), a third sample may be deferred unless additional abnormalities develop on the trace.
- Consultant advice should be sought if there is need for a third FBS.

Contraindications to FBS include:

- prematurity <34 weeks of gestation
- maternal infection, e.g. HIV, hepatitis and herpes simplex virus
- fetal bleeding disorders, e.g. haemophilia, maternal thrombocytopaenia (ITP) where fetal platelet count cannot be predicted

Risk management issues

- One should take into account the time that it would take to achieve birth by both caesarean section and instrumental vaginal delivery when the fetus is compromised and needs delivery.
- FHR traces should be kept for 25 years.
- FHR traces should be photocopied and stored indefinitely in case of possible adverse outcomes.
- If the CTG traces are stored separately from the woman's case notes, tracer systems should be available to locate them.

National Institute for Health and Clinical Excellence. Guidelines on intrapartum care (CG55). NICE, 2007.

Chapter 14

Urogynaecology

1. **The following are complications of surgical management of stress incontinence:**
   A Retention of urine
   B Bleeding
   C Enterocele
   D Sexual problems
   E Detrusor instability

2. **Antimuscarinic drugs are contraindicated in women with:**
   A Myasthenia gravis
   B Glaucoma
   C Ulcerative colitis
   D Gastrointestinal obstruction
   E Asthma

3. **With regards to sacrospinous ligament fixation:**
   A The vaginal vault is fixed to the sacral promontory
   B It is usually done on left side
   C Following surgery, the vagina aligns vertically with the body in standing position
   D This can cause damage to pudendal nerve and vessels
   E Sufficient vaginal length and mobility are prerequisites for undertaking the above operation

4. **The complications of sacrocolpopexy include:**
   A Sacral osteopaenia
   B Enterocele
   C Ureteric obstruction
   D Mesh erosion
   E Injury to pudendal artery

5. **With regards to incontinence terminologies:**
   A Stress incontinence is a leakage of urine in response to a decrease in intra-abdominal pressure
   B Urodynamic stress incontinence is a clinical diagnosis
   C Urgency is a strong desire to void and can be due to increased bladder sensitivity
   D Detrusor instability is an urodynamic diagnosis
   E Urge incontinence is a strong desire to void along with involuntary leakage of urine

Answers

1. A True.

    B True.

    C True.

    D True.

    E True.

    Urinary incontinence (UI)

    The International Continence Society defines urinary incontinence as 'the complaint of any involuntary leakage of urine':

    - Stress UI is an involuntary urine leakage upon effort or exertion or while sneezing or coughing.
    - Urge UI is an involuntary urine leakage accompanied or immediately preceded by urgency.
    - Mixed UI is an involuntary urine leakage associated with both urgency and exertion, as well as effort, sneezing and coughing.
    - Overactive bladder syndrome (OAB) is defined as urgency that occurs with or without (urge) UI and usually with frequency and nocturia.
    - OAB that occurs with (urge) UI is known as 'OAB wet'.
    - OAB that occurs without (urge) UI is known as 'OAB dry'.

    Surgeries for urodynamic stress incontinence

    Surgery is offered to women following failed conservative management. Any woman who is offered surgical therapy should be informed about the pros and cons of surgical management.

    Different operations used to treat stress incontinence include:

    - Retropubic mid-urethral tape with macroporous (type 1) polypropylene meshes are used.
    - Open colposuspension and an autologous rectus fascial sling are the recommended alternatives when clinically appropriate.
    - Synthetic slings are recommended as an alternative treatment option for stress UI if conservative management has failed, provided that women are made aware of the lack of long-term outcome data.
    - Synthetic slings using materials other than polypropylene are not recommended for the treatment of stress UI.
    - Intramural bulking agents (glutaraldehyde cross-linked collagen, silicone, carbon-coated zirconium beads or hyaluronic acid/dextran co-polymer) should be considered for the management of stress UI if conservative management has failed. Women should be made aware of the need for repeated injections to achieve efficacy. Diminution of efficacy with time and surgery is superior to intramural bulking agents.

- An artificial urinary sphincter should be considered in women only if previous surgery has failed. Lifelong follow-up is recommended.
- Laparoscopic colposuspension is not routinely recommended. If used, it should be performed by an experienced laparoscopic surgeon working in a multidisciplinary team.
- Anterior colporrhaphy, needle suspensions, paravaginal defect repair and the Marshall–Marchetti–Krantz procedure are not recommended for the treatment of stress UI.

Complications following surgical management of stress incontinence:

- detrusor instability (17% after burch colposuspension and 3–15% after transvaginal tape [TVT])
- developing enterocele (10–20%)
- retention of urine (10% after Burch colposuspension and 4% after TVT) following operation and the need for short-term or long-term catheterisation including clean intermittent self-catheterisation (CISC)
- bleeding, infection and injury to the bladder
- erosion of the mesh
- vaginal shortening and narrowing
- dyspareunia
- recurrence
- the need for repeat surgery if symptoms recur

National Institute for Health and Clinical Excellence. Guideline on the management of urinary incontinence in women (CG40). NICE, 2006.
Royal College of Obstetricians and Gynaecologists. Surgery for stress incontinence: information for you (patient information leaflet). London: RCOG, 2005.

2. A **True.**

    B **True.**

    C **True.**

    D **True.**

    E **False.**

Anticholinergic drugs are mainly used in urogynaecology for the treatment of detrusor instability. Side effects include dry mouth, dry skin, blurred vision, constipation, drowsiness, headache, restlessness, nausea and vomiting, palpitation, arrhythmia, tachycardia and hot flushes. They should be used with caution in women with arrhythmia, coronary artery disease, hypothyroidism, congestive cardiac failure, gastro-oesophageal reflux disease and renal impairment.

Certain drugs like darifenacin and solifenacin should be avoided in women with severe hepatic impairment.

Abboudi H, Fynes MM, Doumouchtsis SK. Contemporary therapy for the overactive bladder. The Obstetrician and Gynaecologist 2011; 13:98–105.

3. A **False.** Sacrospinous ligament fixation is the surgery used for treating vaginal vault prolapse. The vault is fixed to the sacrospinous ligament and is usually done on one side rather than both sides. The success rate is approximately 90%.

B False. It is usually done on the right side to avoid injury to the sigmoid colon on the left side. There is no evidence that bilateral fixation has any advantage over unilateral sacrospinous fixation.

C False. After operation, the vagina is horizontal in a standing position and therefore when intra-abdominal pressure is increased, the vagina closes against the pelvic floor.

D True. Pudendal nerve injury can lead to claudication of the right buttock. Other complications include bleeding, infection, haematoma, urinary retention, dyspareunia, recurrence of prolapse and the need to repeat surgery if symptoms recur.

E True. This facilitates access to the sacrospinous ligament.

Operative management of vaginal vault prolapse

Operations must be carefully chosen and women appropriately counselled beforehand:

- Both abdominal sacrocolpopexy and sacrospinous ligament fixation are used to treat vaginal vault prolapse.
- Sacrocolpopexy is an effective operation for post-hysterectomy vaginal vault prolapse, compared to sacrospinous fixation.
- Sacrospinous ligament fixation has a lower postoperative morbidity compared to sacrocolpopexy, but a higher failure rate.
- Sacrospinous ligament fixation requires an adequate vaginal length and vault width to enable the sacrospinous ligament to be reached.
- Coexistent anterior and/or posterior vaginal wall prolapse can easily be managed by anterior and/or posterior repair while performing vaginal sacrospinous ligament fixation.
- Vaginal sacrospinous ligament fixation is more suitable for physically frail women because of the morbidity associated with abdominal surgery. However, the operative morbidity associated with sacrocolpopexy is reduced when the procedure is done laparoscopically.
- Abdominal sacrocolpopexy is more suitable for sexually active women, as sacrospinous ligament fixation is associated with an exaggerated retroversion of the vagina, leading to a less physiological axis than following sacrocolpopexy.
- Vaginal length is well maintained after sacrocolpopexy whereas sacrospinous ligament fixation can cause vaginal narrowing and/or shortening, especially when carried out alongside repair of anterior and/or posterior vaginal wall defects, leading to dyspareunia.

Sacrocolpopexy is an operation which lifts the vagina back to its natural position by attaching a synthetic mesh from the top and back of the vagina to the periosteum of the sacral promontory. The point of fixation is the sacrospinous ligament in sacrospinous ligament fixation or suspension surgery.

Royal College of Obstetricians and Gynaecologists. Green-top Guideline No. 42. The management of post hysterectomy vaginal vault prolapsed. London: RCOG Press, 2007.

4. **A False.** It can cause sacral osteomyelitis as the mesh is attached to the longitudinal ligament of the sacral promontory.

   B True. Therefore Moschcowitz operation (obliteration of the cul-de-sac) is advised along with sacrocolpopexy.

   C False. It can cause bowel obstruction and injury to the bowel, bladder and ureter.

   D True.

   E False. It can cause injury to presacral vessels and result in excessive bleeding.

   Royal College of Obstetricians and Gynaecologists. Green-top Guideline No. 42. The management of post hysterectomy vaginal vault prolapsed. London: RCOG Press, 2007.

5. **A False.** Stress incontinence is a leakage of urine in response to an increase in intra-abdominal pressure.

   B False. Urodynamic stress incontinence is an urodynamic diagnosis. It is associated with an involuntary loss of urine when the bladder pressure exceeds the urethral pressure in the absence of detrusor contraction.

   C True. Urgency can be motor (due to an overactive bladder) or sensory.

   D True. Detrusor instability is associated with spontaneous detrusor contractions during filling phase or due to provocation when the patient is actively making an effort to stop micturition.

   E True. Urge urinary incontinence is an involuntary urine leakage accompanied or immediately preceded by urgency.

   National Institute for Health and Clinical Excellence. Guideline on the management of urinary incontinence in women (CG40). NICE, 2006.

Chapter 15

Women's sexual and reproductive health

1. **With regards to long-acting reversible contraception (LARC):**
   - A Levonorgestrel IUS (intrauterine system) must be replaced every 4 years
   - B Etonogestrel subdermal implants must be replaced every 5 years
   - C Levonorgestrel IUS can be used in the context of emergency contraception
   - D Women presenting at 14 weeks from the date of previous injection (depot medroxyprogesterone acetate) should receive it immediately
   - E Epilepsy is a an absolute contraindication for the insertion of levonorgestrel IUS

2. **Bacterial vaginosis is associated with:**
   - A An excess growth of anaerobic organisms in the vagina
   - B An excess growth of *Gardnerella vaginalis* in the vagina
   - C A low pH in the vagina
   - D A positive amine test
   - E An overgrowth of lactobacilli in the vagina

3. *Chlamydia trachomatis:*
   - A Is an obligate intracellular virus
   - B Can cause conjunctivitis in the newborn
   - C Can cause pneumonia in the newborn
   - D Is the causative organism for lymphogranuloma venereum
   - E Is the most common cause of non-gonococcal urethritis in women

4. **With regards to genital herpes simplex:**
   - A It is the most common cause of reported vulval ulceration in the UK
   - B Most genital infections are caused by type 2 herpes simplex
   - C It typically causes multiple shallow painless ulcers on the vulval region
   - D Recurrent infections occur in 80% of the patients
   - E Recurrent infections tend to be more severe

5. **With regards to female sterilisation:**
   - A Risk of failure is 1 in 2000 women
   - B Risk of failure is 1 in 200 women
   - C The risk of ectopic pregnancy is high in cases where the woman gets pregnant
   - D The risk of failure rate is slightly higher with sterilisation during caesarean section than interval sterilisation
   - E Risk of failure is 0.5%

6. The absolute contraindications to combined oral contraceptive pills (COCPs)
    include:
    A   Blood pressure (<140/90)
    B   Smoking cigarettes (40/day)
    C   Diabetic retinopathy
    D   Migraine with aura
    E   Body mass index >40

7. The failure rate of female sterilisation is:
    A   2%
    B   1.5%
    C   2.5%
    D   1%
    E   0.5%

8. Candida infection:
    A   Is more common in sexually active women
    B   Is a sexually transmitted disease
    C   Is more common in pregnant women
    D   Is more common in women with diabetes
    E   Is more common in women with a copper intrauterine contraceptive device
         (IUCD)

9. *Neisseria gonorrhoeae:*
    A   Is a gram-negative organism
    B   Is an intracellular diplococcus
    C   Needs Amies transport medium for transport
    D   Is sensitive to ciprofloxacin
    E   Is sensitive to ampicillin

10. Regarding bacterial vaginosis:
    A   It is a sexually transmitted disease
    B   Most women are asymptomatic
    C   On wet microscopy, bacteria surround the epithelial cells
    D   It is important to treat the partner to avoid recurrence of infection
    E   Clindamycin cream 2% can be used for treatment during pregnancy

11. With regards to syphilis:
    A   It is caused by a virus
    B   The primary chancre is raised, round, indurated and painful
    C   The primary chancre resolves in 3–8 weeks
    D   Secondary syphilis is associated with painless lymphadenopathy
    E   Tertiary syphilis can involve the cardiovascular system

12. The immediate management of women with sexual assault includes:
    A   Screening for sexually transmitted diseases
    B   Referral to the police without consent

C   Emergency contraception
D   Mouth swab
E   Post-exposure human immunodeficiency virus (HIV) prophylaxis

13. **With regards to levonorgestrel IUS:**
    A   It reduces menstrual loss by an average of 50% after 3 months
    B   Breakthrough bleeding is common post-insertion
    C   It increases blood pressure in non-hypertensive women
    D   It increases weight gain when used for contraceptive use
    E   It can cause mastalgia in 4% of women

14. **Copper IUCD:**
    A   Prevents fertilisation
    B   Is contraindicated in women when breastfeeding
    C   Increases menstrual blood loss by an average of 80%
    D   Is useful in women with Asherman syndrome to keep the uterine cavity open
    E   Increases the risk of pelvic inflammatory disease (PID) in the first 3 weeks post-insertion

15. **Amenorrhoea is often seen in women using:**
    A   Desogestrel
    B   Combined oral contraceptive pill
    C   Depot medroxyprogesterone acetate
    D   Oestrogen transdermal patch (EVRA)
    E   Etonogestrel subdermal implant (Implanon)

16. **The following act mainly by reduction in the sperm penetrability of cervical mucus:**
    A   Ethinylestradiol/levonorgestrel
    B   Levonorgestrel
    C   Norethisterone 350 µg
    D   Ethynylestradiol/norethisterone
    E   Oestrogen transdermal patch (EVRA)

17. **The following cardiac conditions are absolute contraindications to COCP use:**
    A   Previous arterio-venous thromboembolism
    B   Atrial fibrillation
    C   Pulmonary hypertension
    D   Pulmonary arteriovenous malformation
    E   Dilated cardiomyopathy

18. **The following should be used with caution in women with a previous history of ectopic pregnancy and who wish to conceive in the future:**
    A   Copper intrauterine device
    B   Desogestrel
    C   Combined oral contraceptive pill
    D   Depot medroxyprogesterone acetate
    E   Conventional progestogen-only pill

19. **The following are contraindications to the use of levonorgestrel IUS:**
    A Unexplained uterine bleeding
    B Suspected pregnancy
    C Current breast cancer
    D Postcoital contraception
    E Past history of pelvic infection

20. **The following are modalities used in the treatment of woman with anogenital warts:**
    A Podophyllotoxin – local application
    B Trichloroacetic acid – oral route
    C Podophyllin – local application
    D 5-fluorouracil – local application
    E Gentian violet – local application

Answers

1. A False.

    B False.

    C False.

    D False.

    E False.

    Levonorgestrel IUS (Mirena) must be replaced every 5 years and etonogestrel subdermal implants must be replaced every 3 years. Levonorgestrel IUS is not licensed for emergency contraception as it is not effective. Women with epilepsy are normally on antiepileptic drugs which are liver enzyme-inducing drugs. Levonorgestrel IUS is unlikely to be affected (as it acts locally on the endometrial lining) by enzyme-inducing drugs unlike the other contraceptive methods, e.g. COCP. However, levonorgestrel and etonogestrel subdermal implants have a high discontinuation rate due to menstrual irregularity and breakthrough bleeding.

    Women presenting for medroxyprogesterone acetate injection should undertake a urine pregnancy test and should receive their next injection only if the pregnancy test is negative. They also need to be advised to use additional contraceptive protection in the form of condoms.

    Guillebaud J. Your Questions Answered: Contraception (4th edn). Edinburgh: Churchill Livingstone, 2004.

2. A True.

    B True.

    C False.

    D True.

    E False.

    Bacterial vaginosis (BV) is a polymicrobial infection caused by an overgrowth of anaerobic organisms in the vagina and is the most common cause of vaginal discharge. *Gardnerella vaginalis* is a facultative, non-flagellated, non-spore-forming anaerobic bacteria, recognised as one of the organisms responsible for causing bacterial vaginosis. The other organisms involved in this pathology are bacteroides, *Peptostreptococcus, Fusobacterium, Mycoplasma hominis*, Mobiluncus and *Veillonella*.

    Anaerobes replace the normal commensal lactobacillus and thereby increase the pH (>4.5) of the vagina. Women present with an offensive vaginal discharge which is typically homogenous although there are no other associated symptoms such as itching or pain.

    BV is diagnosed by using Amsel criteria:

    *   thin grey-white, homogenous discharge
    *   clue cells on microscopy (these are epithelial cells that are coated with bacteria)
    *   vaginal pH >4.5

- release of a fishy odour on adding 10% potassium hydroxide (KOH) solution

At least three of the four criteria should be present to confirm the diagnosis.

The drug of choice for treatment is metronidazole and this can be safely used during pregnancy. It can be used in the form of tablets (400 mg twice a day for 7 days) or a vaginal gel. Intravaginal clindamycin cream 2% (nocte for 7 days) has also shown to give good results. Women taking metronidazole (not applicable to clindamycin) should be warned to avoid alcohol during treatment and at least 48 hours following the last dose of the treatment course as it may cause a disulfiram-like effect. This is true for both vaginal and oral treatment.

Magowan B. Infections: Pelvic inflammatory disease. Churchill's Pocketbook of Obstetrics and Gynaecology (3rd edn). Edinburgh: Churchill Livingstone, 2005.

3. A **False.** It is not a virus.

B **True.**

C **True.**

D **True.**

E **False.**

Chlamydia trachomatis

Chlamydia trachomatis is an obligate intracellular pathogen (gram-negative) and cannot grow outside a living cell or cell culture media. The infectious particle is an elementary body which attaches to susceptible host cells and is engulfed by phagocytosis. The intracellular body is now known as a reticulate body (non-infectious) and cannot survive outside the tissues. The intracellular body multiplies by binary fission to produce intracellular inclusions.

Classification and pathology

Chlamydia trachomatis is a sexually transmitted disease in humans. There are 15 serovariants that exhibit tropism for different organs in the body (e.g. the eye or urogenital tract). Trachoma biovariants consist of serovars A, B, Ba, C, D, E, F, G, H, I, J and K. Serovars A, B, Ba and C strains of *Chlamydia trachomatis* are associated with trachoma (a major cause for blindness worldwide). Serovars L1, L2 and L3 are associated with lymphogranuloma venereum. Serovars D to K cause non-specific urethritis and epididymitis in men and perihepatitis, cervicitis, urethritis, endometritis, salpingitis (infection of the upper genital tract, leading to PID) in women. It can cause Reiter syndrome in both men and women (conjunctivitis, mucosal ulceration and reactive seronegative arthritis), although this is rare in women.

Diagnosis and treatment

Chlamydia is the commonest bacterial sexually transmitted infection (0.5–15%) in the UK. The incubation period is 1–3 weeks. Women are generally asymptomatic and 20–40% of sexually active women have antibodies to *Chlamydia trachomatis*. It causes salpingitis, PID, bartholinitis and neonatal conjunctivitis (1–2 weeks postnatal). PID associated with perihepatitis is known as Fitz-Hugh–Curtis syndrome.

It is sensitive to doxycycline and erythromycin. Azithromycin (1 g orally, single dose) has also been used. Cervical or urethral swabs (the first sample of urine in men) are collected for culture of the organism and a nucleic acid amplification test for its diagnosis. Test of cure is not necessary as swabs may be positive for up to 4 weeks despite adequate treatment. It is important to screen and treat other people involved in the chain (contact tracing) and advise them to avoid unprotected intercourse for 2 weeks.

Long-term sequelae of Chlamydia infection

The long-term sequelae of this infection include chronic pelvic pain, infertility and ectopic pregnancy. It is also associated with increased rates of HIV transmission.

It can be transmitted to the neonate during its passage through the birth canal and may cause conjunctivitis and pneumonia.

Previous tubal surgery, previous ectopic pregnancy, PID and *in vitro* fertilisation are known risk factors for developing subsequent ectopic pregnancy. However, women should be informed that more than 50% of ectopic pregnancies occur in women without previous predisposing factors.

Magowan B. Infections: Pelvic inflammatory disease. Churchill's Pocketbook of Obstetrics and Gynaecology (3rd edn). Edinburgh: Churchill Livingstone, 2005.

4. A **True.**

    B **True.**

    C **False.**

    D **False.**

    E **False.**

Genital herpes is caused by a DNA-containing virus which belongs to the herpes virus family (other viruses in the family include Varicella-Zoster, Cytomegalovirus and Epstein–Barr virus).

Genital herpes is the most commonly reported cause of vulval ulceration in genitourinary medicine departments across the UK. Genital and oral infections can be caused by both type 1 and 2 herpes simplex (type 1 herpes simplex virus [HSV] usually causes cold sores and ocular lesions and can also cause genital lesions in 50% of cases), however most genital infections are caused by type 2 herpes simplex. They typically present with multiple shallow, flat, painful ulcers on the genital region. Secondary infections occur in 50% of patients and tend to be less severe.

The Tzanck test is used to demonstrate multinucleate giant cells. Swabs can also be taken from vesical fluid for cultures, which can then be used for diagnosis. The antiviral drug acyclovir (200 mg five times daily for 5 days) reduces the severity of symptoms when given during an acute primary attack.

One should bear in mind that herpes can be transmitted to the newborn during childbirth and that this generally occurs following primary infection of the mother near term. The risk of transmission is lower with recurrent herpes (around 3%)

due to the transfer of passive immunity. The Royal College of Obstetricians and Gynaecologists recommends a caesarean section for women if the primary attack of genital HSV infection is within 6 weeks of labour or if lesions are visible at the time of labour (there is no benefit to a caesarean section if the membranes have been ruptured for more than 4 hours).

Paediatricians should follow-up on the newborn as there is a possibility of serious infections in the neonatal period, including disseminated herpes disease (mortality rate 70–80%). Herpes infection can cause life-threatening pneumonia and encephalitis (mortality rate >90%) in the newborn with long-term sequelae.

Royal College of Obstetricians and Gynaecologists. Green-top Guideline No. 30. Management of genital herpes during pregnancy. London: RCOG Press, 2007.
Nunns D and Scott IV. Ulcers and erosions of the vulva. Personal assessment in continuing education. Reviews, questions and answers. Volume 3. London: RCOG Press, 2003.
Magowan B. Infections: Pelvic inflammatory disease. Churchill's Pocketbook of Obstetrics and Gynaecology (3rd edn). Edinburgh: Churchill Livingstone, 2005.

5. A False.

B True.

C True.

D True.

E True.

Female sterilisation is permanent and women need to be counselled appropriately prior to the procedure. It has failure rate of 1 in 200 (failure leading to pregnancy may be due to re-canalisation, poor surgical technique and conception could have occurred at the time of the procedure) while male sterilisation has a failure rate of 1 in 2000.

Tubal occlusion can be performed at any time during the menstrual cycle provided that the woman has used effective contraception up until the day of the operation. If this is not the case, the operation should be deferred until the next follicular phase of the cycle. In any case, a pregnancy test must be performed before the operation to exclude a pre-existing pregnancy. Bear in mind that a negative pregnancy test cannot exclude a luteal phase pregnancy (routine curettage at the time of operation to prevent luteal phase pregnancy is not recommended).

Tubal occlusion should be performed after an appropriate interval following pregnancy (term or abortion). They should be warned about the high regret rate and increased failure rate following tubal sterilisation during the postpartum period and after abortion. If tubal sterilisation is performed at the same time as caesarean section, appropriate counselling should have been given at least 1 week before the procedure.

All women should be warned about the increased risk of ectopic pregnancy following tubal sterilisation in the event a woman gets pregnant and she should report immediately if there is a missed period.

Male sterilisation is more effective than the female sterilisation procedure and has fewer complications associated with it. Women should also be offered alternative forms of contraception before being offered female sterilisation as they may be safer options.

Royal College of Obstetricians and Gynaecologists. Male and female sterilisation. Evidence-based Guideline No. 4. London: RCOG, 2004.
Royal College of Obstetricians and Gynaecologists. Sterilisation for men and women: what you need to know (patient information leaflet). London: RCOG, 2004.
StratOG.net. www.stratog.net
Guillebaud J. Your Questions Answered: Contraception (4th edn). Edinburgh: Churchill Livingstone, 2004.

6. A False.

    B True.

    C True.

    D True.

    E True.

The World Health Organization (WHO) classifies contraindications into four categories:

- WHO 1 – medical condition for which there is no restriction for the use of contraceptive method
- WHO 2 – medical condition where the benefits of the method generally outweigh the theoretical or proven risks
- WHO 3 – medical condition where the theoretical or proven risks usually outweigh the benefits
- WHO 4 – medical condition that represents an unacceptable health risk (absolute contraindication)

The absolute contraindications to COCPs include:

- age >51 years
- cigarette smoking 40/day
- severe or diabetic complications present (e.g. retinopathy, retinal damage)
- family history of a defined thrombophilia or an idiopathic thrombotic event in a parent
- personal history of thrombosis
- blood pressure (BP) 160/100 mmHg on repeated readings
- identified clotting abnormalities of any kind
- identified atherogenic lipid profile (family history of atherogenic lipid disorder or of an arterial cerebrovascular event in a sibling or parent)
- Wolff–Parkinson–White syndrome

Guillebaud J. Your Questions Answered: Contraception (4th edn). Edinburgh: Churchill Livingstone, 2004.

7. A False.

    B False.

    C False.

    D False.

    E True.

The failure rate for female sterilisation is around 1 in 200 or 0.5%. However, it is quoted to be slightly higher if performed in pregnant women at the time of caesarean section, during the postpartum period or immediately after an abortion. There are various reasons for failure, which include re-canalisation, poor surgical technique and conception prior to the procedure. Women should be warned that the procedure is permanent and irreversible. Recanalisation is not offered on the NHS and in case of failure of the procedure, the risk of ectopic pregnancy is increased.

Royal College of Obstetricians and Gynaecologists. Consent advice no 3: laparoscopic tubal occlusion. London: RCOG, 2004.
Royal College of Obstetricians and Gynaecologists. Male and female sterilisation. Evidence-based Guideline No. 4. London: RCOG, 2004.
Royal College of Obstetricians and Gynaecologists. Sterilisation for men and women: what you need to know (patient information leaflet). London: RCOG, 2004.
Guillebaud J. Your Questions Answered: Contraception (4th edn). Edinburgh: Churchill Livingstone, 2004.

8.   A True.

     B False.

     C True.

     D True.

     E False.

Candida albicans causes 80% of all cases of vulvovaginitis. It is mainly related to an alteration in the vaginal environment and is not considered a sexually transmitted disease. The precipitating factors include the use of broad spectrum antibiotics, diabetes, pregnancy and the use of COCPs. A definitive diagnosis can be made by microscopy (yeasts and pseudohyphae) or by culture of a high vaginal swab (Sabouraud medium). Treatment is with imidazoles (a stat dose of 500 mg clotrimazole pessary or 200 mg pessaries, one a day for 3 days). In women with a recurrent infection, treating the partner has shown no benefit.

Magowan B. Infections: Pelvic inflammatory disease. Churchill's Pocketbook of Obstetrics and Gynaecology (3rd edn). Edinburgh: Churchill Livingstone, 2005.

9.   A True.

     B True.

     C True.

     D True.

     E True.

Neisseria gonorrhoeae is a gram-negative intracellular diplococcus. Gonorrhoea is a sexually transmitted infection with an incubation period of 2–5 days in men. Women are usually asymptomatic but may present with PID, urethritis and polyarthralgia. It can also cause disseminated infection, septic arthritis and cutaneous lesions. Pharyngeal and rectal infection may be asymptomatic. Neonatal conjunctivitis manifests 2–7 days after birth. Swabs should be taken from both the urethra and cervix, and sent in a transport medium for culture. Definitive diagnosis is by culture as gram staining reveals intracellular diplococci in only 50% of cases.

In the UK, there is some resistance to azithromycin. Ceftriaxone is used for treatment.

Magowan B. Infections: Pelvic inflammatory disease. Churchill's Pocketbook of Obstetrics and Gynaecology (3rd edn). Edinburgh: Churchill Livingstone, 2005.

10. A False.

   B True.

   C True.

   D False.

   E True.

Bacterial vaginosis is a condition which occurs due to the replacement of *Lactobacillus* by anaerobes in the vagina. This raises the vaginal pH and gives a fishy odour upon addition of KOH solution to vaginal discharge (amine test). Wet microscopy shows bacteria attached to epithelial cells. Metronidazole (oral 200 mg twice daily for 7 days) and clindamycin cream 2% are the main forms of treatment. Oral ampicillin can be used for its treatment during pregnancy. Treating partners has shown no benefit.

Magowan B. Infections: Pelvic inflammatory disease. Churchill's Pocketbook of Obstetrics and Gynaecology (3rd edn). Edinburgh: Churchill Livingstone, 2005.

11. A False.

   B False.

   C True.

   D True.

   E True.

Syphilis is caused by the spirochete *Treponema pallidum*. The primary chancre is usually a solitary painless ulcer on the vulval region. Secondary syphilis is associated with a rash on the body, fever, painless lymphadenopathy, headache, bone and joint pain, and condylomata lata. The central nervous system and cardiovascular system can be involved in tertiary syphilis. During pregnancy, it can cause congenital syphilis leading to mid-trimester loss, intrauterine death, fetal growth restriction and pre-term labour. The newborn can show signs of syphilis in the form of Hutchinson triad. Penicillin injection is the treatment of choice, however if the patient is allergic to penicillin, erythromycin should be used.

Magowan B. Infections: Pelvic inflammatory disease. Churchill's Pocketbook of Obstetrics and Gynaecology (3rd edn). Edinburgh: Churchill Livingstone, 2005.

12. A False.

   B False.

   C True.

   D True.

   E True.

Victims of sexual assault can access specialist centres called havens, e.g. Whitechapel haven at Royal London Hospital, which offer both physical and emotional support for all people (women and men, young people and children of all ages) who have been raped or sexually assaulted in the last 12 months.

The management of women who have been sexually assaulted include short-term as well as long-term measures to reduce morbidity (physical, social and psychological). Emergency contraception should be offered to everybody and the method of use depends on the time of presentation, e.g. single dose of levonorgestrel 1.5 mg (up to 72 hours following intercourse) and a copper coil can be fitted (up to 5 days following intercourse). Infection screen for sexually transmitted infections can be postponed until 2–3 weeks after the assault as infections such as chlamydia have an incubation period of 14–21 days. Women should be assessed for the risk of contracting HIV and if assigned high risk, should be offered post-exposure prophylaxis.

The police should be involved only if the woman wishes to do so and has the capacity to make informed decisions. However, if you feel that there are broader issues such as the involvement of children, confidentiality can be breached in line with the General Medical Council guidelines.

A mouth swab should be ideally taken before the person cleans the mouth or has a drink. This is important for DNA analysis, to allow detection of the perpetrator.

The Havens. http://www.thehavens.co.uk/

13. **A False.** The levonorgestrel IUS acts locally to reduce endometrial proliferation and reduces menstrual blood loss by 90% after 3 months.

   B True. Breakthrough bleeding is common in the first couple of months post-insertion and usually settles down after 5 or 6 months.

   C False. It does not increase blood pressure.

   D False. It does not cause weight gain.

   E True. It can also cause abdominal discomfort (10%) and skin problems (5%).

   Guillebaud J. Your Questions Answered: Contraception (4th edn). Edinburgh: Churchill Livingstone, 2004.

14. **A True.** It reduces the number of viable gametes and implantation.

   B False. Copper IUCDs do not have any systemic side effects and can be used in women when breastfeeding.

   C False. It increases menstrual blood loss by an average of 40%.

   D True. Oral oestrogens are also used in the treatment of Asherman syndrome to promote endometrial proliferation and prevent adhesions.

   E True. It is contraindicated in women who are pregnant, have a history of previous tubal pregnancy, recurrent PID, Wilson disease, a previous history of bacterial endocarditis or a prosthetic valve replacement. Routine antibiotic prophylaxis (a single dose of oral azithromycin 1 g) is recommended for women who wish to have an IUCD.

   Guillebaud J. Your Questions Answered: Contraception (4th edn). Edinburgh: Churchill Livingstone, 2004.

15. A **True.** Periods are often irregular and amenorrhoea is common.

    B **False.** Periods are usually regular and amenorrhoea is rare.

    C **True.** Periods are very irregular and amenorrhoea is very common.

    D **False.** Periods are usually regular and amenorrhoea is rare.

    E **True.** Periods are often irregular and amenorrhoea is common.

    Guillebaud J. Your Questions Answered: Contraception (4th edn). Edinburgh: Churchill Livingstone, 2004.

16. A **False.**

    B **True.**

    C **True.**

    D **False.**

    E **False.**

    The primary action of the COCP is inhibition of ovulation. Reduction in the sperm penetrability of cervical mucus and of the receptivity of the endometrium to the blastocyst are back up mechanisms. Progesterone-only pills (POPs) mainly act by reducing the sperm penetrability of the cervical mucus via alteration of the cervical mucus. However, they can also inhibit ovulation in 50–60% of cases.

    Desogestrel (Cerazette) is a POP which contains 75 µg desogestrel. The big difference between this and other POPs is the safety margin for administration (12 hours instead of 3 hours for conventional POPs). It is also more effective in inhibiting ovulation (97–99% of menstrual cycles, unlike other POPs which do this in only 50–60% of cycles).

    Guillebaud J. Your Questions Answered: Contraception (4th edn). Edinburgh: Churchill Livingstone, 2004.

17. A **True.**

    B **True.**

    C **True.**

    D **True.**

    E **True.**

    The WHO classifies risks into four categories (contraception):

    - WHO 1 – no contraindication to COCPs
    - WHO 2 – advantages outweigh risks
    - WHO 3 – risks outweigh benefits
    - WHO 4 – absolute contraindication

    The following are absolute contraindications to COCP use:

    - age >51 years
    - body mass index >39
    - cigarette smoking >40/day
    - hypertension with blood pressure >160/100 mmHg on repeated readings

- diabetes with retinopathy or nephropathy
- migraine with aura
- identified atherogenic lipid profile
- pulmonary vascular disease
- pulmonary hypertension
- pulmonary arteriovenous malformations
- previous coronary arteritis (Kawasaki disease)
- previous cardiomyopathy with residual left ventricular dysfunction
- Fontan procedure
- Bjork–Shiley and Starr–Edwards heart valves
- cyanotic heart disease
- family history of thrombophilia
- current superficial thrombosis in upper thigh

Guillebaud J. Your Questions Answered: Contraception (4th edn). Edinburgh: Churchill Livingstone, 2004.

18. A True. Copper intrauterine devices (IUDs) act by blocking fertilisation. They cause an inflammatory reaction and inflammatory cells of the fluid in the genital tract appear to impede sperm transport and fertilisation. Phagocytosis of sperm has been reported and copper is directly toxic to sperm and ova. Implantation blocking effect acts as a backup mechanism.

B False. Desogestrel (Cerazette) is a POP which contains 75 µg desogestrel. The main difference between this and conventional POPs is that the administration or safety window is greater (12 hours), instead of the 3 hours for conventional POPs, and it inhibits ovulation in 97–99% of menstrual cycles, unlike other POPs which do this only in 50–60% of cycles and more so in older women.

C False. Its main action is anovulation by inhibition of gonadotrophins and steroidogenesis.

D False.

E True.

The WHO classifies IUCDs as WHO 1 (no contraindication) and POPs as WHO 2 (benefits outweigh risks) in women with a history of previous ectopic pregnancy.

A new concept is presented in the book 'Contraception: Your Questions Answered' by Professor John Guillebaud, an expert in contraception. The author suggests that the WHO should be cautious and that patients with past ectopic pregnancies should always be prescribed WHO 1 (IUCDs) or WHO 2 (POPs).

The author classifies the use of copper IUCDs and levonorgestrel IUSs as WHO 3 (risks outweigh benefits) in women with a previous history of ectopic pregnancy (especially nulliparous women). He advises the use of an effective anovulant, which would give maximum protection to prevent a second ectopic pregnancy, in order to preserve fertility (COCP, depot medroxyprogesterone acetate, desogestrel or etonogestrel subdermal implant) and advises against using older POPs or the mini pill which inhibit ovulation in only 50–60% of menstrual cycles.

Guillebaud J. Your Questions Answered: Contraception (4th edn). Edinburgh: Churchill Livingstone, 2004.

19. **A True.** The use of levonorgestrel IUS is recommended in women with a definitive history of menorrhagia but without intermenstrual or postcoital bleeding. Abnormal bleeding should be investigated before any therapy as there may be an underlying pathology.

    B True. Pregnancy should be ruled out before using IUCDs or IUSs.

    C True. The use of levonorgestrel IUS becomes WHO 3 when the disease is in remission and is defined by the WHO as more than 5 years.

    D True. Levonorgesterel IUS is not effective in the use of postcoital contraception and therefore is not to be used. It does not act as quickly as a copper IUCD for postcoital contraception.

    E False.

    Guillebaud J. Your Questions Answered: Contraception (4th edn). Edinburgh: Churchill Livingstone, 2004.

20. **A True.**

    B False. Trichloroacetic acid is used locally.

    C True.

    D False. 5-fluorouracil is not used in the treatment of genital warts.

    E False.

Anogenital warts

Anogenital warts are caused by the human papillomavirus (HPV) 6 and 11 and usually involve the genital and peri-anal region. The virus is transmitted via close skin-to-skin contact, although sharing toys may also pass on the infection in children. Rarely, it can be passed to the baby during childbirth. It can take a long time before it manifests clinically as warts. Most people carry the virus without developing genital warts.

Anogenital warts are one of the most common sexually transmitted infections in the UK (1–2 in 100 people with HPV infection develop anogenital warts).

Treatment of anogenital warts

No treatment:

- Some people prefer not to have any treatment. One third of cases resolve themselves in 6 months.

Chemical treatments:

- Podophyllotoxin (cream or lotion): can be applied twice daily for 3 days followed by 4 days rest (generally the whole treatment cycle lasts about 4 to 5 weeks). However, one should not use it if pregnant, on broken skin or open wounds. It is important to avoid sexual contact immediately after local application as it may cause genital irritation for the partner.
- Imiquimod cream is an immune response modifier. It can be applied at bedtime and washed off 10–12 hours later. This can be repeated three times per week

for up to 16 weeks. It is important to use effective contraception while using the cream as this can weaken condoms and diaphragms. Women should not use it if they are pregnant, have broken skin or open wounds.

- Trichloroacetic acid: is applied once a week for several weeks.

Physical treatments:

- cryotherapy
- surgical removal of warts
- electrocautery
- laser therapy

Soft warts respond well to local application of podophyllin, podophyllotoxin, trichloroacetic acid and imiquimod.

Thickened and keratinised warts should be treated with cryotherapy or surgical excision. Almost all treatments have high failure and relapse rates. Therefore women should be appropriately counselled before treatment. The side effects include local discomfort, pain and allergic reactions. Contact tracing and treatment is recommended, especially for any current partners.

Anogenital warts. http://www.patient.co.uk/health/Anogenital-Warts.htm

Section B

EMQs

Chapter 16

Adolescent gynaecology

Questions 1–5

Options for Questions 1–5

A Autoimmune ovarian failure
B Constitutional delay
C Craniopharyngioma
D Etoposide
E Galactosaemia
F Iatrogenic
G Irradiation
H Kallmann syndrome

I Laurence–Moon–Bardet–Biedl syndrome
J Langerhans cell histiocytosis
K McCune–Albright syndrome
L Noonan syndrome
M Rubella
N Turner syndrome
O Tuberculosis

Instructions: For each clinical scenario described below, choose the **single** most appropriate diagnosis from the list of options above. Each option may be used once, more than once, or not at all.

1. A 16-year-old girl attends her general practitioner centre with her mother as she has not attained menarche. Clinical examination reveals a short stature, cubitus valgus and coarctation of the aorta. Ultrasound scan shows streak gonads.

2. A 15-year-old girl attends the paediatric emergency department with a fall. Clinical examination reveals a short stature, hypertelorism, downward slanting of the eyes and a right-sided heart murmur.

3. A 14-year-old girl attends her general practitioner centre with her mother as she has not attained menarche. She has a history of an unknown cancer at the age of 10 years and had received chemotherapy in Pakistan.

4. A 7-year-old girl attends the paediatric emergency department with her mother as she started to have monthly vaginal bleeding. Clinical examination reveals incomplete sexual precocity and café-au-lait spots with irregular borders.

5. A 6-year-old girl is brought to her general practitioner by her mother as she started to have vaginal bleeding. Clinical examination is normal. She was prescribed steroid hormonal cream by a local general practitioner in Pakistan, to be applied in the vulval area, as she had itching 6 months ago.

Questions 6–10

Options for Questions 6–10

A	Angelman syndrome	I	Mayer–Rokitansky–Küster–Hauser
B	Androgen insensitivity syndrome		syndrome
C	Congenital adrenal hyperplasia	J	Fragile X syndrome
D	Gonadal dysgenesis	K	Pituitary tumour
E	Hypothyroidism	L	Pituitary prolactinoma
F	Hyperprolactinaemia	M	Turner syndrome (45XO)
G	Noonan syndrome	N	Turner mosaic (45XO/46XX)
H	Klinefelter syndrome	O	von Hippel–Lindau disease

Instructions: For each scenario described below, choose the **single** most appropriate diagnosis for amenorrhoea from the list of options above. Each option may be used once, more than once, or not at all.

6. A 16-year-old tall girl presents with primary amenorrhoea. On clinical examination there is normal breast development, sparse axillary and pubic hair, blind vaginal pouch and an absent uterus.

7. A 16-year-old young girl is referred to the gynaecology clinic by her general practitioner with primary amenorrhoea. She gives a history of excessive weight gain and lethargy. Secondary sexual characters are normal on clinical examination. Investigations reveal raised serum thyroid-stimulating hormone (TSH) and prolactin levels.

8. A 16-year-old tall girl presents with primary amenorrhoea. She has been taking medication for psychosis since the age of 13 years.

9. A 16-year-old tall girl presents with primary amenorrhoea. She gives a history of visual disturbance for the last year. She has changed her glasses twice in the last year and her blood sugars are normal. Clinical examination reveals bitemporal hemianopia.

10. A 16-year-old girl is referred to the gynaecology clinic by her general practitioner with primary amenorrhoea. She has recently been unwell, hospitalised and diagnosed with coarctation of aorta and a renal abnormality. Blood tests' results are suggestive of autoimmune hypothyroidism.

Questions 11–15

Options for Questions 11–15

A	Adrenal adenoma	I	Hypothyroidism
B	Adrenal carcinoma	J	Hyperthyroidism
C	Anorexia nervosa	K	Hyperprolactinaemia
D	Bulimia nervosa	L	Late onset congenital adrenal
E	Cushing disease		hyperplasia
F	Cushing syndrome	M	Polycystic ovary syndrome
G	Gynandroblastoma	N	Premature menopause
H	Hypothalamic cause	O	Sheehan syndrome

Instructions: For each clinical scenario described below, choose the **single** most appropriate cause of amenorrhoea from the list of options above. Each option may be used once, more than once, or not at all.

11. A 22-year-old woman, who is studying at university, presents to her general practitioner with amenorrhoea during the last 6 months. She has a body mass index of 15 but she thinks she is overweight and goes to the gym every day. Her urine pregnancy test is negative. A blood test reveals slightly low follicle-stimulating hormone (FSH) and luteinising hormone (LH) levels.

12. A 30-year-old woman presents to her general practitioner with amenorrhoea (lasting a year). She gives a history of an intraductal carcinoma of the breast (T2L2M1) 18 months previously. Subsequently, she received three cycles of chemotherapy followed by a left-sided mastectomy. Four weeks later she received radiotherapy for the left breast and axilla. She has one child and wants to conceive.

13. A 20-year-old woman is referred to the gynaecology clinic having had amenorrhoea for the past 6 months and a negative pregnancy test. She has recently noticed an increased growth of hair on the face, chin and chest with clitoromegaly. Her blood test results show very high levels of 17-hydroxyprogesterone.

14. A 25-year-old woman presents to her general practitioner with a history of amenorrhoea for the last 6 months. She is an athlete and has recently participated in the Olympics. Her serum FSH and LH levels are normal.

15. A 20-year-old woman presents to her general practitioner with facial hirsutism and irregular periods for the past year. She has recently put on weight and her body mass index is 28.

Answers

1. N Turner syndrome

Turner syndrome is the most common cause of gonadal failure in young girls. Short stature is the most common clinical presentation in childhood; however, young girls may present with primary amenorrhoea during pubertal age. The most common chromosomal abnormality is 45XO, followed mosaicism and by X isochromosomes.

2. L Noonan syndrome

Noonan syndrome is an autosomal dysmorphic syndrome. It is characterised by hypertelorism (an increase in distance between the inner canthi of eyes), downward slanting of the eyes, low set posteriorly rotated ears, short stature and right-sided cardiac anomalies. The incidence is 1 in 2500 live births.

3. D Etoposide

Chemotherapy is one of the most common causes of ovarian failure in peripubertal children. Etoposide, procarbazine and nitrosourea can cause permanent ovarian failure while transient ovarian failure is associated with vincristine.

4. K McCune–Albright syndrome

Breast development corresponding to Tanner stage 2 before the age of 8 years in a girl is considered as precocious puberty in the UK. It is also known as central precocious puberty and is caused by the premature activation of the hypothalamic-pituitary-gonadal axis.

McCune–Albright syndrome is caused by a somatic activating mutation of the alpha subunit of G proteins. Most cases are sporadic but autosomal dominant inheritance has been reported. It is characterised by incomplete sexual precocity, café-au-lait pigmentation and polyostotic fibrous dysplasia. The sexual precocity in this condition is independent of gonadotrophins.

5. F Iatrogenic

Exogenous steroids are a well-known cause of sexual precocity. The most common drugs used are oestrogen–containing creams and pills. Other potential sources of oestrogens include soy formulas and ginseng cream (phyto-oestrogens).

Banerjee K. Puberty delayed. In: Hollingworth T (ed). Differential Diagnosis in Obstetrics and Gynaecology: An A–Z. London: Hodder Arnold, 2008.
Banerjee K. Puberty precocious. In: Hollingworth T (ed). Differential Diagnosis in Obstetrics and Gynaecology: An A–Z. London: Hodder Arnold, 2008.
Balen A. Chapter 14: Disorders of puberty. In: Shaw RW, Luesley D, Monga A (eds). Gynaecology (4th edn). Edinburgh: Churchill Livingstone, 2011.

Critchley HOD, Horne A, Munro K. Chapter 16: Amenorrhoea and oligomenorrhoea, and hypothalamic–pituitary dysfunction. In: Shaw RW, Luesley D, Monga A (eds). Gynaecology (4th edn). Edinburgh: Churchill Livingstone, 2011.

6. B Androgen insensitivity syndrome

Androgen insensitivity syndrome is an X-linked recessive inherited disorder. The karyotype is 46XY (male genotype) and external genitalia usually appear female. Breast development is normal with sparse axillary and pubic hair. Genital examination will reveal a short, blind vaginal pouch with an absent uterus. Cases with partial androgen insensitivity syndrome can present with ambiguous genitalia at birth and this poses real difficulty in gender assignment. The gonads should be removed after puberty in view of the high incidence of developing malignancy (gonadoblastoma) in the future (approximately 5%).

7. E Hypothyroidism

Hypothyroidism can be associated with hyperprolactinaemia in 3–5% of cases.

8. F Hyperprolactinaemia

Drugs used to treat psychosis (e.g. haloperidol, reserpine) can cause hyperprolactinaemia (pharmacological therapy is associated with hyperprolactinaemia in 1–2% of cases). Other drugs that can cause hyperprolactinaemia include metoclopramide, methyldopa, phenothiazines (trifluoperazine, prochlorperazine, chlorpromazine, thioridazine) and cimetidine.

Hyperprolactinaemia is characterised by abnormally high levels of prolactin that is normally down-regulated by dopamine in the hypothalamus. Hence, dopamine agonists are the mainstay of treatment.

Hyperprolactinaemia can be caused by reduced dopamine levels, increased production of prolactin from a prolactinoma or compression of the pituitary stalk by non-prolactin secreting tumours such as craniopharyngiomas, chromophobe adenomas or growth hormone secreting tumours. Prolactinomas can be microadenomas or macroadenomas. Two per cent of patients with microadenomas develop symptoms or signs of tumour progression during pregnancy, while 15% do so with macroadenomas.

Drugs used in the treatment of hyperprolactinaemia

Bromocriptine:

- dopamine agonist
- dose: start with the lowest dose of 1.25 mg at bedtime and gradually increase to 7.5 mg in divided doses daily
- common side effects: nausea, vomiting, headache and postural hypotension
- may cause adverse psychiatric effects at the beginning of therapy
- the side effects can be minimised by taking the tablets at bedtime

Cabergoline:

- long-acting dopamine agonist
- dose: start with 0.25–1 mg twice weekly and this can be increased to 1 mg daily
- fewer side effects compared to bromocriptine
- can be used in women who cannot tolerate bromocriptine due to its side effects
- may cause adverse psychiatric effects
- it is not licensed for use in pregnancy
- a single dose (1 mg) can be used for breast milk suppression in women with fetal loss

Quinagolide:

- long-acting dopamine agonist
- dose: 25–150 µg daily in divided doses
- fewer side effects compared to bromocriptine
- can be used in women who cannot tolerate bromocriptine due to its side effects
- may cause adverse psychiatric effects
- it is not licensed for use in pregnancy

9. L Pituitary prolactinoma

The most common causes of hyperprolactinaemia are pituitary prolactinomas (found in 40–50% of cases) and idiopathic hypersecretion. Pituitary prolactinomas can present with visual disturbances especially visual field defects as the prolactinoma presses on the optic chiasma (nasal fibres which represent the temporal field are affected). In view of this, visual field testing will reveal bitemporal hemianopia. Blood tests will reveal hyperprolactinaemia and computed tomography (CT) or magnetic resonance imaging (MRI) will show a pituitary tumour.

10. M Turner syndrome

Turner syndrome (XO) is associated with congenital heart defects (coarctation of the aorta).

Critchley HOD, Horne A, Munro K. Chapter 16: Amenorrhoea and oligomenorrhoea, and hypothalamic–pituitary dysfunction. In: Shaw RW, Luesley D, Monga A (eds). Gynaecology (4th edn). Edinburgh: Churchill Livingstone, 2011.
Balen A. Chapter 14: Disorders of puberty. In: Shaw RW, Luesley D, Monga A (eds). Gynaecology (4th edn). Edinburgh: Churchill Livingstone, 2011.

11. C Anorexia nervosa

Anorexia nervosa is more commonly seen in adolescent females than males. It is an eating disorder characterised by a low body weight, distortion of the body image and an obsessive fear of gaining weight. It can involve the hypothalamic-pituitary-gonadal axis causing hypothalamic amenorrhoea (usually if body mass index <18).

12. N Premature menopause

Chemotherapy drugs used in the treatment of breast cancer are toxic to the ovary and can cause premature menopause.

13. L Late onset congenital adrenal hyperplasia

An increase in the growth of hair on the face, chin and chest, deepening of the voice clitoromegaly, male pattern hair loss and an increase in muscle bulk are symptoms of virilisation (excessive androgen levels). These can be symptoms of virilising adrenal adenoma, adrenal carcinoma, adrenal hyperplasia and some ovarian tumours. Serum levels for androgens such as testosterone, dehydroepiandrosterone sulphate and urinary 17-ketosteroid excretion, are generally well above the normal range in virilising adrenal tumours. Failure to suppress androgen secretion after the administration of dexamethasone is normally indicative of a virilising adrenal tumour. An MRI scan of the abdomen and pelvis should be arranged to rule out virilising adrenal and ovarian tumours.

Congenital adrenal hyperplasia (CAH) is a form of adrenal insufficiency. About 95% of cases of CAH are caused because of the lack of enzyme 21-hydroxylase, resulting in the inadequate production of two vital hormones; cortisol and aldosterone; but an increase in the production of androgens via alternative pathways in hormone synthesis. CAH can present at birth, early childhood, late childhood and adulthood. The late onset, or non-classical, form is usually milder and may manifest during adolescence or even later in women. It can present with hirsutism, acne, anovulation and infertility. The diagnosis is usually made from very high levels of serum 17-hydroxyprogesterone. The treatment is low dose glucocorticoids.

14. H Hypothalamic cause

Amenorrhoea due to weight loss, excessive exercise and stress are usually due to a hypothalamic cause.

15. M Polycystic ovary syndrome

Polycystic ovaries are commonly seen in 25% of women in the reproductive age. It is defined as polycystic ovary syndrome (PCOS) when associated with symptoms such as menstrual irregularity, hirsutism and anovulation.

PCOS: definition by the Rotterdam European Society for Human Reproduction and Embryology (ESHRE) and the American Society of Reproductive Medicine (ASRM) PCOS Consensus Workshop Group.

Two of the three following criteria should be present to diagnose PCOS:

- polycystic ovaries (either 12 or more peripheral follicles or increased ovarian volume (>10 cm^3)

- clinical and/or biochemical signs of hyperandrogenism
- oligo- or anovulation

Women who are overweight or obese should be advised to lose weight (5–10% weight loss can correct menstrual irregularity) as this corrects hormonal imbalance, reduces insulin resistance and initiates ovulation in such women. However, one should treat patients symptomatically (e.g. hirsutism, irregular periods, infertility). All women should be counselled about the short-term (infertility, menstrual irregularity and hirsutism) and the long-term implications (hypertension, type 2 diabetes, ischaemic heart disease and endometrial cancer) of PCOS.

Royal College of Obstetricians and Gynaecologists. Green-top Guideline No. 33. Long-term consequences of polycystic ovarian syndrome. London: RCOG Press, 2007.
Critchley HOD, Horne A, Munro K. Chapter 16: Amenorrhoea and oligomenorrhoea, and hypothalamic–pituitary dysfunction. In: Shaw RW, Luesley D, Monga A (eds). Gynaecology (4th edn). Edinburgh: Churchill Livingstone, 2011.

Chapter 17

Antenatal care

Questions 1–5

Options for Questions 1–5

A	Bursitis of the knee joint
B	Dislocation of the hip
C	Fracture of sacral promontory
D	Fracture of the pubic bone
E	Lumbosacral disc prolapse
F	Mechanical back pain
G	Osteitis pubis
H	Osteomyelitis of pubis
I	Osteomyelitis of the hip
J	Osteoma of the hip
K	Pregnancy-induced osteomalacia
L	Symphysis pubis dysfunction
M	Sciatica
N	Subluxation of the sacral promontory
O	Transient osteoporosis of pregnancy affecting the hip joint
P	Tuberculosis of the spine or Pott disease

Instructions: For each clinical scenario described below, choose the **single** most appropriate diagnosis from the list of options above. Each option may be used once, more than once, or not at all.

1. A 42-year-old woman attends her antenatal appointment at 28 weeks of gestation. A waddling gait is seen on entering the examination room. She complains of a burning pain in the pubic region during walking, standing on one leg and parting her legs. Clinical examination reveals tenderness on the sacroiliac joint and restriction of the abduction and lateral rotation of hip.

2. A 42-year-old woman attends the obstetric day assessment unit at 28 weeks of gestation with low grade pyrexia and reduced hip movements due to severe pain. Clinical examination reveals tenderness over the pubic symphysis and pubic rami, painful abduction of the hip and pain on lateral compression of the pelvis. She gives a history of recurrent urinary tract infection in the past and recently had stenting of the ureters for ureteric stricture. X-ray of the pelvis shows widening as well as bony erosions of the symphysis pubis.

3. A 42-year-old woman attends the obstetric day assessment unit at 28 weeks of gestation. A waddling gait is seen on entering the examination room. She complains of pain in the pubic region which is radiating to the groin and thigh. She also explains that the pain is aggravated on climbing stairs and lying on one side in bed. The other aggravating factors for pain include coughing and sneezing. Examination of her hips reveals tenderness on compression of the right as well as left trochanters.

4. A 42-year-old Asian woman, para 5, attends her antenatal appointment at 28 weeks of gestation. She complains of non-specific pain in the lumbosacral and pubic

regions. Blood tests reveal low serum calcium but raised alkaline phosphatase. Pseudofractures (Looser zones) are reported on the X-ray of the pubic bone.

5. A 42-year-old Asian woman, para 3, attends the obstetric day assessment unit at 28 weeks of gestation. She complains of pain in her left hip and the anterior aspect of her left knee (especially during walking). Clinical examination reveals no tenderness on pubic symphysis and an ultrasound scan of the left hip joint shows effusion.

Questions 6–10

Options for Questions 6–10

A Amniocentesis and viral culture	acyclovir to the neonate
B Fetal blood sampling	J Administer intravenous ganciclovir to
C Intravenous acyclovir	the neonate
D Offer termination following thorough	K Administer intravenous zidovudine to
counselling	the neonate
E Offer rubella immunoglobulin	L Vaccinate the mother against rubella
F Refer to fetal medicine unit for special	M Vaccinate the newborn against
scan	rubella
G Refer to virology department	N Vaccinate the mother against
H Reassure	chickenpox
I Administer prophylactic intravenous	O Vaccinate the fetus against chickenpox

Instructions: For each clinical scenario described below, choose the **single** most appropriate management option from the list of options above. Each option may be used once, more than once, or not at all.

6. A 40-year-old woman, para 4, had a forceps delivery and is very excited about her baby. She was about to be discharged on postnatal day 2 but finds out from her husband that her first child has developed rubella. She is really worried about taking her newborn baby home. Her virology results at booking (her first midwife appointment) reveal that she is immune to rubella.

7. A 30-year-old woman, para 10, presents to the early pregnancy assessment unit (EPAU) for advice as she recently had a rash (2 weeks ago) and was found to have rubella. She gives a history of a positive urine pregnancy test and has mild spotting. Clinically, the diagnosis is a threatened miscarriage and an ultrasound scan reveals an 8 week, single, viable, intrauterine pregnancy.

8. A 35-year-old woman, para 0, calls a heath service helpline at 35 weeks of gestation. She is very anxious as she had contact with her nephew who developed a rubella rash 1 week ago. She wants to know if her baby will be affected. Her booking virology tests results show an immunity to rubella.

9. A 40-year-old woman, para 3, has suffered from epilepsy for the last 20 years. She comes to her general practitioner for preconception counselling. Currently she is on carbamazepine 400 mg per day and has read about the risks to the baby if she gets pregnant. She has recently started taking folic acid (5 g) daily as she is

planning to conceive. She gives a history of vaccination against rubella in the past. However, her booking blood tests reveal that she is not immune to rubella.

10. A 30-year-old woman, para 4, had a normal vaginal delivery 6 hours ago. She possibly does not want to have more children in the future but is currently considering using reliable contraception. She is about to be discharged home and the midwife finds out that her booking blood tests revealed IgG antibodies to rubella.

Questions 11–15

Options for Questions 11–15

A   Commence intravenous prophylactic unfractionated heparin

B   Change to prophylactic intravenous unfractionated heparin

C   Change to heparinoid danaparoid sodium

D   Change to low-molecular weight heparin (LMWH)

E   Commence prophylactic low molecular heparin

F   Commence dalteparin

G   Monitor anti-Xa levels

H   Remove catheter 3 hours after giving heparin

I   Remove catheter 8 hours after giving the last dose of heparin

J   Remove catheter 12 hours after giving the last dose of heparin

K   Remover catheter 24 hours after giving the last dose of heparin

L   Withhold heparin for 12 hours before giving spinal anaesthesia

M   Withhold heparin 24 hours before giving spinal anaesthesia

N   Withhold heparin for 24 hours before giving epidural anaesthesia

O   Withhold heparin for 48 hours before giving epidural anaesthesia

Instructions: For each scenario described below, choose the **single** most appropriate management option from the list of options above. Each option may be used once, more than once, or not at all.

11. A 43-year-old woman, para 3, presents to the EPAU at 12 weeks of gestation with mild vaginal bleeding. She gives a history of unprovoked deep venous thrombosis (DVT) 1 year prior to this pregnancy and was treated with warfarin for 6 months. Currently, the general practitioner has started her on aspirin in view of a previous history of pre-eclampsia.

12. A 40-year-old woman, para 2, presents to the obstetric day assessment unit at 28 weeks of gestation with reduced fetal movements (normal cardiotocograph [CTG]). Her notes indicate that she had DVT at 20 weeks of gestation during her current pregnancy and is on 80 mg LMWH twice daily. Her booking blood results were normal. However, her recent blood test reveals a platelet count of 60×10^9/L.

13. A 30-year-old woman, para 1 (delivered 8 hours ago), gives a history of previous thrombophilia. Her mode of delivery was caesarean section for a prolonged second stage of labour. She had a massive postpartum haemorrhage and her current haemoglobin level is 8 g/dL. The midwife comes to you to inform you about the minimal soakage of the caesarean section wound dressing.

14. A 33-year-old woman, para 3, is reviewed by the senior house officer in the postnatal ward. She had a caesarean section for failure to progress and has been using an epidural for pain relief for the last 4 hours following caesarean section. The midwife has just given her the first dose of prophylactic LMWH postnatally.

15. A 38-year-old woman, gravid 3, para 2, is admitted to the antenatal ward for an elective caesarean section for breech presentation. She had a pulmonary embolism during this pregnancy and has been on a therapeutic dose of LMWH (90 mg twice daily) for the last 3 months. She took her last dose just before coming into the ward.

Questions 16–20

Options for Questions 16–20

A   LMWH plus low dose heparin
B   LMWH not recommended
C   LMWH during antenatal period
D   Low dose aspirin only
E   Prophylactic LMWH during labour
F   Prophylactic LMWH postnatally for 7 days
G   Prophylactic LMWH postnatally for 6 weeks
H   Prophylactic LMWH antenatally plus postnatally for 6 weeks
I   Prophylactic LMWH antenatally plus postnatally for 5 days
J   Therapeutic dose of LMWH antenatally
K   Therapeutic dose of LMWH antenatally and postnatally
L   Therapeutic dose of LMWH antenatally and prophylactic dose postnatally
M   Unfractionated heparin all through the antenatal period
N   Unfractionated heparin during the postnatal period
O   Unfractionated heparin during labour

Instructions: For each scenario described below, choose the **single** most appropriate management from the list of options above. Each option may be used once, more than once, or not at all.

16. A 36-year-old obese nulliparous woman (body mass index >30) attends the maternal medicine obstetric clinic for a review at 38 weeks of gestation to discuss mode of delivery, as her ultrasound scan shows a breech presentation. Subsequently, she undergoes an elective caesarean section at 39 weeks of gestation and was discharged home on the second postoperative day.

17. A 36-year-old nulliparous woman attends the early pregnancy assessment unit at 10 weeks of gestation with minimal vaginal bleeding. A transvaginal scan reveals triplets. Medical history unveils that she had single episode of axillary venous thrombosis 3 years ago. She was investigated adequately but no cause was found.

18. A 36-year-old obese nulliparous woman attends the antenatal clinic for her first consultation with the doctor at 20 weeks of gestation (her ultrasound scan shows a low lying placenta). A further review was done at 34 weeks of gestation as her repeat scan also showed a low lying placenta. Subsequently, she undergoes an elective caesarean section at 38 weeks of gestation because of the increased vaginal bleeding (She loses 2000 mL of blood). She recovers well following 3 units of blood

transfusion. The senior house officer discharges her on postnatal day 3. However, 5 days later she presents to the emergency department with a spiking temperature due to caesarean section wound infection and is admitted to the gynaecology ward for intravenous antibiotic therapy.

19. A 36-year-old woman, para 5, attends the antenatal clinic for a review at 20 weeks of gestation. A general examination reveals a body mass index of 41 and varicose veins. Her anomaly scan and booking bloods are normal.

20. A 31-year-old woman attends the antenatal clinic for review at 20 weeks of gestation. She suddenly remembers to tell you that she had superficial thrombophlebitis 6 months prior to pregnancy which resolved with no residual signs.

Questions 21–25

Options for Questions 21–25

A   Anti-D immunoglobulin 50 IU
B   Anti-D immunoglobulin 100 IU
C   Anti-D immunoglobulin 200 IU
D   Anti-D immunoglobulin 250 IU
E   Anti-D immunoglobulin 500 IU
F   Anti-D immunoglobulin 1000 IU
G   Anti-D immunoglobulin 1500 IU
H   Anti-D immunoglobulin 2000 IU
I   Anti-D immunoglobulin is not recommended or indicated
J   Anti-D immunoglobulin is indicated in next pregnancy
K   Anti-D immunoglobulin is not indicated in next pregnancy
L   Anti-D immunoglobulin is indicated in all future miscarriages
M   Anti-D immunoglobulin is indicated in all future pregnancies
N   Anti-D immunoglobulin to all her family members
O   Anti-D immunoglobulin to all her siblings

Instructions: For each scenario described below, choose the **single** most appropriate action from the list of options above. Each option may be used once, more than once, or not at all.

21. A 20-year-old woman presents to her general practitioner requesting a termination of an unwanted pregnancy. She had some vaginal bleeding 1 week ago and attended the EPAU at her local hospital. A scan showed a single viable intrauterine pregnancy of 11 weeks gestation. The general practitioner refers her to a clinic for a termination of pregnancy. She undergoes abortion 2 weeks later. However, her blood tests reveal that she is Rhesus (RhD)-negative and positive for antibodies to Rhesus D antigen.

22. A 20-year-old woman attends the EPAU with mild vaginal bleeding. She has just missed her period and the urine pregnancy test is positive. An ultrasound scan shows a single viable intrauterine pregnancy of 5 weeks gestation. Her blood group is 'AB' negative and has anti-Kell antibodies.

23. A 20-year-old woman attends the obstetric day assessment unit at 21 weeks of gestation with minimal vaginal bleeding. Clinically, her abdomen is soft with no

contractions. Her cervix, vagina and vulva are normal. An obstetric ultrasound scan reveals a 22-weeks fetus with anterior low lying placenta. Her booking blood tests reveal 'O' negative blood group with no antibodies.

24. A 20-year-old woman attends the EPAU at 8 weeks of gestation. She complains of very minimal lower abdominal pain and mild vaginal bleeding. An ultrasound scan shows a left-sided ectopic pregnancy (2 × 2 cm in size) with no free fluid in the pelvis. Clinically, she is stable and comfortable. Following appropriate counselling, she decides to have medical management by methotrexate and is willing to be followed up closely by the EPAU to review her symptoms and test for βhCG. Her blood tests reveal haemoglobin 14 g% and 'B' negative blood group. There are antibodies to Duffy antigen.

25. A 20-year-woman attends the obstetric day assessment unit at 36 weeks of pregnancy with an antepartum haemorrhage. She had received anti-D immunoglobulin at 32 weeks of gestation as her blood group is 'O' negative with no antibodies. Clinically, she is stable and speculum examination reveals minimal vaginal bleeding but closed cervical os. An ultrasound scan reveals a viable baby with normal growth, liquor and placental location.

Questions 26–30

Options for Questions 26–30

A Anti-D immunoglobulin injection	I ECV not indicated
B Allow vaginal breech delivery	J Offer ECV at 36 weeks gestation
C Abandon external cephalic version	K Offer ECV at 37 weeks gestation
D Conduct vaginal breech delivery	L Follow up in 1 week in the antenatal
E Elective caesarean section	clinic
F Emergency caesarean section	M Repeat ECV in 1 week
G Emergency caesarean section not	N Repeat ECV after tocolysis
indicated	O Vaginal breech delivery
H External cephalic version (ECV)	contraindicated
contraindicated	

Instructions: For each clinical scenario described below, choose the **single** most appropriate intervention with regards to breech presentation from the list of options above. Each option may be used once, more than once, or not at all.

26. A 39-year-old multiparous woman presents to the antenatal clinic at 36 weeks of gestation for a routine review. Abdominal examination reveals breech presentation and an ultrasound scan reveals footling breech presentation with normal amniotic fluid.

27. A 39-year-old nulliparous woman presents to the antenatal clinic at 36 weeks of gestation for a routine review. Clinical examination reveals breech presentation. An ultrasound reveals extended breech with normal amniotic fluid.

28. A 39-year-old multiparous woman comes into the labour ward at 39 weeks of gestation for an ECV. After 15 minutes of abdominal manipulation, the ECV is

successful. However, post-ECV, the CTG reveals bradycardia which recovers to baseline after 3 minutes followed by a normal trace. Clinically, her abdomen is soft with no tenderness.

29. A 39-year-old nulliparous woman presents to the obstetric day assessment unit at 36 weeks of gestation with mild to moderate vaginal bleeding. Clinical examination reveals a soft abdomen with a normal cervix and vagina, with no active vaginal bleeding. A formal departmental ultrasound scan shows breech presentation with normal growth and liquor with a posterior low lying placenta. She is admitted for 24 hours for observation and is then discharged home. Three days later she attends the labour ward as she is booked for an ECV. You are the registrar on call for the labour ward on that day.

30. A 39-year-old multiparous woman presents to the labour ward at 40 weeks of gestation with contractions. You are called to review the woman as the midwife is not sure about the presentation. A clinical examination reveals 4 cm cervical dilatation and footling breech presentation. She has a history of precipitous delivery with her last two deliveries.

Questions 31–35

Options for Questions 31–35

A	*Actinomyces*	I	*Plasmodium vivax*
B	*Bacillus anthracis*	J	*Plasmodium ovale*
C	*Chlamydia trachomatis*	K	*Plasmodium falciparum*
D	*Escherichia coli*	L	*Staphylococcus aureus*
E	*Gardnerella vaginalis*	M	*Treponema pallidum*
F	Group B streptococcus	N	Tuberculosis
G	*Molluscum contagiosum*	O	Yaws
H	*Mycoplasma hominis*		

Instructions: For each fact described below, choose the **single** most likely organism from the list of options above. Each option may be used once, more than once, or not at all.

31. Afro-Caribbeans with a Duffy negative blood group antigen are less susceptible to this particular bacterial infection.

32. Women with sickle cell trait are less susceptible to this particular bacterial infection.

33. Fetal ingestion of infected fluid, aspiration of infected amniotic fluid and haematogenous infection via umbilical vein are proposed mechanisms of infection.

34. Antibiotic prophylaxis is recommended for pregnant women during the intrapartum period with this particular infection.

35. This particular organism can cause neonatal conjunctivitis and pneumonia.

Questions 36–40

Options for Questions 36–40

A	Aortic dissection	I	Mitral valve prolapse
B	Aortic stenosis	J	Peripartum cardiomyopathy
C	Aortic regurgitation	K	Patent ductus arteriosus
D	Coarctation of the aorta	L	Rheumatic heart disease
E	Epstein anomaly	M	Transposition of aorta
F	Eisenmenger syndrome	N	Tricuspid regurgitation
G	Hypertrophic cardiomyopathy	O	Ventricular septal defect
H	Mitral regurgitation		

Instructions: For each scenario described below, choose the **single** most appropriate diagnosis from the list of options above. Each option may be used once, more than once, or not at all.

36. A 42-year-old Bangladeshi woman presents to the emergency department at 32 weeks of gestation with distension of the abdomen. An abdominal scan reveals a congested liver and minimal ascites. An echocardiogram shows left ventricular dilatation with an ejection fraction of 15%. Clinical examination reveals a respiratory rate of 26 breaths/minute and an oxygen saturation of 95%. She is para 10 with all normal vaginal deliveries. She speaks no English.

37. A 28-year-old woman is brought to the emergency department at 25 weeks of gestation with acute severe chest pain radiating to the back. She has a lifelong history of Marfan syndrome but has remained well for the last 18 years. She is hypertensive and currently on methyldopa 250 mg three times a day. General examination reveals a blood pressure of 180/80 mmHg, pulse 120 beats/minute and respiratory rate 22 breaths/minute.

38. A 20-year-old Asian woman presents to the obstetric day assessment unit at 24 weeks of gestation with palpitations. A cardiovascular system examination reveals a mid systolic click and late systolic murmur.

39. A 42-year-old Asian woman presents to the emergency department 4 weeks post delivery with increasing shortness of breath while lying flat. On cardiovascular examination the apical impulse is diffuse and displaced downwards. A chest radiograph shows cardiomegaly and a respiratory system examination reveals vesicular breath sounds with fine basal crepitations.

40. A 35-year-old woman, para 1, presents with syncope at 20 weeks of gestation. A cardiovascular examination reveals an ejection systolic murmur, double apical pulsation and arrhythmia. She was started on beta-blockers following which her symptoms improved gradually. She gives a history of the sudden death of her cousin who was 18 years old.

Answers

1. L Symphysis pubic dysfunction

Symphysis pubis dysfunction is common during pregnancy and results from instability of the pelvic girdle owing to laxity or diastasis of the pubic symphysis joint. The incidence varies from 1 in 36 to 1 in 300 pregnancies in the UK (this is related to a deficiency in objective criteria for diagnosing this condition). Symptoms include pubic bone pain (burning, stabbing or shooting) during walking, turning over in bed, standing on one leg and lifting and parting of legs. The pain can also radiate to the lower abdomen, perineum, groin, thigh, leg and lower back.

Clinical examination usually reveals tenderness over the pubic symphysis or sacroiliac joint, positive Trendelenburg sign (sagging of the opposite buttock when the patient is asked to stand on one leg) and positive Patrick's Fabere sign. (With one iliac spine held in a fixed position by the doctor who is examining, the woman lies in a supine position, placing her opposite heel on the ipsilateral knee with the leg falling passively outwards. The test is positive if pain occurs in either sacroiliac joint.) A waddling gait is seen in extreme cases.

2. H Osteomyelitis of the pubis

Osteomyelitis of the pubis is a rare condition and is caused by low grade infection of the pubic bone. It may occur following gynaecological surgery (2–12 weeks later), urogenital procedures or operative delivery. Common symptoms include tenderness over the pubic rami or symphysis pubis, reduced painful hip movements (especially abduction) and pain on the lateral compression of the pelvis. Low grade pyrexia is a systemic feature. Haematological investigations reveal normocytic normochromic anaemia, increased white blood cell count and C-reactive protein. Blood and urine cultures are positive in 50% of cases.

Radioisotope bone scans show an increase in uptake but are not recommended for use during pregnancy.

3. G Osteitis pubis

Osteitis pubis is a painful inflammatory condition involving the pubic region in a symmetrical fashion. The cause is mostly idiopathic although it can be associated with pregnancy, seronegative spondyloarthritis, urogenital procedures and trauma. The symptoms are pain in the pubic region, which is aggravated by climbing stairs, kicking and pivoting (rotating or spin) on one leg. X-rays of the pubic bone reveal erosions, cystic changes and rarefaction of the medial margins of the pubic rami. Also, when the patient is asked to stand on one leg, diastasis of the pubic symphysis with displacement is seen on a pelvic X-ray. Blood tests usually reveal normal inflammatory markers.

4. K Pregnancy-induced osteomalacia

Pregnancy-induced osteomalacia is a metabolic disorder caused by vitamin D deficiency. The increased requirements of vitamin D during pregnancy are normally met by an increased dietary intake. If this is not the case, it can result in osteomalacia. The woman presents with vague symptoms (aches and pains) and these may lead to misdiagnoses. The pain described is usually in the spinal area and localised pain in the pubic area can occur due to pseudo fractures (Looser zones seen in pubic bone and ischial rami). A waddling gait may be seen due to proximal myopathy. Low serum calcium and a raised alkaline phosphatase are invariably seen in almost all patients. A reduced serum vitamin D level confirms the diagnosis. Biochemistry is normalised following replacement of vitamin D orally. If there is no improvement with this treatment, malabsorption needs to be ruled out.

5. O Transient osteoporosis of pregnancy affecting the hip joint

Transient osteoporosis of pregnancy affecting the hip joint is a rare condition of the hip. It typically affects the left hip in pregnant women although the right hip and other joints may be involved. Symptoms include pain in the hip, localised either to the groin or referred to the anterior aspect of knee. Pain is elicited especially during walking or on weight bearing. Lack of tenderness on pressure on the pubic symphysis distinguishes this condition from other painful conditions affecting the pubic bone.

Haematological tests reveal marginally raised inflammatory markers.

X-rays of the hip reveal osteopenia that is localised and involves the femoral head and acetabulum.

Williams S. Pubic pain during pregnancy. In: Hollingworth T (ed). Differential Diagnosis in Obstetrics and Gynaecology: An A–Z. London: Hodder Arnold, 2008: 297–301.
Jain S, Eedarapalli P, Jamjute P, Sawdy R. Symphysis pubis dysfunction: a practical approach to management. The Obstetrician and Gynaecologist 2006; 8:153–158.

6. H Reassure

The mother is immune and passive transfer of immunity (antibodies) is expected from mother to baby. Therefore reassure the mother.

7. D Offer termination following thorough counselling

The incubation period for rubella is 14–21 days. Most women (50–70%) with rubella will present with maculopapular rash, lymphadenopathy and arthritis. The period of infectivity is 7 days before and 7 days after the appearance of the rash.

Maternal infection affects most fetuses during the first trimester of pregnancy. The risk is small at 13–16 weeks of gestation and very small after 16 weeks of gestation. The major fetal effects include congenital heart defects (patent ductus arteriosus), ocular defects (cataract, glaucoma and microphthalmia), hearing problems (sensorineural deafness) and mental retardation. It also causes haemolytic anaemia, thrombocytopenia, viraemia, jaundice, transient hepato-splenomegaly, purpura and diabetes.

8. H Reassure

The mother has been in contact with a person who had rubella but she is immune to rubella so reassurance is all that is required.

9. L Vaccinate the mother against rubella

Women should be advised routinely about rubella vaccination during preconception counselling. In this scenario she can be offered and vaccinated against rubella as she would be at risk of developing rubella and also wants to get pregnant. However, women should be advised to avoid pregnancy until 1 month post vaccination as the fetus is at risk in view of the live virus in the vaccine (Center for Disease Control recommendations).

10. H Reassure

This woman is immune to rubella and therefore no further action is necessary. Reassure the woman.

Nelson-Piercy C. Handbook of Obstetric Medicine (4th edn). London: Informa Healthcare, 2010.

11. E Commence prophylactic low molecular heparin

She had a previous history of DVT and therefore warrants commencement of prophylactic LMWH during pregnancy. It should be started in early pregnancy or as soon as the risk is identified and continued for 6 weeks during puerperium.

12. C Change to heparinoid danaparoid sodium

Pregnant women who develop heparin-induced thrombocytopenia and require further anticoagulant therapy, can be managed by changing LMWH to heparinoid danaparoid sodium during the antenatal period. During the postnatal period LMWH can be changed to warfarin therapy.

13. A Commence intravenous prophylactic unfractionated heparin

If there is need for heparin treatment in a woman considered to be at increased risk of bleeding, intravenous unfractionated heparin can be given while awaiting the resolution of risk factors for bleeding (because unfractionated heparin is short acting).

14. J Remove catheter 12 hours after giving the last dose of heparin

At least 12 hours should pass after the last prophylactic dose of LMWH and the introduction or removal of epidural or spinal catheter.

15. M Withhold heparin 24 hours before giving spinal anaesthesia

A therapeutic dose of heparin should be withheld 24 hours before spinal or epidural anaesthesia is given. The woman in this scenario has just received a therapeutic dose and will be at risk of bleeding and epidural haematoma if a spinal or epidural anaesthesia is given to her now. Thus, it is recommended to withhold the heparin for 24 hours before spinal anaesthesia is given. In case of emergency before 24 hours, general anaesthesia is preferred.

Letsky E, Murphy MF, Ramsay JE, Walker I. Haemorrhagic Disease and Hereditary Bleeding Disorders. London: RCOG Press, 2005.
Royal College of Obstetricians and Gynaecologists. Green-top Guideline No. 37. Reducing the risk of thrombosis and embolism during pregnancy and the puerperium. London: RCOG Press, 2009.

16. F Prophylactic LMWH postnatally for 7 days

All women who have had an elective caesarean section (category 4) and have one or more additional risk factors (such as age over 35 years, body mass index >30) should be considered for thromboprophylaxis with LMWH for 7 days after delivery.

All women who have had an emergency caesarean section (category 1, 2 or 3) should be considered for thromboprophylaxis with LMWH for 7 days after delivery.

A daily dose of 40 mg clexane is recommended for women who have had a caesarean section. However, a higher thrombo-prophylactic dose (enoxaparin sodium 40 mg twice daily) needs to be considered with a body mass index >35. In the Confidential Enquiry into Maternal Deaths, the majority of morbidly obese women who died of thromboembolism did not receive thromboprophylaxis and those who did either had an inadequate dose or received it for an insufficient amount of time post-caesarean section.

17. H Prophylactic LMWH antenatally plus postnatally for 6 weeks

Women with previous recurrent venous thromboembolism (VTE), a previous unprovoked, oestrogen or pregnancy-related VTE, a previous VTE and a history of VTE in a first-degree relative (or a documented thrombophilia) or other risk factors should be offered antenatal thromboprophylaxis with LMWH. Also recommended is the use of graduated elastic compression stockings in all women with a previous VTE or thrombophilia during pregnancy and for 6–12 weeks postpartum.

Women with a previous single provoked (excluding oestrogen-related) VTE and no other risk factors require close surveillance; antenatal LMWH is not routinely recommended.

18. G Prophylactic LMWH postnatally for 6 weeks

Any woman with two or more current persisting risk factors shown (other than previous VTE or thrombophilia) should be considered for prophylactic LMWH for at least 7 days postpartum. Women with three or more current or persisting risk factors (other than VTE or thrombophilia) should be considered for prophylactic LMWH before giving birth and this is usually continued for 6 weeks postpartum.

In women who have additional persistent risk factors (lasting more than 7 days postpartum), such as prolonged admission or wound infection, thromboprophylaxis should be extended for up to 6 weeks or until the additional risk factors are no longer present.

19. H Prophylactic LMWH antenatally plus postnatally for 6 weeks

The incidence of pulmonary embolism reported during the antenatal period is 1.3 in 10,000 maternities with a case fatality rate of 3.5%. It remains the leading direct cause of maternal death in the UK (1.56 in 100,000 maternities). However, according to the recent Confidential Enquiry into Maternal Deaths, it is the second most common cause of overall maternal deaths (11% of maternal deaths). Seventy-nine per cent of women who died from pulmonary embolism in the UK (2003–2005) had identifiable risk factors. Therefore, it is possible to prevent VTE in obstetric patients with appropriate thromboprophylaxis.

RCOG recommendations (Table 17.1)

Table 17.1 RCOG recommendations for women with previous VTE with or without thrombophilia

Scenario	Recommendations
Women with previous recurrent VTE	Antenatal and 6 weeks postnatal prophylactic LMWH
Women with previous VTE + family history of VTE	
Women with previous VTE + thrombophilia	
Women with thrombophilia: anti-thrombin deficiency or more than one thrombophilia defect (homozygous factor V Leiden deficiency, prothrombin gene defect, compound heterozygotes) or presence of other risk factors	
Women with thrombophilia (other than above): asymptomatic and no other risk factors or family history	7 days postnatal LMWH
Women with thrombophilia (other than above): asymptomatic with other risk factors or family history	Postnatal thromboprophylaxis with LMWH should be extended to 6 weeks

Table 17.1 *Continued.*

Scenario	Recommendations
Single previous provoked VTE without thrombophilia, family history and other factors	Close surveillance antenatally and thromboprophylaxis with LMWH for 6 weeks postpartum
Women with previous VTE and on long-term warfarin	Antenatal high dose prophylactic or therapeutic LMWH and postnatal warfarin

Women should be reassessed before or during labour for risk factors for VTE. Age over 35 years and body mass index >30 or body weight >90 kg are important independent risk factors for postpartum VTE even after vaginal delivery.

Any woman with three or more current or persisting risk factors (other than previous VTE or thrombophilia) should be considered for prophylactic LMWH antenatally and will usually require prophylactic LMWH for 6 weeks postnatally.

Any woman with two or more current or persisting risk factors shown (other than previous VTE or thrombophilia) should be considered for prophylactic LMWH for at least 7 days postpartum.

20. B LMWH not recommended

A past history of superficial thrombophlebitis is not an indication for the administration of LMWH during pregnancy.

Royal College of Obstetricians and Gynaecologists. Green-top Guideline No. 37. Reducing the risk of thrombosis and embolism during pregnancy and the puerperium. London: RCOG Press, 2009. Calderwood CJ and Thanoon OI. Thromboembolism and thrombophilia in pregnancy. Obstet Gynecol Reprod Med 2009; 19:339–343.

21. I Anti-D immunoglobulin is not recommended or indicated

Anti-D immunoglobulin should be given to all non-sensitised RhD-negative women having a therapeutic abortion or termination of pregnancy, whether surgical or medical regardless of gestational age. It is not recommended for women who are already sensitised.

22. I Anti-D immunoglobulin is not recommended or indicated

The diagnosis in this case is threatened miscarriage and she is less than 12 weeks pregnant. She has antibodies to Kell antigen which are entirely unrelated to antibodies to D antigen. Hence, if she continues with this pregnancy uneventfully, she would need prophylactic anti-D immunoglobulin at 28 weeks and 34 weeks of gestation.

The Royal College of Obstetricians and Gynaecologists (RCOG) does not recommend the routine administration of anti-D immunoglobulin before 12 weeks of pregnancy. However, anti-D immunoglobulin should be given to all non-sensitised RhD-negative women diagnosed with threatened miscarriage after 12 weeks of pregnancy. Where bleeding continues intermittently after 12 weeks of gestation, anti-D immunoglobulin should be given at 6-weekly intervals.

Anti-D immunoglobulin should be given to all non-sensitised RhD-negative women who have a spontaneous complete or incomplete miscarriage after 12 weeks of pregnancy.

It is not indicated for women who have a spontaneous miscarriage before 12 weeks of pregnancy or for women with minimal vaginal bleeding before 12 weeks of pregnancy.

Anti-D immunoglobulin administration should be considered in non-sensitised Rhesus-negative women if there is heavy or repeated bleeding or associated with abdominal pain as gestation approaches 12 weeks.

23. E Anti-D immunoglobulin 500 IU

A dose of 250 IU is recommended for prophylaxis following sensitising events up to 20 weeks of pregnancy. For all events after 20 weeks, at least 500 IU anti-D immunoglobulin should be given followed by a test to identify fetomaternal haemorrhage (FMH) greater than 4 mL red cells; additional anti-D immunoglobulin should be given as required.

24. D Anti-D immunoglobulin 250 IU

Anti-D immunoglobulin should be given to all non-sensitised RhD-negative women who have an ectopic pregnancy.

25. E Anti-D immunoglobulin 500 IU

Anti-D immunoglobulin should be given to all non-sensitised RhD-negative women after the following potentially sensitising events during pregnancy:

- amniocentesis, chorionic villus sampling, cordocentesis
- other intrauterine procedures (e.g. insertion of shunts, embryo reduction)
- antepartum haemorrhage
- external cephalic version for breech presentation
- closed abdominal injury
- intrauterine death

Royal College of Obstetricians and Gynaecologists. Green-top Guideline No. 22. The use of anti-D immunoglobulin for rhesus D prophylaxis. London: RCOG Press, 2011.

26. K ECV offer for 37 weeks

ECV before 36 weeks of gestation is not associated with a significant reduction in non-cephalic births or caesarean section. ECV should be offered from 36 weeks in nulliparous women and from 37 weeks in multiparous women. The overall success rate of ECV has been described to be 50% (30–80%), 40% in nulliparous women and 60% in multiparous women. The spontaneous reversion rate to breech presentation is 5%.

27. J ECV offer for 36 weeks

Spontaneous version rates for nulliparous women are approximately 8% after 36 weeks but less than 5% after unsuccessful ECV. Success rates of ECV are 30–80%. Spontaneous reversion to breech presentation after successful ECV occurs in less than 5% of cases. Therefore, ECV from 36 weeks of gestation in nulliparous women seems reasonable; however, there is no upper time limit on the appropriate gestation for ECV. Successes have been reported at 42 weeks of gestation and can be performed in early labour provided that the membranes are intact.

28. G Emergency caesarean section not indicated

ECV is associated with alterations in fetal parameters. Fetal bradycardia and a non-reactive cardiotocograph can occur but are usually transient findings. One should not rush to theatre if the bradycardia recovers within a few minutes. Alterations in the umbilical and middle cerebral artery waveforms have been reported and also an increase in amniotic fluid volume. However, the significance of these changes is unknown.

While taking consent, women should be warned about a 0.5% risk of emergency caesarean section associated with complications (e.g. fetal distress, abruption placenta and uterine rupture) during ECV.

29. H ECV contraindicated

RCOG guidelines describe antepartum haemorrhage within 7 days as an absolute contraindication to ECV.

The absolute contraindications to ECV include:

- where caesarean delivery is necessary
- abnormal CTG
- major uterine anomaly
- ruptured membranes
- multiple pregnancies (except delivery of second twin)
- placenta praevia

Relative contraindications to ECV include:

- fetal growth restriction
- proteinuric pre-eclampsia
- oligohydramnios
- major fetal anomalies
- scarred uterus
- unstable lie

30. F Emergency caesarean section

Footling breech presentation in labour is an indication for caesarean section. The feet normally enter the vagina with less than full dilatation of the cervix and it is more likely to be associated with cord prolapse (7%) than otherwise. Also, it is almost impossible to deliver the aftercoming fetal head with less than full dilatation of the cervix.

Royal College of Obstetricians and Gynaecologists. Green-top Guideline No. 20a. External cephalic version (ECV) and reducing the incidence of breech presentation. London: RCOG Press, 2006.

31. I *Plasmodium vivax*

A Duffy blood group antigen acts as an erythrocyte receptor for *Plasmodium vivax* merozoites. This is absent in certain Afro-Caribbean populations and therefore they are less susceptible to *Plasmodium vivax* infection.

32. K *Plasmodium falciparum*

Women with haemoglobinopathies (e.g. sickle cell trait) and erythrocyte enzyme defects (glucose-6-phosphate dehydrogenase deficiency) are less susceptible and resistant to severe and complicated malaria. If they acquire *Plasmodium falciparum* infection, the disease is less severe because the parasite is less able to divide in the abnormal erythrocyte. This may be due to the physical characteristics of the HbAS erythrocytes or due to the acquisition of natural immunity.

33. N Tuberculosis

Congenital tuberculosis is rare but carries a high mortality rate (around 50%). It is frequently under-diagnosed and is more common in the offspring of a mother if she has miliary tuberculosis with involvement of the endometrium.

The following women should be screened for tuberculosis prior to pregnancy:

- women with human immunodeficiency virus (HIV)
- women in close contact with a person having or suspected to have tuberculosis
- women born in countries with a high prevalence of tuberculosis, e.g. Asia and Africa
- women of low socioeconomic status including certain racial and ethnic minority populations
- women with certain medical disorders which are known to increase the risk of infection
- alcoholics and intravenous drug users (IVDU)
- residents of long-term and residential care facilities

34. F Group B streptococcus

Streptococci are facultative anaerobic gram-positive cocci (usually arranged in chains) and may be cultured from the genital tract in up to 30% (6–30%) of pregnant women at some point during pregnancy. It causes no problems most of the time. In view of this, screening all women means treating 30% of women and two maternal deaths every year due to penicillin allergy.

Overall 3–12% of all neonates are colonised with group B streptococcus (GBS) in the first week of life. It can cause severe neonatal sepsis in 1 in 1000 deliveries and is also a recognised cause of neonatal infection (meningitis) and postpartum endometritis. The pregnancies at risk include: (a) vaginal swab culture positive for GBS infection in the current pregnancy; and (b) a previous baby affected by neonatal GBS infection. Therefore, prophylactic benzylpenicillin (if given more than 4 hours before delivery it decreases the risk of neonatal infection by 70%) has been recommended to be given during the intrapartum period for pregnant women identified as GBS carriers, GBS bacteriuria in the current pregnancy and previous neonate with GBS infection or delivering before 37 weeks of gestation irrespective of maternal GBS colonisation. If no treatment is given or if there is less than 4 hours of treatment before delivery, then the baby should have swabs taken and the paediatricians should be informed.

In women without GBS colonisation or unknown status, prophylactic antibiotics should be offered if the following risk factors are present (risk factors for developing early onset neonatal GBS infection):

- prolonged rupture of membranes >18 hours
- premature delivery (<37 weeks of gestation)
- intrapartum fever (>38°C)

35. C *Chlamydia trachomatis*

The baby can acquire Chlamydia infection during the passage through the birth canal. This can cause neonatal conjunctivitis (5–14 days postnatally) and neonatal pneumonia.

James D, Steer PJ, Weiner CP, Gonik B, Crowther C, Robson S (eds). High Risk Pregnancy: Management Options (4th edn). St Louis: Saunders, 2011.
Magowan B. Churchill's Pocketbook of Obstetrics and Gynaecology (3rd edn). Edinburgh: Churchill Livingstone, 2005.
Royal College of Obstetricians and Gynaecologists. Green-top Guideline No. 36. Group B streptococcal disease: Early onset. London: RCOG Press, 2003.

36. J Peripartum cardiomyopathy

The aetiology of peripartum cardiomyopathy is unclear. Women usually present late in pregnancy or early in the postpartum period (it can occur up to 6 months postpartum). It is more common in older multiparous Afro-Caribbean women but is also associated with multiple pregnancies, hypertension and pre-eclampsia. Women may present with symptoms and signs of biventricular failure (tachycardia, pulmonary oedema and peripheral oedema).

The above diagnosis should be considered in pregnant or puerperal women presenting with worsening breathlessness especially while lying flat or at night. It can be confused with pre-eclampsia as 25% of affected women will be hypertensive. RCOG recommends all such women should have an electrocardiogram and a chest X-ray. The treatment aims at reducing the preload and afterload (beta-blockers, diuretics and angiotensin-converting enzyme inhibitors).

Fifty per cent of women will have a spontaneous recovery. The prognosis is related to left ventricular size and function within 6 months after delivery. The maternal mortality rate is reported to be 25–50%, although a 95% survival rate after 5 years has been recently reported. Also, 25% of the maternal deaths due to cardiac causes are associated with cardiomyopathy.

37. A Aortic dissection

Marfan syndrome is inherited as an autosomal dominant disease. The majority of patients (80%) with Marfan syndrome will have cardiac involvement, the most common being mitral valve prolapse, mitral regurgitation and aortic root dilatation.

During pregnancy, Marfan syndrome carries a risk of aortic dissection and aortic rupture. The predictors for dissection and rupture include systolic hypertension, pre-existing aortic root dilatation (10% if the size of the root is more than 4 cm) or if there is a strong family history of rupture or dissection. Pregnancy is contraindicated in women with an aortic root that is more than 4–4.5 cm.

As systolic hypertension has been a key factor in the majority of deaths from aortic dissection, there has been an emphasis on monitoring and adequate control of hypertension with antihypertensive therapy during pregnancy.

In women who are at high risk, aortic root replacement should be offered prior to pregnancy. Beta-blockers used in these women (with aortic dilatation or hypertension) have been shown to reduce the rate of aortic dilatation and the risk of adverse effects in patients with Marfan syndrome. Repeated echocardiograms are advocated in order to assess aortic root dilation.

Planned caesarean section is usually recommended for women with progressive aortic root dilatation of more than 4.5 cm.

Aortic dissection is a serious complication and one should have a high index of suspicion in women with a history of Marfan syndrome. The presentation is usually acute with central chest pain radiating to the back. It is diagnosed by a computed tomography (CT) scan of the chest.

The other risk factors for aortic dissection include coarctation of aorta and Ehlers–Danlos syndrome type IV.

38. I Mitral valve prolapse

If a woman with mitral valve prolapse is asymptomatic she should be left alone. However, if she is symptomatic one should consider mitral valve repair (balloon valvuloplasty).

39. J Peripartum cardiomyopathy

Peripartum cardiomyopathy can present late in the pregnancy or in the first 6 months of the postpartum period. If the woman presents with increasing shortness of breath on lying down flat or at night the above diagnosis should seriously be considered.

40. G Hypertrophic cardiomyopathy

Hypertrophic cardiomyopathy is a rare disease with an incidence of 0.1–0.5% in women. The spectrum of presentation is broad and is associated with sudden death. Seventy per cent are familial with autosomal dominant inheritance. There is usually a family history of sudden death in a first-degree relative following which other family members are screened or the woman is investigated for a murmur or symptoms during pregnancy.

Signs and symptoms

The symptoms and signs are mainly due to a left ventricular outflow obstruction. These include:

- syncope
- chest pain
- ejection systolic murmur
- pan-systolic murmur
- heart failure
- arrhythmias

Effect of pregnancy on hypertrophic cardiomyopathy

Women usually tolerate this condition well in pregnancy (due to an increase in left ventricular size and stroke volume). If the woman is symptomatic, beta-blockers should be commenced. One should avoid hypotension and hypovolaemia as this would increase left ventricular outflow obstruction. Therefore, be overcautious if considering regional anaesthesia and treat hypovolaemia immediately and adequately.

Royal College of Obstetricians and Gynaecologists. Good Practice Series No. 13. Cardiac disease and pregnancy. London: RCOG Press, 2011.

Nelson-Piercy C. Handbook of Obstetric Medicine (4th edn). London: Informa Healthcare, 2010.

Knight M, Kurinczuk JJ, Spark P, Brocklehurst P. United Kingdom Obstetric Surveillance System (UKOSS) Annual Report 2007. National Perinatal Epidemiology Unit, 2007.

Lewis G (ed). The Confidential Enquiry into Maternal and Child Health (CEMACH). Saving Mothers' Lives: reviewing material deaths to make motherhood safer: 2003–2005. The seventh report on confidential enquiries into maternal deaths in the United Kingdom. CEMACH, 2007.

Roth A and Elkayam U. Acute myocardial infarction associated with pregnancy. Ann Int Med 1996; 125:751–762.

Webber MD, Halligan RE, Schumacher JA. Acute infarction, intracoronary thrombolysis, and primary PTCA in pregnancy. Cathet Cardiovasc Diag 1997; 42:28–43.

Chapter 18

Benign gynaecology

Questions 1–5

Options for Questions 1–5

A   Aphthous ulcers
B   Behcet disease
C   Group B streptococcus
D   Candidial vulvovaginits
E   Chanchroid
F   Eczema
G   Genital herpes simplex
H   Lichen planus

I   Lichen sclerosus
J   Pemphigoid
K   Pemphigus
L   Syphilis
M   Lymphogranuloma venereum
N   Molluscum contagiosum
O   Acanthosis nigricans

Instructions: For each scenario described below, choose the **single** most appropriate diagnosis from the list of options above. Each option may be used once, more than once, or not at all.

1. A 55-year-old woman presents with redness and itching in the vulval region. Clinical examination reveals an inflamed labia associated with oedema, scaling and fissuring. She expresses that this has been an ongoing symptom for the last 6 months. She also gives a recent history of a flare-up of systemic lupus for which she is receiving treatment. She is worried that this could be cancer as her sister died of liposarcoma of the thigh.

2. A 20-year-old woman went to Amsterdam for summer vacation. She attends a sexual health clinic after her return to UK with complaints of a small ulcer on her vulva. Clinical examination reveals a solitary ulcer on the left labia, with a well-defined margin and indurated base. It is non-tender to touch and is associated with painless inguinal lymphadenopathy.

3. A 58-year-old woman is referred to the vulval clinic by her general practitioner. She complains of vulval itching and pain for the last 2 years. Examination reveals a labial fusion, pale atrophic vulva and lichenification in the vulval and perineal region. She is a known diabetic who has been on 40 units of insulin per day for the last 20 years.

4. A 55-year-old woman is referred to a joint vulval/dermatology clinic with blisters and erosions on the vulval region. Examination reveals subepidermal blisters, vulval scarring and introital narrowing. Immunofluorescence studies on biopsies showed antibody deposits at the dermoepidermal junction. She was prescribed steroids following her consultation.

5. A 22-year-old woman presents to a sexual health clinic with a painful vulval ulcer. It is tender on touch and is associated with inguinal lymphadenopathy.

Questions 6–10

Options for Questions 6–10

A   Combined oral contraceptive pill (COCP)

B   Cimetidine

C   Ciprofloxacin

D   Cyproterone acetate

E   Dexamethasone

F   Depot medroxyprogesterone acetate

G   Desmopressin

H   Gonadotropin-releasing hormone analogues

I   Eflornithine

J   Finasteride

K   Flutamide

L   Ketoconazole

M   Progesterone only pill (POP)

N   Spironolactone

O   Spiramycin

Instructions: For each mechanism of action described below, choose the **single** most appropriate drug used in the treatment of hirsutism from the list of options above. Each option may be used once, more than once, or not at all.

6.   A 28-year-old woman is referred to an endocrinologist for an increase in facial hair and acne with bloating during her periods. She has been prescribed an aldosterone antagonist which also has a diuretic action.

7.   A 30-year-old woman is referred to an endocrinologist for an increase in facial hair which she describes as embarrassing as she has to shave almost every week. Investigations so far have been normal. She has been prescribed a drug which reduces 5α reductase enzyme activity.

8.   A 40-year-old woman is referred to an endocrinologist for an increase in facial hair. She has been prescribed a non-steroidal anti-androgen which acts directly on the hair follicles.

9.   A 20-year-old woman is referred to an endocrinologist for an increase in facial hair and acne. She has been prescribed an anti-androgenic which has weak progestational activity.

10.   A 20-year-old woman presents to her general practitioner with an increase in facial hair. Clinical examination reveals a mild increase in facial hair with no major concerns. The general practitioner prescribes her a facial cream which inhibits ornithine decarboxylase.

Questions 11–15

Options for Questions 11–15

A	Aromatase inhibitor	I	Prostaglandin inhibitor
B	Anti-glucocorticoid and anti-progestogenic	J	Progestogenic and anti-androgenic
C	Anti-progestogen, anti-oestrogen and weak androgen	K	Reduces endometrial tissue plasminogen activator
D	Endometrial atrophy	L	Reduces endometrial thromboplastin
E	Endometrial proliferation	M	Reduces and blocks oestrogen receptors at pituitary level
F	Endometritis		
G	Pituitary down regulation	N	Stimulates endothelial growth factor
H	Pituitary up regulation	O	Vasopressin analogue

Instructions: For each drug used in management in gynaecology, choose the **single** most appropriate mechanism of action for the following drugs from the list of options above. Each option may be used once, more than once, or not at all.

11. Danazol

12. Gestrinone

13. Luteal phase progestogens (days 15–25)

14. Tranexamic acid

15. Combined oral contraceptive pill (COCP)

Questions 16–20

Options for Questions 16–20

A	Cryotherapy	I	Microwave ablation of endometrium
B	Cold knife conisation of cervix	J	Radio frequency endometrial ablation
C	Electrode ablation	K	Roller ball ablation of endometrium
D	Endometrial laser ablation	L	Transcervical resection of endometrium
E	Hydrothermal endometrial ablation		
F	Laparoscopic uterine artery clipping	M	Transcervical resection of fibroid
G	Laparoscopic myolysis	N	Transcervical resection of polyp
H	Laparoscopic internal artery ligation	O	Uterine artery embolisation

Instructions: For each action described below, choose the **single** most appropriate method of treatment for menorrhagia from the list of options above. Each option may be used once, more than once, or not at all.

16. This reduces menstrual blood loss, pressure effects, size of fibroids and dysmenorrhoea.

17. This burns the endometrial lining following introduction of hot fluid into the endometrial cavity.

18. It causes collagen denaturation and programmed cell death by heating.

19. A procedure where the endometrium is available for histopathological analysis.

20. It causes severe postoperative adhesions and sepsis.

Answers

1. D Candidal vulvovaginitis

Candidal vulvovaginitis typically presents with vulval redness, oedema and scaling with scratch marks and fissuring on the vulva. It is also associated with an erythematous vagina and thick white non-offensive discharge. Microscopy of the vaginal discharge will reveal hyphae.

Imidazoles are the drugs of choice for treating this condition.

2. L Syphilis

Syphilis is rare in the UK.

Primary chancre: a macule forms at the site of entry (cervix, vagina, vulva and anal canal) of the organism into the body and is followed by ulceration (which is single, indurated and painless). It is often associated with painless inguinal lymphadenopathy. If not treated, secondary syphilis occurs 3–8 weeks later and manifests with genital mucosal ulceration, rash, malaise and condylomata lata. The drug of choice is penicillin. Erythromycin is recommended during pregnancy if the woman is allergic to penicillin.

3. I Lichen sclerosus

Vulval disorders typically involve the perineal area in an hourglass pattern.

Lichen sclerosus is a common, inflammatory condition of the vulval region which is associated with pale atrophic vulva. It is also associated with scratch marks and lichenification on the vulval and perineal region. An underlying malignancy should be ruled out if this is suspected, although this is an uncommon finding.

Highly potent short-term local steroid application (0.05% Clobetasol propionate or Dermovate) is recommended for treatment. Local emollients are also prescribed to prevent dryness.

4. J Pemphigoid

Pemphigoid and pemphigus rarely affect the vulva. Their differences are summarised in **Table 18.1**.

Systemic immunosuppressive therapy and oral corticosteroids are usually required to prevent scarring.

Table 18.1 Differences between pemphigoid and pemphigus	
Pemphigoid	**Pemphigus**
Occurs in older women	Occurs in younger women
Subepidermal blistering	Intraepidermal blistering
Lesions heal with scarring	Lesions heal without scarring
Immunofluorescence studies on biopsies of lesions show antibody deposits at dermoepidermal junction	Immunofluorescence studies on biopsies of lesions show antibody deposits at intercellular spaces of the epidermis

5. E Chanchroid

Chanchroid is caused by *Haemophilus ducreyi*. The ulcer is typically painful, unlike the ulcers in syphilis which are painless. Both are associated with inguinal lymphadenopathy.

Nunns D and Scott IV. Ulcers and erosions of the vulva. Personal assessment in continuing education. Reviews, questions and answers. Volume 3. London: RCOG Press, 2003.

6. N Spironolactone

Spironolactone is a potassium-sparing diuretic. It has a variable effect on the ovaries and adrenals by mainly reducing androstenedione levels. It causes competitive inhibition of the 5α reductase enzyme. The side effects include fatigue, increased frequency of micturition due to diuresis and hyperkalaemia due to the potassium-sparing effect. However, it should be used with caution as it can cause demasculinisation of a male fetus if the woman is pregnant.

7. J Finasteride

Finasteride is an anti-androgen which is rarely used in the management of hirsutism. It inhibits 5α reductase enzyme activity, and therefore blocks the conversion of testosterone to dihydrotestosterone. However, it should be used with caution as it can cause demasculinisation of a male fetus if the woman is pregnant.

8. K Flutamide

Flutamide is an anti-androgen which acts at the receptor level. It acts directly on the hair follicles and has few side effects. These include hepatotoxicity and dry skin. Like finasteride, it should be used with caution as it can cause demasculinisation of a male fetus.

9. D Cyproterone acetate

Cyproterone acetate is a synthetic derivative of 17-hydroxyprogesterone which is an androgen receptor antagonist with weak progestational and glucocorticoid activity. It suppresses actions of both testosterone and its metabolite dihydrotestosterone on tissues by blocking androgen receptors. It also suppresses luteinising hormone (LH) which in turn reduces testosterone levels. The pharmacological actions of this drug are mainly attributed to the acetate form (cyproterone acetate has three times the anti-androgenic activity of cyproterone).

The side effects include mastalgia, weight gain and fluid retention causing oedema and fatigue. In high doses (200–300 mg/day) it can cause liver toxicity and hence should be monitored with liver enzymes. However, the low doses (2 mg) used in gynaecology are unlikely to cause any major problems.

10. I Eflornithine

Eflornithine hydrochloride (Vaniqa cream) inhibits the enzyme (ornithine decarboxylase) in the dermal papillae required for hair growth. It slows hair growth and softens it when applied locally twice daily. It is recommended for facial hair but can cause acne as it blocks the glands.

Barth J. Chapter 26: Hirsutism and virilisation. In: Shaw RW, Luesley D, Monga A (eds). Gynaecology (4th edn). Edinburgh: Churchill Livingstone, 2011.

11. C Anti-progestogen, anti-oestrogen and weak androgen

Danazol has various actions. These include:

- anti-gonadotrophin
- anti-oestrogen
- anti-progestogen
- also a weak androgen

It is effective in the treatment of menorrhagia (it reduces menstrual blood loss by 85%) but the side effects preclude its use. Contraception should be used when using this drug as it can cause masculinisation of a female fetus. The dose used is 200 mg once daily.

The side effects are mainly androgenic which include:

- irreversible voice change
- terminal hair growth
- frontal baldness
- increase in muscular mass
- osteoporosis due to anti-oestrogen action
- weight gain

12. C Anti-progestogen, anti-oestrogen and weak androgen

Gestrinone has similar actions to danazol but with better compliance. Contraception should be used during its use as it can cause masculinisation of a female fetus.

13. D Endometrial atrophy

Luteal phase progestogens (days 15–25) are not effective in reducing menstrual blood loss and therefore should be avoided in the management of menorrhagia.

14. K Tranexamic acid

Tranexamic acid is an antifibrinolytic agent (it reduces endometrial tissue plasminogen activator) which reduces menstrual blood loss by 54%. It is used as second line therapy for menorrhagia and is considered safe, effective and less expensive. Side effects include headache, nausea and dizziness. It should be avoided in women with a previous history of thromboembolism as there is small risk of venous thromboembolism (VTE).

15. D Endometrial atrophy

The COCP reduces menstrual blood loss by 50%. It is effective in treating menorrhagia and also provides contraception for women who want it. It inhibits LH and therefore ovarian hormones and thus causes endometrial atrophy. Side effects can be minor (nausea, headache, mastalgia) or major (thromboembolism).

National Institute of Health and Clinical Excellence. NICE guideline on heavy menstrual bleeding (CG44). NICE, 2007.
Sen S and Lumsden MA. Chapter 31: Menstruation and menstrual disorder. In: Shaw RW, Luesley D, Monga A (eds). Gynaecology (4th edn). Edinburgh: Churchill Livingstone, 2011.
Letsky E, Murphy MF, Ramsay JE, Walker I. Haemorrhagic Disease and Hereditary Bleeding Disorders. London: RCOG Press, 2005.

16. O Uterine artery embolisation

Uterine artery embolisation (UAE) requires interventional radiology and needs to be done in specialist centres. The main purpose of this method is to obliterate the blood flow in both uterine arteries by using a substance (polyvinyl alcohol) which causes emboli in these arteries until flow ceases. This is done by passing a catheter through the femoral vessels in a retrograde fashion to reach the uterine vessels to facilitate the introduction of these substances to block the vessels.

UAE causes shrinkage of the fibroids and reduces menstrual blood loss by 80–96%. Side effects include post-embolisation syndrome (seen in 8–10% and manifests with fever, chills and pain abdomen), sepsis (due to infection in the necrotic fibroid), bowel perforation and fibroid expulsion. Some women may need a hysterectomy in view of the ongoing complications. It rarely causes death.

There is risk of ovarian failure in 1% of cases and therefore its use is not suggested for women who wish to preserve their fertility. Recent reports have suggested an increased risk of miscarriage and pre-term labour in women who have had uterine artery embolisation in the past.

17. E Hydrothermal endometrial ablation

Hydrothermal endometrial ablation reduces menstrual blood loss by 75% (it burns the endometrium after introduction of hot fluid into the uterine cavity).

Other ablative methods include:

- Fluid balloon reduces menstrual blood loss by 73–88%.
- Radiofrequency ablation of the endometrium reduces menstrual blood loss by 84%. In this procedure, a sheath with a bipolar radiofrequency electrode is introduced into the uterine cavity. On pulling the sheath back, the electrode conforms to the shape of the uterine cavity and then emits radiofrequencies. The electrode is subsequently withdrawn into the sheath and removed from the uterus. The disadvantage is there is no specimen for histopathological examination.
- Microwave ablation of the endometrium reduces menstrual blood loss by 83%. It involves insertion of a probe into the endometrial cavity to heat the endometrium. During the procedure the temperature is maintained between 75 and 80°C to destroy the endometrium. Lack of histopathological specimens for examination is one of its disadvantages.

18. G Laparoscopic myolysis

Myolysis: the evidence is limited to anecdotal reports. It may be useful in a selected group of women (fibroid <8 cm). Heating at 40–60°C causes programmed cell death and at 60–65°C causes collagen denaturation. It causes shrinkage of fibroids by 30–50% and causes no postoperative pain or regrowth of fibroids.

19. L Transcervical resection of endometrium

Transcervical resection of the endometrium (TCRE) is the resection of the endometrial lining up to a depth of 5 mm (including stratum basalis which normally regenerates endometrium). This leads to amenorrhoea. The most common fluid medium used is glycine. It is a non-conducting fluid but can cause dilutional hyponatraemia and glycine emboli. One also needs to be cautious due to the increased risk of uterine perforation with this procedure.

20. G Laparoscopic myolysis

Myolysis may cause extensive postoperative adhesions and sepsis.

De Souza N and Cosgrove D. Chapter 5: Imaging techniques in gynaecology. In: Shaw RW, Luesley D, Monga A (eds). Gynaecology (4th edn). Edinburgh: Churchill Livingstone, 2011.
National Institute of Health and Clinical Excellence. Microwave endometrial ablation. NICE, 2003.
National Institute of Health and Clinical Excellence. NICE guideline on heavy menstrual bleeding (CG44). NICE, 2007.

Chapter 19

Core surgical skills

Questions 1–5

Options for Questions 1–5

A   Up to 1 woman in 10
B   Up to 1 woman in 100
C   Up to 5 women in 100
D   Up to 1 woman in 1000
E   Up to 2 women in 1000
F   Up to 5 women in 1000
G   Up to 4–8 women in 1000
H   Up to 7–8 women in 1000

I   Up to 1 woman in 12,000
J   Up to 1 woman in 100,000
K   Up to 3–8 women in 100,000
L   Up to 10 women in 100,000
M   Up to 100 women in 100,000
N   Up to 1000 women in 100,000
O   Up to 10,000 women in 100,000

Instructions: For each condition described below, choose the **single** most likely quoted risk from the list of options above. Each option may be used once, more than once, or not at all.

1. A 24-year-old woman complains of pelvic pain for the last 8 months. She has been booked for diagnostic laparoscopy. A specialist registrar is obtaining consent for the surgery and informing about the risk of serious complications in this procedure.

2. A 40-year-old woman is booked for an elective caesarean section for breech presentation. She goes into labour before the planned operation date at 38 weeks of gestation. She is concerned about the possibility of losing her womb during caesarean section.

3. A 34-year-old woman, para 1, presents to the labour ward at 40 weeks of gestation with regular contractions every 3 minutes. Abdominal examination reveals ballotable head and vaginal examination reveals early labour. Thirty minutes later she has a spontaneous rupture of membranes and cord prolapse. She is pushed to theatre for crash caesarean section. She wants to know her risk of bladder injury.

4. A 20-year-old woman presents to the early assessment unit at 9 weeks of gestation with mild vaginal bleeding. An ultrasound scan reveals a missed miscarriage. The doctors discuss with her these options: (1) conservative, (2) medical and (3) surgical management. The woman prefers to have surgical management for missed miscarriage but is concerned about the risk of uterine perforation.

5. A 28-year-old woman is admitted to the day surgery unit for diagnostic laparoscopy. She has been suffering from dysmenorrhoea which has outlasted her periods for the last 2 years. An ultrasound scan reveals normal ovaries and an endometrial polyp. She is scared that she may die while asleep.

Answers

1. E Up to 2 women in 1000

The risks associated with diagnostic laparoscopy are divided into frequent (wound bruising, shoulder tip pain, wound gaping and wound infection) and serious risks (serious complications in up to 2 women in every 1000 undergoing laparoscopy – damage to the bowel, bladder, uterer or major blood vessels which would require immediate repair by laparoscopy, or laparotomy, failure to gain entry to abdominal cavity and to complete intended procedure, hernia at site of entry, death); 3–8 women in every 100,000 undergoing laparoscopy die as a result of complications.

Additional procedures which may be necessary during the procedure include laparotomy, repair of damage to the bowel, bladder, uterer or blood vessels and blood transfusion.

2. H Up to 7–8 women in 1000

Risks of caesarean section

Serious risks: maternal

- emergency hysterectomy, 7–8 women in every 1000 undergoing caesarian section
- need for further surgery at a later date, including curettage, 5 in 1000 women
- admission to intensive care unit (highly dependent on the reason for caesarean section), 9 in 1000 women
- thromboembolic disease, 4–16 in 10,000 women
- bladder injury, 1 in 1000 women
- ureteric injury, 3 in 10,000 women
- death, approximately 1 in 12,000 women

Frequent risks: maternal

- persistent wound and abdominal discomfort in the first few months after surgery, 9 in 100 women
- increased risk of a repeat caesarean section when vaginal delivery is attempted in subsequent pregnancies, 1 in 4 women
- readmission to hospital, 5 in 100 women
- haemorrhage, 5 in 1000 women
- infection, 6 in 100 women

Frequent risk: fetal

- lacerations, 1–2 in 100 babies

Risks for future pregnancies include:

- increased risk of uterine rupture during subsequent pregnancies/deliveries, 2–7 in 1000 women

- increased risk of ante partum stillbirth, 2–4 In 1000 women
- increased risk in subsequent pregnancies of placenta praevia and placenta accreta, 4–8 in 1000 women

Additional procedures during caesarean section which may become necessary include hysterectomy, repair of injured organs and blood transfusion.

3. D Up to 1 woman in 1000

Serious risks associated with caesarean section are:

- bladder injury, 1 in 1000 women
- ureteric injury, 3 in 10,000 women

4. F Up to 5 women in 1000

Serious risks include:

- uterine perforation, up to 5 in 1000 women
- significant trauma to the cervix
- there is no substantiated evidence in the literature of any impact on future fertility

Frequent risks include:

- bleeding that lasts for up to 2 weeks is very common but blood transfusion is uncommon (1–2 in 1000 women)
- need for repeat surgical evacuation, up to 5 in 100 women
- localised pelvic infection, 3 in 100 women

The additional procedures that may be necessary during the procedure include laparoscopy or laparotomy to diagnose or repair organ injury, or uterine perforation.

5. K Up to 3–8 women in 100,000

Death; 3–8 women in every 100,000 undergoing laparoscopy die as a result of complications.

Royal College of Obstetricians and Gynaecologists. Consent Advice No. 2. Diagnostic laparoscopy. London: RCOG Press, 2008.
Royal College of Obstetricians and Gynaecologists. Consent Advice No. 7. Caesarean section. London: RCOG Press, 2009.
Royal College of Obstetricians and Gynaecologists. Consent Advice No. 10. Surgical evacuation of uterus for early pregnancy loss. London: RCOG Press, 2010.

Chapter 20

Drug therapy in obstetrics and gynaecology

Questions 1–5

Options for Questions 1–5

A	Adriamycin	H	Imiquimod
B	Carboplatin	I	Methotrexate
C	Cisplatin	J	Melphalan
D	Chlorambucil	K	Paclitaxel
E	Cyclophosphamide	L	Topotecan
F	Etoposide	M	Treosulfan
G	5–Fluorouracil	N	Vincristine

Instructions: For each side effect of chemotherapy described below, choose the **single** most appropriate drug from the list of options above. Each option may be used once, more than once, or not at all.

1. A 49-year-old woman presents with haematuria. She has recently been diagnosed with ovarian cancer and has received two cycles of chemotherapy. Cystoscopy reveals haemorrhagic cystitis.

2. A 40-year-old woman presents with palpitations, numbness and tingling in the legs, and alopecia involving all body hair. She has recently been diagnosed with ovarian cancer and has received three cycles of chemotherapy. Clinical examination reveals pulse of 180 beats/minute and normal blood pressure. She is booked for debulking surgery in 10 days.

3. A 20-year-old woman is having treatment for a high-risk gestational trophoblastic disease. She has just finished her second cycle of chemotherapy. One week later she presents with feeling unwell with motor weakness, double vision and sore throat. Clinical examination reveals lower limb power of 3/5, lateral rectus palsy of right eye and blood results show myelosuppression.

4. A 40-year-old woman has recently been diagnosed with ovarian cancer and has received two cycles of chemotherapy. She presents with decreased urine output, tingling in the lower limbs and is hard of hearing following completion of the second cycle. Her blood results show high creatinine and low magnesium.

5. A 20-year-old woman had medical treatment for an ectopic pregnancy 15 days ago. She has been told not to get pregnant for at least 1 month following this injection as the drug has an antifolate action.

Questions 6–10

Options for Questions 6–10

A	Intravenous artesunate	H	Oral quinine
B	Antiemetic plus repeat oral quinine	I	Oral clindamycin
C	Antiemetic plus repeat oral quinine and clindamycin	J	Oral quinine plus oral clindamycin
		K	Oral chloroquine for 3 days
D	Intravenous quinine	L	Oral chloroquine 300 mg weekly until
E	Intravenous clindamycin		delivery
F	Intravenous quinine plus oral clindamycin	M	Pyrimethamine
		N	Primaquine
G	Intravenous quinine plus intravenous clindamycin	O	Sulphadiazine

Instructions: For each scenario described below, choose the **single** most appropriate treatment from the list of options above. Each option may be used once, more than once, or not at all.

6. A 28-year-old Afro-Caribbean woman, para 4, presents to the obstetric day assessment unit with these vague symptoms: malaise, fever and headache. She had travelled to Ghana 4 weeks ago and was perfectly fine. She is currently 30 weeks pregnant and has good fetal movements. Her blood tests and peripheral smear reveal anaemia, thrombocytopenia, and hyperparasitaemia with *Plasmodium falciparum*.

7. A 28-year-old Afro-Caribbean woman, para 2, presents to the day assessment unit at 29 weeks of gestation with fever, malaise and musculoskeletal pain. She gives a history of malaria 4 years ago during her visit to Nigeria. A peripheral blood smear shows *Plasmodium falciparum*. Clinically, haematologically and biochemically there are no symptoms or signs of severe complications.

8. A 28-year-old African woman, para 1, presents to the day assessment unit at 37 weeks of gestation with fever, malaise and muscle pain. She gives a history of malaria during childhood and has been a fit person so far. Peripheral blood smear shows *Plasmodium falciparum*. Clinically, haematologically and biochemically there are no symptoms or signs of severe complications. She vomits after receiving the first dose of oral quinine and clindamycin.

9. A 28-year-old Asian woman, para 0, presents to the day assessment unit at 20 weeks of gestation with fever, malaise and muscle pain. She returned to the UK 2 weeks ago from India. A peripheral blood smear shows *Plasmodium vivax*. She receives anti-malarial treatment for 7 days and is cured. Four weeks later, she comes to see her general practitioner for advice as she is about to go on holiday to Africa.

10. A 28-year-old Afro-Caribbean woman, para 3, presents to the day assessment unit at 37 weeks of gestation with fever, malaise and muscle pain. Her peripheral smear

shows *Plasmodium ovale*. Clinically, haematologically and biochemically there are no symptoms or signs of severe complications.

Questions 11–15

Options for Questions 11–15

A	Vitamin A	I	Vitamin B12
B	Vitamin B1	J	Vitamin C
C	Vitamin B2	K	Vitamin D
D	Vitamin B3	L	Vitamin E
E	Folic acid	M	Vitamin K
F	Vitamin B5	N	Vitamin M
G	Vitamin B6	O	Vitamin I
H	Vitamin B7		

Instructions: For each action described below, choose the **single** most appropriate vitamin from the list of options above. Each option may be used once, more than once, or not at all.

11. A water soluble vitamin which is involved in myelin formation, synthesis of neurotransmitters, and also reduces total plasma homocysteine concentrations.

12. A lipid soluble vitamin acting on the lipid membrane and with synergistic interaction with vitamin C.

13. A vitamin photosynthesised by ultraviolet radiation in the epidermis.

14. A lipophilic vitamin important in post-translational modifications of proteins, particularly those involved in blood coagulation.

15. An essential water-soluble vitamin which has important roles in collagen synthesis, wound healing, absorption of non-haem iron and antioxidant action.

Questions 16–20

Options for Questions 16–20

A Angiotensin-converting-enzyme (ACE) inhibitors
B Amitriptyline
C Amiodarone
D Bendroflumethiazide
E Citalopram
F Cabergoline
G Change therapy to oral carbimazole
H Change therapy to oral propylthiouracil
I Commence 5 mg folic acid/day
J Commence 0.4 mg folic acid/day
K Commence 10 mg oral vitamin K
L Commence thyroxine
M Frusemide
N Increase the dose of thyroxine
O Propylthiouracil
P Propranolol

Instructions: For each scenario described below, choose the **single** most appropriate therapy from the list of options above. Each option may be used once, more than once, or not at all.

16. A 29-year-old woman, para 1, presents to the early pregnancy assessment unit at 6 weeks of gestation with mild vaginal bleeding. She has a history of diabetes with well-controlled blood glucose levels. An ultrasound scan reveals a single intrauterine viable pregnancy. Currently, the only medication she is taking is insulin.

17. A 29-year-old woman, para 1, presents to the early pregnancy assessment unit at 6 weeks of gestation with mild vaginal bleeding. She has a history of epilepsy controlled by sodium valproate and carbamazepine. An ultrasound scan reveals a single intrauterine viable pregnancy.

18. A 29-year-old woman, para 1, attends the antenatal clinic at 16 weeks of pregnancy for review of booking (her first midwife appointment) blood tests. She suffers from hypothyroidism and is currently on 75 μg of thyroxine. Her haematological, biochemical and virology results are normal. Her thyroid-stimulating hormone (TSH) is 6.5 mU/mL and T4 is 14 pmol/L.

19. A 29-year-old woman, para 1, attends the obstetric day assessment unit at 34 weeks of gestation with itching. Fetal cardiotocograph (CTG) is normal. Her blood tests reveal raised alanine aminotransferase (48 U/L) and a normal autoimmune screen. A diagnosis of obstetric cholestasis is made.

20. A 29-year-old woman, para 1, attends the antenatal clinic at 18 weeks of gestation for review. She gives a history of Graves' disease prior to pregnancy and had discontinued prophythiouracil as she developed a severe sore throat and agranulocytosis. At present her haematological results are normal. Her TSH is 0.5 mU/L.

Answers

1. E Cyclophosphamide

Alkylating agents bind covalently to DNA side chains and cause cross-linkage and strand breaks. They act on multiple phases of the cell cycle (therefore they kill both slowly and rapidly proliferating cells). Alkylating drugs include melphalan, chlorambucil, cyclophosphamide, ifosfamide and treosulfan. Cyclophosphamide is an alkylating agent which is inactive in itself and has to be converted to an active drug (4-hydroxy cyclophosphamide) in the liver. It then decomposes within the cells to form phosphoramide mustard and acrolein (this is excreted in the urine and is toxic to bladder epithelium). It is less myelotoxic compared to other alkylating agents (melphalan causes leukaemia in the long run).

It causes haemorrhagic cystitis (ifosfamide also causes this side effect) which can be neutralised by administering acetylcysteine or mesna (it neutralises the effects of acrolein). It can also cause alopecia. It is not currently used as first line treatment for ovarian cancer.

2. K Paclitaxel

Paclitaxel belongs to the taxane group of drugs and acts by binding to microtubules (it prevents depolymerisation into tubulin dimmers), thereby disrupting mitosis. When administered intravenously, it is 95% protein bound and is metabolised in the liver by the cytochrome P450 enzyme system. However, 5–10% is excreted in the kidneys.

Side effects include neutropaenia, arrhythmias, sensory peripheral neuropathy and alopecia. It is also associated with hypersensitivity reactions which can be reduced by the administration of glucocorticoids and H1 and H2 antagonists prior to infusion.

3. N Vincristine

Vincristine belongs to the vinca alkaloids and acts by binding to tubulin (it prevents polymerisation), thus causing mitotic arrest in the G2 and M phases of the cell cycle. It is highly protein bound (like paclitaxel) and is metabolised in the liver. Side effects include neurotoxicity (paraesthesia, motor weakness and cranial nerve palsy) and myelosuppression.

4. C Cisplatin

Cisplatin and carboplatin belong to the platinum group of drugs (they act by cross-linking with DNA strands). Conventionally, cisplatin was used as a first line treatment alone or in combination therapy for the treatment of ovarian cancer.

Cisplatin is administered intravenously and is 90% protein bound. It is mainly excreted by the kidneys and is highly nephrotoxic (dose limiting toxicity). This can be reduced to some extent by forced diuresis. The newer drug carboplatin is much less nephrotoxic than cisplatin and has therefore replaced it in modern chemotherapy for ovarian cancer. Cisplatin also causes peripheral neuropathy and is toxic to the middle ear causing high frequency hearing loss and tinnitus.

5. I Methotrexate

Methotrexate is an antimetabolite and acts by inhibiting dihydrofolate reductase. It is excreted mainly in the kidneys. It is used in the treatment of gestational trophoblastic disease and also ectopic pregnancy. Side effects include mucositis, nausea, vomiting, photosensitivity, nephrotoxicity and hepatotoxicity.

Shafi MI, Luesley DM, Jordan JA. Handbook of Gynaecological Oncology. Edinburgh: Churchill Livingstone, 2001.

6. A Intravenous artesunate

Malaria can present with non-specific flu-like illness. The symptoms include headache, fever with chills, nausea, vomiting, diarrhoea, coughing and general malaise. The signs include raised temperature, splenomegaly, jaundice, pallor, sweating and respiratory distress.

The features of complicated or severe malaria include prostration, impaired consciousness, respiratory distress (acute respiratory distress syndrome), pulmonary oedema, convulsions, collapse, abnormal bleeding, disseminated intravascular coagulation, jaundice and haemoglobinuria.

Laboratory findings include severe anaemia, thrombocytopenia, hypoglycaemia, acidosis, renal impairment, hyperlactataemia, hyperparasitaemia, algid malaria (gram-negative septicaemia) and meningitis.

Microscopic diagnosis allows for species identification and estimation of parasitaemia. Pregnant women with 2% or more parasitised red blood cells are at higher risk of developing severe malaria and should be treated by following the severe malaria protocol.

The Royal College of Obstetricians and Gynaecologists (RCOG) recommends:

- admission of women with uncomplicated malaria to hospital
- admission of women with complicated malaria to the intensive care unit
- intravenous artesunate as first line for the treatment of severe falciparum malaria
- intravenous quinine if artesunate is not available
- to use quinine and clindamycin to treat uncomplicated P. falciparum (or mixed, such as P. falciparum and P. vivax)
- use chloroquine to treat P. vivax, P. ovale or P. malariae
- primaquine use should be avoided in pregnancy
- involve infectious diseases specialists, especially for severe and recurrent cases
- if vomiting persists, oral therapy should be stopped and intravenous therapy should be instituted
- treat the fever with antipyretics
- screen for anaemia and treat appropriately
- follow-up to ensure detection of relapse

7. J Oral quinine plus oral clindamycin

Uncomplicated falciparum malaria

Uncomplicated malaria in the UK is defined as fewer than 2% parasitised red blood cells in a woman with no signs of severity and no complicating features.

The treatment is one of the following:

- oral quinine 600 mg 8-hourly and oral clindamycin 450 mg 8-hourly for 7 days (they can be given together) or
- artemether with lumefantrine (Riamet) four tablets/dose for weight >35 kg, twice daily for 3 days (with fat) or
- atovaquone-proguanil (Malarone) four standard tablets daily for 3 days

8. C Antiemetic plus repeat oral quinine and clindamycin

Vomiting is a known adverse effect of quinine and is associated with malarial treatment failure. Use an antiemetic if the patient vomits and repeat the antimalarial medication. Repeat vomiting after an antiemetic is an indication for parenteral therapy.

Uncomplicated falciparum malaria with vomiting:

- Quinine 10 mg/kg dose intravenous in 5% dextrose over 4 hours every 8 hours plus intravenous clindamycin 450 mg every 8 hours.
- Once the patient stops vomiting she can be switched to oral quinine 600 mg three times a day to complete 5–7 days and if needed oral clindamycin can be switched to 450 mg three times a day for 7 days.

9. L Oral chloroquine 300 mg weekly till delivery

Preventing relapse during pregnancy:

- chloroquine oral 300 mg weekly until delivery

10. K Oral chloroquine for 3 days

Non-falciparum malaria *P. vivax, P. ovale* and *P. malariae*:

- Oral chloroquine (base) 600 mg followed by 300 mg 6 hours later. Then 300 mg on day 2 and again on day 3.

Royal College of Obstetricians and Gynaecologists. Green-top guideline No. 54B. The diagnosis and treatment of malaria in pregnancy. London: RCOG Press, 2010.

11. G Vitamin B6

Vitamins are organic compounds essential for normal cell function, growth and development. The essential vitamins include vitamins A, C, D, E, K and the B series including B1 (thiamine), B2 (riboflavin), B3 (niacin), B5 (pantothenic acid), B6 (pyridoxine), B7 (biotin), B9 (folic acid) and B12 (cobalamin).

Vitamin B6 decreases in the third trimester of pregnancy (it is uncertain whether this is due to volume expansion or true deficiency). Vitamin B6 alleviates the severity of nausea but not vomiting in the first trimester. It is also associated with a statistically significant decrease (by 16%) in the risk of dental decay in pregnant women, particularly when given in lozenge form, suggesting a local effect.

The effect of vitamin B6 supplementation on outcomes such as eclampsia, pre-eclampsia, low birth weight and breast milk production are inconclusive. Current evidence is not strong enough to support routine supplementation in pregnancy.

12. L Vitamin E

Vitamin E is an antioxidant. However, recent evidence (supplementation of vitamin E and vitamin C in pregnancy) showed no difference in the effect on pre-eclampsia, pre-term birth, small-for-gestational-age infants or any baby death. Current evidence does not support routine supplementation of these vitamins during pregnancy.

13. K Vitamin D

Vitamin D deficiency is more common in Asians than Caucasians as they require longer exposure to the sun to produce the same amounts of the vitamin. It is also more common in women who are fully covered and stay indoors.

A significant increase in infantile rickets is reported with decreased transfer of vitamin D to the fetus during pregnancy and breastfeeding by vitamin D-deficient mothers. Approximately 15% of all adults may be deficient in vitamin D in the UK and the prevalence is said to increase to 90% in South Asian adults. Obesity before pregnancy is also associated with a significant increase in maternal and neonatal vitamin D deficiency independent of factors like ethnicity.

A systematic review showed that antenatal vitamin D supplementation is effective in improving the vitamin D status of Asian and Caucasian women and promotes growth in the first year of life in South Asian babies. The current National Institute of Health and Clinical Excellence (NICE) guidelines on antenatal care support the importance of maintaining adequate vitamin D stores in pregnancy, especially for those at highest risk of vitamin D deficiency (women of South Asian, African, Caribbean or Middle Eastern family origin, women who have limited exposure to sunlight, women who eat a diet particularly low in vitamin D and women with a pre-pregnancy body mass index >30 kg/m^2). The recommended dose is 10 µg/day.

14. M Vitamin K

Vitamin K is required for the synthesis of coagulation factors II, VII, IX and X (synthesised in the liver). This can be deficient in women taking anticonvulsants (carbamazepine and phenytoin which are liver enzyme inducers). Therefore, there is a potential risk of periventricular haemorrhage in babies born to these mothers. The current evidence suggests no significant decrease in periventricular haemorrhage with vitamin K supplementation during pregnancy and therefore the evidence to support routine supplementation is not strong.

15. J Vitamin C

Vitamin C is an essential vitamin which is abundant in fruit and vegetables. It is important in wound healing and also promotes the absorption of non-haem iron in food. Multivitamin preparations for pregnancy generally contain low doses of vitamin C.

Royal College of Obstetricians and Gynaecologists. Vitamin supplementation in pregnancy. Scientific Advisory Committee opinion paper 16. London: RCOG, 2009.
Walker SP, Permezel M and Berkovic SF. The management of epilepsy in pregnancy. BJOG 2009; 116:758–767.

16. I Commence 5 mg folic acid/day

Diabetic women during pregnancy are at high risk of congenital anomalies. NICE recommends 5 mg folic acid supplementation for these women during the first trimester instead of 0.4 mg.

17. I Commence 5 mg folic acid/day

Epilepsy and pregnancy

It is the most common neurological disorder in pregnant women with an incidence of 3–4 in 1000 pregnancies. Most women will not have problems with regards to seizures (60%). However, the seizure frequency can either decrease (10%), increase (30%) or remain the same during pregnancy (the risk of seizure is highest during labour and in the first 24 hours postpartum) (1–2%). The increase in seizure frequency is attributed to non-compliance with medication, hyperemesis, weight gain and altered pharmacokinetics.

The risk of congenital anomalies increases due to the antifolate action of anti-convulsants (phenytoin, phenobarbitone, sodium valproate and carbamazepine). Therefore, the principle of treatment during pregnancy is to maintain the lowest possible dose to control the seizures and mono-drug therapy instead of high doses and polydrug therapy. However, routine monitoring of drug levels in pregnancy is not recommended (monitor only if seizure frequency increases).

Sodium valproate particularly increases the risk of neural tube defects, orofacial clefts and congenital heart defects. The newer drugs levetiracetam, gabapentin and tiagabine are not teratogenic in animals. However, human data are sparse. Lamotrigine has a weak antifolate action (it inhibits dihydrofolate reductase) and therefore caries similar risk of teratogenesis to other mono-drug therapies. Benzodiazepines (clonazepam) as an add-on therapy are not said to be teratogenic if used in monotherapy.

To avoid some of these risks to the fetus, it is recommended that these women take 5 mg folic acid daily during pregnancy.

Risks to the fetus

- congenital malformations

- fetal growth restrictions
- increased perinatal mortality
- increased risk of epilepsy (4–5% if one parent affected, 15–20% if both parents affected and 10% if one sibling affected)
- neurodevelopment delay

Women with epilepsy should have consultant-led care in the hospital and should be seen in specialist clinics (neurology/obstetric joint clinic). Pain and anxiety should be avoided during labour with early recourse to epidural anaesthesia. Vaginal delivery is not contraindicated and a caesarean section should be offered only for obstetric indications.

Breast feeding is not contraindicated and the baby should receive vitamin K at birth to prevent haemorrhagic disorders.

18. N Increase the dose of thyroxine

Hypothyroidism

- Incidence: affects 1% of pregnancies.
- Aetiology: is more common in women than men, with a positive family history in most women.
- Most cases are due to autoimmune destruction of the thyroid gland (autoimmune thyroiditis and Hashimoto thyroiditis) indicated by the presence of antimicrosomal antibodies.
- It may be due to radioiodine therapy, surgical thyroidectomy or drug therapy (amiodarone, lithium, iodine and antithyroid drugs).
- Subacute de Quervain thyroiditis and postpartum thyroiditis are causes of transient hypothyroidism.
- It is also associated with other autoimmune diseases such as type 1 diabetes mellitus, vitiligo and pernicious anaemia.
- Most women are already on treatment before conception.
- Fetus: the fetus depends on maternal thyroid hormones until 12 weeks of gestation. Hence, adequate thyroid replacement therapy in early pregnancy is important. If pregnant women remain untreated, it increases the risk of miscarriage, fetal loss and low birth weight. Reduced intelligence quotient (IQ) and neurodevelopmental delay have also been reported in the offspring of undertreated mothers (especially in the first and second trimesters).
- Neonatal hypothyroidism: is a rare condition (incidence 1 in 80,000) caused by transplacental transfer of TSH receptor-blocking antibodies. It is more commonly seen in women with atrophic rather than Hashimoto thyroiditis. One should suspect diagnosis in the presence of fetal goitre. The Guthrie heel prick test is used as a screening test to identify the condition in newborn babies.
- Mother: the disease should be optimised or controlled prior to conception, with dose adjustments in the first trimester to ensure adequate treatment (one should be cautious as TSH levels increase in the first trimester and hence thyroxine should not be increased unless treatment is confirmed by low serum T4 levels). If the woman is already on an adequate dose, thyroid function should be checked

at least once in each trimester. However, if the dose is adjusted (increased or decreased) at any time during pregnancy, thyroid function should be checked every 4–6 weeks.

- Overall, women will require an increase in dose by almost 20–30% as the pregnancy progresses. The aim is to achieve a TSH level of 2.5 mU/L or less. If untreated or uncontrolled it can cause anaemia (due to inadequate stimulation of red blood cell development in the bone marrow) and pre-eclampsia.
- Postpartum thyroiditis: It affects 1% of women and usually presents within 1 year of childbirth. Its aetiology is generally unknown although it is attributed to having an autoimmune origin and is more common in diabetics. These women initially present with hyperthyroidism (lasts for 1–3 months) with one third progressing to hypothyroidism (lasts for about 9–12 months). Also, 20% of these will continue to be hypothyroid. The risk of recurrence is reported to be 20%. The treatment for hypothyroidism is thyroxine and treatment for hyperthyroidism is beta-blockers, as this is a temporary phase.

19. K Commence 10 mg oral vitamin K

Daily supplementation of vitamin K until delivery is recommended for women with obstetric cholestasis in view of the theoretical risk of postpartum haemorrhage (PPH) and haemolytic disease in the newborn.

20. G Change therapy to oral carbimazole

Hyperthyroidism

- Incidence: 0.2% of pregnant women.
- Causes: Graves' disease (90%), toxic multinodular goitre, toxic nodule, hyperemesis gravidarum and hydatidiform mole.
- Symptoms: the physiological symptoms of pregnancy (palpitation, heat intolerance and increased metabolic rate) mimic symptoms of hyperthyroidism, making diagnosis difficult. The most sensitive symptoms for diagnosis include failure to gain weight despite adequate appetite, tremor and persistent resting tachycardia.
- Treatment: propylthiouracil or carbimazole block the thyroid hormone synthesis and reduce TSH receptor antibody levels.
- Fetus: both of the above drugs cross the placenta and are secreted in breast milk (propylthiouracil less than carbimazole) and can therefore cause fetal goitre and hypothyroidism in high doses. Neonatal thyrotoxicosis (usually transient) can occur in 1% of babies (if untreated the mortality is 30%) due to stimulation of fetal thyroid by maternal antibodies crossing the placenta. Other risks to the fetus include prematurity, fetal growth restriction and stillbirth.
- Mother: if the condition is not treated or well-controlled, there is an increased risk of pre-eclampsia and heart failure.
- Monitoring: thyroid function should be measured every 4–6 weeks during pregnancy and free T4 levels should be kept at the upper limit of their normal values.

- Role of surgery: surgery is rarely required in pregnancy. It is indicated if there is retrosternal extension of goitre causing pressure symptoms, if women are not responding to medical therapy or if women develop serious adverse effects with medical therapy (surgery should be performed during the second trimester).

Nelson-Piercy C. Handbook of Obstetric Medicine (4th edn). London: Informa Healthcare, 2010.
Anthony K and Nelson-Piercy C. Obstetric cholestatis. Personal assessment in continuing education. Reviews, questions and answers. Volume 3. London: RCOG Press, 2003: 48–49.
Royal College of Obstetricians and Gynaecologists. Green-top Guideline No. 43. Obstetric cholestasis. London: RCOG Press, 2006.

Questions 1–5

Options for Questions 1–5

A   Abdominal cerclage
B   Cerclage for women with a multiple pregnancy
C   Cerclage for women with cervical trauma
D   Cervical cerclage contraindicated
E   Cervical cerclage plus progesterone vaginal pessaries
F   Cut the suture through posterior colpotomy
G   Elective cerclage not indicated
H   Elective cerclage at 12–14 weeks
I   Elective caesarean section
J   Emergency caesarean section
K   Emergency cerclage not recommended
L   History indicated cerclage
M   Hysterotomy
N   Suction evacuation through the suture
O   Rescue cerclage

Instructions: For each clinical scenario described below, choose the **single** most appropriate initial management from the above list of options. Each option may be used once, more than once, or not at all.

1. A 28-year-old woman, para 0+3 (second trimester miscarriage), attends the miscarriage clinic in view of her poor obstetric history. She also gives a history of cervical cerclage in her last pregnancy.

2. A 28-year-old woman presents to the labour ward with a premature rupture of membranes at 24 weeks of gestation. Abdominal examination reveals an absence of contractions and a speculum examination reveals a 2 cm dilated posterior cervix with intact forewaters.

3. A 28-year-old woman attends the early pregnancy assessment unit with vaginal bleeding at 8 weeks of gestation. She gives a history of abdominal cerclage prior to pregnancy in view of two previous mid-trimester miscarriages following vaginal cervical cerclage. An ultrasound scan reveals an absence of fetal heart activity.

4. A 28-year-old woman attends the obstetric day assessment unit with reduced fetal movements at 23 weeks and 3 days of gestation. She gives a history of abdominal cerclage in early pregnancy in view of a previous failed vaginal cerclage. Abdominal examination reveals an absence of uterine activity and an ultrasound examination reveals an absence of fetal heart activity.

5. A 28-year-old woman , para 0, presents to the early pregnancy assessment unit at 15 weeks of gestation with mild vaginal bleeding. She gives a history of large loop excision of the transformation zone of the cervix 2 years ago. An ultrasound

examination reveals the presence of fetal heart activity. Bicornuate uterus and funnelling of cervix are also noted on the scan report.

Questions 6–10

Options for Questions 6–10

A   Antibiotics
B   Antenatal low molecular weight heparin (LMWH)
C   Close surveillance and LMWH postnatally for 6 weeks
D   Low dose aspirin only during first trimester
E   Low dose aspirin plus steroids
F   Low dose aspirin until 36 weeks of gestation
G   Low dose aspirin antenatally plus LMWH postnatally for 7 days
H   Low dose aspirin plus LMWH plus steroids

I   Prophylactic antenatal LMWH plus postnatal for 6 weeks
J   Prophylactic antenatal enoxaparin sodium plus postnatal enoxaparin sodium for 3–5 days
K   Prophylactic LMWH in the first trimester
L   Reassure the woman
M   Therapeutic antenatal enoxaparin sodium plus prophylactic postnatal enoxaparin sodium
N   Therapeutic antenatal enoxaparin sodium plus therapeutic postnatal enoxaparin sodium
O   Varicose vein stripping

Instructions: For each scenario described below, choose the **single** most appropriate initial management from the list of options above. Each option may be used once, more than once, or not at all.

6. A 40-year-old nulliparous woman attends the maternal medicine clinic for a consultation at 13 weeks of gestation. A dating ultrasound scan at 12 weeks of gestation reveals a single viable intrauterine fetus. She gives a history of a single episode of deep venous thrombosis (DVT) following a road traffic accident 5 years ago. A recent thrombophilia screen prior to pregnancy is negative.

7. A 40-year-old nulliparous woman attends the early pregnancy assessment unit at 12 weeks of gestation with mild vaginal bleeding. A transvaginal scan reveals a viable dichorionic diamniotic twin pregnancy. Medical history reveals that she had an episode of DVT and a pulmonary embolism 2 years and 1 year ago respectively. A recent thrombophilia screen is negative.

8. A 40-year-old woman attends her antenatal appointment at 12 weeks of gestation. She gives history of three miscarriages (<10 weeks) with a single episode of provoked venous thromboembolism (VTE) following major surgery of the hip. Her blood test is positive for anticardiolipin antibody. A vaginal swab shows growth of group B streptococcus.

9. A 40-year-old woman attends her antenatal appointment at 12 weeks of gestation. She gives a history of a stillbirth at 28 weeks of gestation and DVT 7 days following that delivery. Her blood test reveals an antithrombin III deficiency. She has been treated for toxoplasmosis in the past and her blood shows IgG antibodies for toxoplasmosis.

10. A 40-year-old Asian woman attends her antenatal clinic appointment at 12 weeks of gestation. She gives a history of eclampsia in her last pregnancy at 28 weeks of gestation and hence she had a caesarean section. Now her blood pressure is 120/60 mmHg and her urine shows absence of protein.

Questions 11–15

Options for Questions 11–15

A	Evacuation of retained products of conception	J	Laparotomy
B	Mifepristone	K	Laparoscopic salpingectomy
C	Misoprostol followed by mifepristone	L	Repeat ultrasound in 1 week
D	Mifepristone followed by misoprostol	M	Repeat ultrasound scan by a senior member of staff
E	Methotrexate	N	Reassure
F	Hysteroscopy	O	Termination of pregnancy
G	Hysterectomy	P	Ultrasound scan by a fetal medicine consultant
H	KCl injection to stop fetal heart activity		
I	Laparoscopy		

Instructions: For each clinical scenario described below, choose the **single** most appropriate management from the list of options above. Each option may be used once, more than once, or not at all.

11. A 34-year-old woman attends the antenatal clinic for her booking (her first midwife appointment). She had a scan at 9 weeks following vaginal bleeding which showed a fetus with herniation of the gut through the umbilical area. The midwife comes to the registrar for advice as she is worried about the scan report.

12. A 32-year-old woman is referred to the early pregnancy assessment unit at 6 weeks of gestation with mild vaginal bleeding and suprapubic pain. Her urine shows 1 + leucocyte and no nitrates. A transvaginal scan reveals a viable intrauterine pregnancy with subchorionic bleeding.

13. A 28-year-old woman presents to the early pregnancy assessment unit with mild vaginal bleeding. An ultrasound scan shows an intrauterine gestation sac of $14 \times 15 \times 14$ mm with no fetal pole. She is unsure of her last menstrual period.

14. A 34-year-old woman at 7 weeks of gestation is sent to the early pregnancy assessment unit by her general practitioner. Her ultrasound scan confirms a missed miscarriage. She has multiple large fibroids.

15. A 28-year-old woman is referred to the early pregnancy assessment unit with a scan report of a missed miscarriage and she has been clearly informed by the ultrasonographer that the fetal heart beat is absent during the scan. The complete scan report reads as follows:

- patient's name and hospital number
- gestational age 10 weeks and 5 days
- fetal heart action present
- findings suggestive of missed miscarriage

Answers

1. A Abdominal cerclage

A previous failed transvaginal cerclage is an indication of transabdominal cerclage. It can be done prior to pregnancy or during early pregnancy. However, women should be informed about the increased morbidity associated with it (infection bleeding and pregnancy loss).

2. D Cervical cerclage contraindicated

The contraindications for a cervical cerclage include:

- active pre-term labour
- clinical evidence of chorioamnionitis
- continuing vaginal bleeding
- pre-term premature rupture of membranes
- evidence of fetal compromise
- lethal fetal defect
- fetal death

3. N Suction evacuation through the suture

In this case, the woman is eight weeks pregnant and can possibly get away with suction evacuation through the suture.

4. F Cut the suture through posterior colpotomy

Management decisions in cases of delayed miscarriage or fetal death in women with an abdominal cerclage can be difficult and should be made with senior involvement. An experienced doctor should carry out the procedure.

Suction evacuation through the suture up to 18 weeks has been described. Alternatively, the suture may be cut via posterior colpotomy. Failing this, a hysterotomy or caesarean section may be necessary.

5. K Emergency cerclage not recommended

The Royal College of Obstetricians and Gynaecologists (RCOG) does not recommend history or ultrasound indicated cerclage in women classified as other high-risk groups, including women with Müllerian anomalies, previous cervical surgeries (cone biopsy, large loop excision of the transformation zone or a destructive operation such as laser ablation or diathermy) or multiple dilatation and evacuation.

Royal College of Obstetricians and Gynaecologists. Green-top Guideline No. 60. Cervical cerclage. London: RCOG Press, 2011.

6. C Close surveillance and LMWH postnatally for 6 weeks

The Royal College of Obstetricians and Gynaecologists (RCOG) classifies the risk assessment for women with a previous VTE in the categories recurrent or single VTE. The latter can be subclassified into:

- unprovoked VTE
- oestrogen-provoked (oestrogen-containing contraception or pregnancy) VTE
- thrombophilia (heritable or acquired) or family history-associated VTE
- temporary risk factor (e.g. major trauma or surgery) associated VTE

Women with a previous single provoked VTE require close surveillance antenatally and thromboprophylaxis with LMWH for 6 weeks postpartum (to exclude oestrogen-related causes and other risk factors).

7. I Prophylactic antenatal LMWH plus postnatal for 6 weeks

Women with a recurrent VTE in the past, a previous unprovoked VTE, an oestrogen/pregnancy-related VTE or a previous VTE and a history of VTE in a first-degree relative (or a documented thrombophilia), or other risk factors should be offered thromboprophylaxis with LMWH antenatally and for 6 weeks postpartum.

8. I Prophylactic antenatal LMWH plus postnatal for 6 weeks

A previous VTE with a documented thrombophilia warrants antenatal plus postnatal LMWH for 6 weeks.

9. I Prophylactic antenatal LMWH plus postnatal for 6 weeks

Inherited thrombophilia in women who are asymptomatic and do not have other risk factors may be managed with close surveillance antenatally but should be considered for LMWH for at least 7 days postpartum.

However, for women with antithrombin deficiency, more than one thrombophilic defect (including homozygous factor V Leiden, homozygous prothrombin G20210A and compound heterozygotes) or those with additional risk factors, advice of a local expert should be sought and antenatal prophylaxis considered. Any woman receiving antenatal thromboprophylaxis should receive postnatal thromboprophylaxis for 6 weeks.

10. F Low dose aspirin until 36 weeks of gestation

Women with previous pre-eclampsia should be started on low dose aspirin in the subsequent pregnancy. This should be done as soon as the pregnancy is confirmed and continued until 36 weeks of gestation.

Royal College of Obstetricians and Gynaecologists. Green-top Guideline No. 37. Reducing the risk of thrombosis and embolism during pregnancy and puerperium. London: RCOG Press, 2009.
Calderwood CJ and Thanoon OI. Thromboembolism and thrombophilia in pregnancy. Obstet Gynecol Reprod Med 2009; 19:339–343.

11. N Reassure

Physiological gut herniation is a normal phenomenon that occurs during early pregnancy (it usually starts at 8 weeks and returns to the abdominal cavity before 12 weeks).

Physiology

Physiological herniation of the gut occurs as a result of the bowel growing faster than the abdominal cavity during the early gestational period. Subsequently, the intestine moves outside the embryonic abdomen, herniating into the base of the umbilical cord. This usually occurs at 8 weeks of gestation and is presumed to be due to the rapid growth of the cranial end of the midgut and the large size of the developing liver and kidneys. At approximately 10–12 weeks the abdomen enlarges and allows the intestines to return within the abdominal cavity (they should not be present beyond 13 weeks of gestation).

Ultrasound appearance

- herniation of the fetal gut out of the abdomen through the umbilical area
- usually seen in early pregnancy as mentioned above
- should not contain other organs, such as the liver
- the size of the herniation should be comparatively small (usually <10 mm)

If herniation of the gut is seen later in the pregnancy, one of the two differentials should be considered as listed below.

Omphalocele

- it is a defect in the abdominal wall in the midline at the umbilicus
- it occurs due to failure of the midgut to return back into the abdomen
- the bowel and abdominal content herniate through the base of the umbilical cord
- the bowel is covered by fine membranes
- it is usually associated with other defects and chromosomal anomalies, especially trisomy 13 and trisomy 18
- it is associated with a poor prognosis and outcome

Gastroschisis

- it is a defect in the abdominal wall, usually to the right of the umbilicus
- the bowel is freely floating in the amniotic fluid
- the bowel is not covered with any membranes
- the risk of chromosomal abnormality is low
- survival following surgery is 90%

12. N Reassure

Subchorionic bleeding during early pregnancy is not uncommon and usually resolves itself. This woman should be reassured and managed conservatively.

13. L Repeat ultrasound in 1 week

In known cases of intrauterine pregnancy, viability will be uncertain in approximately 10% of women at their first early pregnancy assessment unit (EPAU) visit.

Pregnancy of uncertain viability:

- Intrauterine sac (<25 mm mean diameter) with no obvious fetus or yolk sac

Or:

- Fetal echo <7 mm crown–rump length with no obvious fetal heart activity. In order to confirm or refute viability, a repeat scan at a minimal interval of 1 week is necessary.

14. D Mifepristone followed by misoprostol

This woman has large uterine fibroids and should be managed by medical rather than surgical treatment unless emergency evaluation of retained products is necessary due to excessive bleeding.

15. M Repeat ultrasound scan by a senior member of staff

There is a disparity in the scan report saying fetal heart action present but the final report implies missed miscarriage. Although the woman has been told clearly that the fetal heartbeat is absent, it is important to repeat the scan by seniors (ideally a consultant) just to confirm the viability again as otherwise this may lead to litigation.

Royal College of Obstetricians and Gynaecologists. Green-top Guideline No. 25. The management of early pregnancy loss. London: RCOG Press, 2006.
Buckett W and Regan L. Chapter 23: Sporadic and recurrent miscarriage. In: Shaw RW, Luesley D, Monga A (eds). Gynaecology (4th edn). Edinburgh: Churchill Livingstone, 2011.

Chapter 22

Fetal medicine

Questions 1–5

Options for Questions 1–5

A	Hepatitis B	I	Epstein–Barr virus
B	Hepatitis C	J	Influenza A
C	Hepatitis E	K	Measles
D	Herpes simplex type 1	L	Parvovirus B19
E	Herpes simplex type 2	M	Rubella
F	Human immunodeficiency virus (HIV)	N	Rhinovirus
G	Human papilloma virus	O	Varicella
H	Cytomegalovirus		

Instructions: For each fetal or neonatal condition described below, choose the **single** most appropriate maternal viral infection from the list of options above. Each option may be used once, more than once, or not at all.

1. Laryngeal papilloma in infants.

2. Patent ductus arteriosus.

3. Cutaneous scarring in the fetus.

4. Ventriculomegaly in the fetus.

5. Limb hypoplasia in the fetus.

Questions 6–10

Options for Questions 6–10

A	Amitriptyline	I	Lithium
B	Benzodiazepines	J	Olanzapine
C	Citalopram	K	Paroxetine
D	Clozapine	L	Risperidone
E	Domperidone	M	Sertraline
F	Fluoxetine	N	Sulpiride
G	Haloperidol	O	Venlafaxine
H	Imipramine		

Instructions: For each abnormality described below, choose the **single** most appropriate drug from the list of options above. Each option may be used once, more than once, or not at all.

6. Risk of raised blood pressure on higher dose.

7. Right ventricular outflow tract obstruction.

8. Risk of gestational diabetes and weight gain.

9. Agranulocytosis in the fetus and breastfed infant.

10. Cleft palate.

Questions 11–15

Options for Questions 11–15

A   Avoid amniocentesis in the third trimester
B   Amniocentesis of a single twin sac
C   Biophysical profile
D   Chorionic villus sampling before 10 weeks
E   Chorionic villus sampling after 10 weeks
F   Cordocentesis
G   Detailed fetal anomaly scan and fetal cardiac scan
H   First trimester amniocentesis
I   Fetal growth scan
J   Fetal scalp blood sampling
K   *In utero* fetal blood transfusion
L   Middle cerebral artery doppler
M   Peritoneal shunt
N   Second trimester amniocentesis
O   Third trimester amniocentesis

Instructions: For each clinical scenario described below, choose the **single** most appropriate initial intervention from the list of options above. Each option may be used once, more than once, or not at all.

11. A 29-year-old Asian woman presents to the day assessment unit at 35 weeks of gestation with reduced fetal movements. An anomaly scan performed in another country at 20 weeks gestation was normal. A fetal cardiotocograph (CTG) reveals reduced variability for 60 minutes followed by a normal CTG. A detailed ultrasound scan performed by the fetal medicine department reveals polyhydramnios and double bubble sign with no other abnormality. Booking blood results (her first midwife appointment) show that she is positive for HIV antigen.

12. A 29-year-old Caucasian woman attends the antenatal clinic at 15 weeks for a review of her booking antenatal investigations. Her haematological, biochemical and virology results are normal and she is Rhesus positive with no antibodies. However, her screening (quadruple) tests for trisomies showed an increased risk of trisomy 21 (more than 1 in 100) and an ultrasound at 13 weeks and 5 days revealed an increased nuchal translucency.

13. A 29-year-old European woman, para 1, attends for her dating scan (at 12 weeks) which reveals normal morphological features of the baby but 5 mm nuchal translucency. Her serum screening tests reveal decreased pregnancy-associated plasma protein A (PAPP-A) levels.

14. A 29-year-old Afro-Caribbean woman attends her antenatal booking appointment with the midwife at 15 weeks gestation. Four weeks later she comes in for her

booking blood test results. Her haematological, biochemical and virology results were normal and her blood group was 'O' positive with no antibodies. However, her quadruple test for trisomy 21 showed an increased risk (more than 1 in 100). She refuses to have invasive testing.

15. A 29-year-old Asian woman attends the ultrasound department for her dating scan at 13 weeks and 5 days. It reveals a monochorionic diamniotic twin pregnancy and an increased nuchal translucency of both the twins. She is quite anxious as this is her fifth attempt at an IVF pregnancy. After appropriate counselling, she declines invasive testing and leaves the consultation room. Two weeks later, she returns and decides to have the test.

Questions 16–20

Options for Questions 16–20

A	Twin reversed arterial perfusion (TRAP)	H	Non-immune hydrops
B	Alpha–thalassaemia	I	Idiopathic hydrops
C	Beta–thalassaemia	J	Immune hydrops
D	Congenital toxoplasmosis	K	Down syndrome
E	Congenital heart disease	L	Turner syndrome
F	Congenital adenomatoid malformation of lungs	M	Twin-to-twin transfusion
		N	Sickle cell disease
G	Congenital diaphragmatic hernia	O	Parvovirus infection
		P	Placental insufficiency

Instructions: For each clinical scenario described below, choose the **single** most appropriate diagnosis from the list of options above. Each option may be used once, more than once, or not at all.

16. A 36-year-old Caucasian woman attends the obstetric day assessment unit at 28 weeks of gestation with reduced fetal movement for the last 2 days. An ultrasound scan reveals an absence of fetal heart activity and a hydropic fetus. She delivers 24 hours later following induced labour and agrees to be investigated. At her six-week postnatal follow-up visit, the postmortem results reveal a macerated fetus with ventricular septal defect and oesophageal atresia. Her booking blood tests were normal.

17. A 36-year-old Asian woman attends the obstetric day assessment unit at 37 weeks of gestation with reduced fetal movements for the last 24 hours. A CTG shows fetal tachycardia of more than 200 beats/minute. An ultrasound scan reveals an obvious scalp oedema and ascites. The fetal heart rate normalised following administration of flecainide to the mother. Subsequently, she was delivered by caesarean section and the baby was admitted to the neonatal unit. Her booking blood tests were normal.

18. A 36-year-old Asian woman attends the obstetric day assessment unit at 34 weeks of gestation with reduced fetal movements. Clinical examination reveals she is small for dates and has reduced amniotic fluid. Vital signs show raised blood pressure with normal pulse and temperature. She does not have a history of

ruptured membranes or any recent illness. A fetal cardiotocograph (CTG) reveals a baseline heart rate of 140 beats/minute, variability <5 beats/minute, absence of accelerations and unprovoked shallow decelerations with slow recovery for 40 minutes. A tocograph reveals an absence of uterine activity.

19. A 36-year-old Caucasian woman, para 1, attends the obstetric day assessment unit at 32 weeks of gestation with reduced fetal movements. A CTG reveals baseline heart rate of 150 beats/minute, variability <5 beats/minute, absence of accelerations and two shallow unprovoked decelerations in the last 40 minutes. A repeat CTG 6 hours later shows baseline 150, variability <5, absence of accelerations and occasional repeat decelerations. An ultrasound scan reveals fetal ascites and pleural effusion. Her booking blood tests show her blood group to be 'O' negative with anti-D antibodies (titre 1:16).

20. A 36-year-old Caucasian woman attends the obstetric day assessment unit at 30 weeks of gestation with reduced fetal movements. An ultrasound scan revealed fetal ascites and an absence of fetal heart activity. Her booking blood tests and anomaly scan at 20 weeks of gestation were normal. She had a vaginal delivery and attends for her bereavement appointment and postmortem results 6 weeks later. Her haematological, biochemical and infection screen for hydrops was normal. However, postmortem results revealed hydropic changes in the fetus.

Questions 21–25

Options for Questions 21–25

A	Anencephaly	H	Gastroschisis
B	Adenomatoid malformation of the lung	I	Meconium ileus
		J	Microcephaly
C	Choroid plexus cyst	K	Neural tube defect
D	Cardiac echogenic foci	L	Patau syndrome
E	Diaphragmatic hernia	M	Pelvicaliceal dilatation
F	Down syndrome	N	Ventriculomegaly
G	Exomphalos	O	Virilisation of fetus

Instructions: For each condition described below, choose the **single** most appropriate association from the list of options above. Each option may be used once, more than once, or not at all.

21. A 38-year-old Caucasian woman attends her antenatal clinic appointment for a review of her booking investigations. Her booking blood tests are normal. The anomaly scan at 20 weeks of gestation reveals a hyperechogenic bowel.

22. A 38-year-old Caucasian woman is referred to the fetal medicine unit as her 20-week anomaly scan shows some abnormality of the head. A repeat ultrasound scan by a fetal medicine specialist reveals holoprosencephaly.

23. A 38-year-old Asian woman attends her antenatal clinic appointment at 20 weeks of gestation. The anomaly scan at 20 weeks of gestation reveals pulmonary hypoplasia and mediastial shift to right side. She does not give any history of ruptured membranes.

24. A 38-year-old Afro-Caribbean woman is referred to the day assessment unit by her midwife as her clinical examination revealed a uterine height of 29 cm at 32 weeks of gestation. As the fetus was fine, a growth scan was arranged and she was discharged home. One week later she attends the antenatal clinic with her growth scan report which shows an estimated fetal weight of 1300 g with short long bones.

25. A 38-year-old Asian woman attends her antenatal clinic appointment at 28 weeks of gestation following her growth scan, which showed her to be small for dates. The scan shows normal growth with a double bubble sign.

Answers

1. G Human papilloma virus

Maternal genital warts are caused by human papilloma virus 6 and 11. The presence of genital warts during vaginal birth can transmit the virus to the baby and can cause laryngeal papillomas which obstruct the airway in the infant.

2. M Rubella

Rubella causes a triad of symptoms: (a) cardiac – patent ductus arteriosus, pulmonary artery stenosis, pulmonary valvular stenosis, coarctation of aorta, atrial septal defect and ventricular septal defect (the last two are rare abnormalities); (b) eye – congenital cataract; and (c) ear – sensorineural deafness.

3. O Varicella

Congenital varicella infection causes limb hypoplasia, cutaneous scarring, hypoplastic digits, muscular atrophy, paralysis, seizures, microcephaly, chorioretinitis, chorioretinal scarring, optic disc hypoplasia, Horner syndrome, cataracts, cerebral cortical atrophy, early childhood zoster and psychomotor retardation.

4. H Cytomegalovirus

Cytomegalovirus infection of the fetus can cause abnormalities which manifest in the early or late neonatal period. These include hepatosplenomegaly, jaundice, haemolytic anaemia, thrombocytopenia, growth restriction, microcephaly, chorioretinitis, optic atrophy, seizures, cerebral atrophy, psychomotor retardation, learning disabilities, dental abnormalities, pneumonitis and intracerebral calcifications.

5. O Varicella

Varicella affects the fetus in less than 2% of cases before 20 weeks of gestation. It causes various defects, including limb defects, but it usually manifests weeks later, before it can be identified on the ultrasound scan. Therefore, an ultrasound scan should be arranged 5 weeks after the date of presentation.

James D, Steer PJ, Weiner CP, Gonik B, Crowther C, Robson S (eds). High Risk Pregnancy: Management Options (4th edn). St Louis: Saunders, 2011.
Nelson-Piercy C. Handbook of Obstetric Medicine (4th edn). London: Informa Healthcare, 2010.

6. O Venlafaxine

If taken in high doses venlafaxine is associated with high blood pressure and an increased risk of withdrawal symptoms.

Tricyclic antidepressants

- amitriptyline and imipramine are associated with lower risks in pregnancy
- no increase in incidence of miscarriage or malformation
- associated with neonatal withdrawal syndrome and therefore, if possible, reduce the dose 3–4 weeks prior to delivery
- can have an adverse synergistic effect if taken with multiple drugs or alcohol

Other drugs

- All antidepressants are associated with neonatal withdrawal symptoms. In most cases these effects are mild and self-limiting.
- Imipramine, nortriptyline and sertraline have lower levels in breast milk than other antidepressants.
- Citalopram and fluoxetine have higher levels in breast milk than other antidepressants.

7. K Paroxetine

Selective serotonin reuptake inhibitors (SSRIs)

SSRIs are the most commonly used drugs for the treatment of depression. Data on the safety of SSRIs in human pregnancy are limited, but recently their use during pregnancy has shown to be associated with congenital heart defects in the fetus.

Important points:

- Fluoxetine has the lowest risks.
- Paroxetine is associated with heart defects if taken during the first trimester, hence advise women to stop taking this drug.
- SSRIs can be associated with neonatal withdrawal syndrome, which includes convulsions, irritability, tremors, rigidity and feeding problems.
- Persistent pulmonary hypertension in the neonate if taken after 20 weeks of gestation (persistent pulmonary hypertension occurs in 1–2 infants per 1000 live births and is associated with increased morbidity and mortality. Despite treatment, 10–20% of affected infants will not survive. Newborns with this condition are typically full-term or near-term infants who present shortly after birth with severe respiratory failure requiring intubation and mechanical ventilation).
- SSRIs use in the first trimester is associated with an increased risk of anencephaly, craniosynostosis and omphalocele, specifically with use of paroxetine.
- Sertraline use is associated with omphalocele and septal defects.
- Paroxetine is associated with right ventricular outflow tract obstruction.

8. J Olanzapine

Antipsychotic associations:

- risperidone and sulpiride: raise prolactin levels
- olanzapine: risk of gestational diabetes and weight gain
- are associated with extra pyramidal symptoms in the neonate especially depot preparations. They are usually self-limiting.

9. D Clozapine

Antipsychotics

Clozapine can cause agranulocytosis in the fetus and breastfed infants.

10. B Benzodiazepines

Benzodiazepines:

- used in anxiety disorders and panic attacks
- should not be prescribed routinely except for the short-term treatment of extreme anxiety and agitation
- risk of cleft palate
- floppy baby syndrome in the neonate.

Louik C, Lin AE, Werler MM, Hernández-Díaz S, Mitchell AA. First-trimester use of selective serotonin-reuptake inhibitors and the risk of birth defects. N Engl J Med 2007; 356:2675–2683.

Alwan S, Reefhuis J, Rasmussen SA, Olney RS, Friedman JM. Use of selective serotonin-reuptake inhibitors in pregnancy and the risk of birth defects. N Engl J Med 2007; 356:2684–2692.

Chambers CD, Hernandez-Diaz S, Van Marter LJ, Werler MM, Louik C, Lyons Jones K, Mitchell AA. Selective serotonin-reuptake inhibitors and risk of persistent pulmonary hypertension of the newborn. N Engl J Med 2006; 354:579–587.

11. A Avoid amniocentesis in the third trimester

Testing women with HIV should be avoided, particularly in the third trimester.

If invasive prenatal diagnosis is considered essential in HIV positive women, it should be undertaken under anti-retroviral treatment cover.

Invasive prenatal testing in the first or second trimester can be carried out in women who carry hepatitis B or C. However, the available data are limited and this should be explained to the patient.

The indications for third-trimester amniocentesis include:

- late karyotyping
- amniotic fluid optical density assessments for Rhesus disease
- measure amniotic fluid insulin levels
- lung maturity studies
- detection of indices of infection in suspected pre-term labour or rupture of the membranes

The risk of emergency delivery does not appear to be high with third-trimester amniocentesis. However, complications such as multiple attempts and blood stained fluid are more common compared to mid-trimester procedures.

12. N Second-trimester amniocentesis

Amniocentesis

Early: before 14 completed weeks of gestation

Late: after 15 weeks of gestation

One of the main reasons for amniocentesis is to detect whether or not the fetus has a chromosomal disorder (e.g. Down syndrome). The safest time to do an amniocentesis is after 15 weeks of pregnancy. However, one should counsel the woman about the risks, which include:

- abdominal discomfort and vaginal spotting
- 1% risk of miscarriage, infection and leakage of amniotic fluid
- inadequate first sample and need for reinsertion of the needle: about 8 in every 100 women having amniocentesis
- serious infection: less than 1 in 1000 women who have amniocentesis
- anti-D immunoglobulin injection is recommended for women who are Rhesus negative to prevent formation of antibodies against fetal red blood cells

It is recommended that early amniocentesis (before 14 weeks) should be avoided as it is associated with greater fetal loss compared with late amniocentesis (after 15 weeks) (7.6% vs. 5.9%).

Also, a 10-fold increase in fetal neonatal talipes is reported with early amniocenteses. However, the Royal College of Obstetricians and Gynaecologists (RCOG) recommends that an early amniocentesis is undertaken in exceptional circumstances after the mother is counselled adequately and fully made aware of the potential complications.

There are two types of laboratory test used for the detection of chromosomal abnormalities:

- a full karyotype: usually takes 2–3 weeks for results
- a rapid test to check for specific chromosomes: usually takes 3 working days for results. This is used to detect Down syndrome (trisomy 21), Edwards syndrome (trisomy18), Patau syndrome (trisomy 13) and sex chromosome disorders.

13. E Chorionic villus sampling after 10 weeks

Chorionic villus sampling

Chorionic villus sampling (CVS) is usually performed between 11 and 13 weeks and under ultrasound guidance (performed transvaginally between 11 and 13 weeks and transabdominally from 13 weeks onwards).

CVS before 10 weeks is associated with oromandibular hypoplasia and isolated limb disruption defects (attributed to transient fetal hypoperfusion and vasospastic phenomenon secondary to vascular disruption of the placental circulation). Therefore, CVS is not recommended before 10 completed weeks of gestation.

The risks of CVS include:

- abdominal discomfort and vaginal bleeding
- miscarriage: 2%
- a full karyotype may not give a clear result following CVS: about 1 in 100
- serious infection: less than 1 in 1000 women who have CVS

- anti-D immunoglobulin injection is recommended for women who are Rhesus negative to prevent formation of antibodies against fetal red blood cells

14. G Detailed fetal anomaly scan and fetal cardiac scan

Women should be appropriately counselled to make an informed choice. Following this, one should respect their decision and support her through the pregnancy. A detailed anomaly scan and fetal cardiac scan is important to check for abnormalities (since trisomy 21 is associated with gut and cardiac abnormalities) to inform and prepare them for delivery. Also, a multidisciplinary team should be involved to treat the child with abnormalities at birth (medical as well as surgical treatment).

15. B Amniocentesis of a single twin sac

Nuchal translucency is the screening test for trisomies performed for women with twin pregnancy. In monochorionic and diamniotic twins, amniocentesis of one twin sac is enough to make the diagnosis.

Royal College of Obstetricians and Gynaecologists. Green-top Guideline No. 8. Amniocentesis and chorionic villus biopsy. London: RCOG Press, 2005.
Royal College of Obstetricians and Gynaecologists. Amniocentesis: what you need to know (patient information leaflet). London: RCOG Press, 2006.
Royal College of Obstetricians and Gynaecologists. Chorionic villus biopsy: what you need to know (patient information leaflet). London: RCOG Press, 2006.

16. K Down syndrome

Oesophageal atresia

- Absence of stomach bubble or poor visualisation of the stomach
- Present after 25 weeks of gestation
- It is associated with chromosomal abnormalities in 20% of cases
- Mostly associated with Down syndrome
- It is also associated with cardiac anomalies in 50% of cases

17. H Non-immune hydrops

Fetal tachyarrhythmia is one of the causes for non-immune hydrops. The mother should be urgently referred to a fetal medicine specialist for review as well as for a scan to confirm the findings.

Treatment for the fetus can be started *in utero* with maternal administration of drugs. Also, an urgent fetal echocardiogram should be performed to determine the rate and rhythm, and to rule out any cardiac abnormalities (as a cardiac cause is found in 30% of the cases of non-immune hydrops). The prognosis is better in the absence of structural cardiac abnormalities.

The poor prognosis and risk of intrauterine death if the fetus does not respond to treatment should be explained to the mother.

In this case, she is already at term, therefore delivery can be accomplished.

18. P Placental insufficiency

The clinical findings are suggestive of placental insufficiency. The CTG is pathological as there are recurrent unprovoked decelerations. She needs immediate caesarean delivery as she is not in labour.

19. J Immune hydrops

The investigation reveals that this woman is Rhesus negative and has antibodies. If the antibody titre is 1:4, it is more likely to be due to administration of an anti-D immunoglobulin injection. However, if the titre is more than this (more than 1 in 4), it indicates rhesus isoimmunisation leading to hydrops fetalis.

20. I Idiopathic hydrops

When no cause is found for hydrops, it is labelled as idiopathic which accounts for one third of the cases of hydrops.

Magowan B. Churchill's Pocketbook of Obstetrics and Gynaecology (3rd edn). Churchill Livingstone, 2005. James D, Steer PJ, Weiner CP, Gonik B, Crowther C, Robson S (eds). High Risk Pregnancy: Management Options (4th edn). Saunders Elsevier, 2011.

21. I Meconium ileus

Hyperechogenic bowel is associated with cystic fibrosis, meconium ileus, cytomegalovirus infection, trisomy 21, fetal growth restriction and fetal death. Most cases are not clinically significant. However, it is important to screen for the cystic fibrosis gene (Delta F 508 mutation), serum IgM for cytomegalovirus and karyotyping for aneuploidy. As it is also associated with fetal growth restriction (8%) and intrauterine fetal death (23%), serial scans should be arranged.

22. L Patau syndrome

Holoprosencephaly

It is a disorder in which the prosencephalon or the forebrain of the embryo fails to develop into two hemispheres. Other features include partially or completely fused thalami or ventricles (single ventricle), absence of cavum septi pellucidi, dysgenesis of the corpus callosum and associated midline facial abnormalities (with a single eye and midline proboscis in the region of the nose). The malformations of the brain are very severe and will lead to miscarriage or stillbirth.

It is usually associated with trisomy 13 and 18, triploidy and warfarin use during early pregnancy.

23. E Diaphragmatic hernia

Diaphragmatic hernia (incidence 1 in 2500) is difficult to diagnose on an ultrasound scan. The stomach in the chest or dextrocardia should raise a high suspicion of this condition. It is commonly associated with trisomy 18. In 85% of cases, it occurs on the left side and may cause mediastinal shift and pulmonary hypoplasia. The prognosis is bad when the liver is involved on the right side.

24. F Down syndrome

Shortened long bones

Shortened long bones on ultrasound scan (especially the femur and humerus) are more likely seen in fetuses with Down syndrome. The risk increases 11-fold if both the bones are short. The fetal growth restriction is symmetrical unlike babies with placental insufficiency which have an asymmetrical growth pattern (head sparing). It is important to consider performing karyotyping in the fetus with symmetrical fetal growth restriction to rule out chromosomal abnormalities.

25. F Down syndrome

Duodenal atresia

- Double bubble sign is seen in duodenal atresia
- It is present after 25 weeks of gestation
- It is associated with chromosomal abnormalities in 40% of cases
- It is mostly associated with Down syndrome.
- It is also associated with cardiac anomalies in 50% of cases

Soft markers on the ultrasound scan in the fetus are usually transient features which may indicate a risk to the fetus in the form of chromosomal abnormalities. However, if they are found alone they may not pose any major problem or risk to the fetus. The most common soft markers include echogenic focus in the heart, hyperechogenic bowel, pelvicaliceal dilatation, choroid plexus cyst and short femur.

Choroid plexus cyst

- Incidence: 1–2% of fetuses in the second trimester scan
- Echolucent structures found in the choroid plexus of the lateral ventricles
- If it is an isolated finding, it does not have much significance. The majority (90%) of them disappear by 26 weeks of gestation
- If associated with other soft markers, chromosomal abnormalities need to be ruled out
- It is usually associated with trisomy 18, while the risk for trisomy 21 is not increased

Increased nuchal translucency

- It can be simple or septated
- The risk is higher with a septated pattern
- It is associated with increased risk of chromosomal abnormalities
- It is also associated with Turner syndrome, Noonan syndrome and Robert syndrome

- It is associated with fetal cardiac abnormalities
- it is associated with increased perinatal mortality

Cardiac echogenic foci

- Hyperechogenicity is located in the chordate tendineae
- It resolves spontaneously in most cases
- The risk of chromosomal abnormalities is low
- If it is an isolated finding and there are no other risk factors, there is no need for invasive testing

Ventriculomegaly

- Incidence: 1% of pregnancies
- Lateral ventricular dilatation >10 mm
- It can be unilateral or bilateral
- It can be associated with chromosomal or congenital anomalies or may be an acquired condition due to infection and haemorrhage or may be unexplained
- Prognosis depends on associated chromosomal abnormalities or other defects.

James D, Steer PJ, Weiner CP, Gonik B, Crowther C, Robson S (eds). High Risk Pregnancy: Management Options (4th edn). St Louis: Saunders, 2011.
Connor JM. Medical Genetics for MRCOG and Beyond. London: RCOG Press, 2005.

Chapter 23

Gynaecological oncology

Questions 1–5

Options for Questions 1–5

A	Stage IA	G	Stage IIIA
B	Stage IB	H	Stage IIIB
C	Stage IC	I	Stage IIIC1
D	Stage II	J	Stage IIIC2
E	Stage IIA	K	Stage IVA
F	Stage IIB	L	Stage IVB

Instructions: For each scenario described below, choose the **single** most appropriate the International Federation of Gynecology and Obstetrics (FIGO) stage for endometrial cancer from the list of options above. Each option may be used once, more than once, or not at all.

1. A 60-year-old woman presents with postmenopausal bleeding (PMB) to the gynaecology oncology clinic. An endometrial pipelle biopsy reveals an endometrioid adenocarcinoma. She is further investigated with a magnetic resonance imaging (MRI) scan which reveals uterine myometrial invasion of less than 50% and enlarged pelvic nodes. She subsequently undergoes a total abdominal hysterectomy, bilateral salpingo-oophorectomy and sentinel lymph node biopsy. You review her in the clinic at 2 weeks follow-up with a histology report of endometrial cancer with myometrial invasion of more than 50% and pelvic lymph node involvement.

2. A 44-year-old woman presents to the emergency department with heavy vaginal bleeding and intermenstrual bleeding for the last 6 months. Following a gynaecology review a hysteroscopy and endometrial biopsy were arranged. Two weeks after her hysteroscopy she attends the gynaecology oncology clinic and the histology reveals a papillary serous carcinoma. A computed tomography (CT) scan of the chest is reported as normal while the MRI scan reveals a large uterine tumour infiltrating the serosal surface of the uterus and also involving the pelvic nodes. Subsequently, she undergoes a total abdominal hysterectomy, bilateral salpingo-oophorectomy and pelvic lymphadenectomy in an oncology centre. The final histology confirms the MRI findings.

3. An 82-year-old woman presents to the emergency department with postmenopausal heavy bleeding and her haemoglobin is 7 g/dL. She receives 2 units of blood transfusion and undergoes hysteroscopy and an endometrial biopsy on an emergency basis, as she continued to bleed heavily. An endometrial

biopsy reveals clear cell carcinoma. She subsequently undergoes a total abdominal hysterectomy, bilateral salpingo-oophorectomy and pelvic lymphadenectomy. The histology reveals clear cell carcinoma involving the uterine cervix and serosal surface.

4. A 55-year-old woman is referred to a rapid access clinic with PMB. She returns to the clinic for her pipelle biopsy results which reveal endometrial cancer. She then undergoes a total abdominal hysterectomy and bilateral salpingo-oophorectomy. The final histology reveals tumour infiltration of less than 50% of the myometrium and involvement of the cervical stroma. Also, peritoneal washings are reported to be positive for malignant cells.

5. A 58-year-old woman attends the rapid access clinic with PMB, following which she has outpatient hysteroscopy and endometrial biopsy. The histology revealed an endometrioid adenocarcinoma. She subsequently undergoes a total abdominal hysterectomy and bilateral salpingo-oophorectomy. The final histology is reported as endometrioid adenocarcinoma involving the endometrium and peritoneal washings were positive for malignant cells.

Questions 6–10

Options for Questions 6–10

A	Benign teratoma	G	Granulosa cell tumour
B	Choriocarcinoma	H	Gynandroblastoma
C	Dysgerminoma	I	Gonadoblastoma
D	Endodermal sinus tumour	J	Leydig cell tumour
E	Embryonal carcinoma	K	Malignant teratoma
F	Epithelial ovarian tumour	L	Sertoli cell tumour

Instructions: For each scenario described below, choose the **single** most appropriate tumour type from the list of options above. Each option may be used once, more than once, or not at all.

6. A 19-year-old girl is referred to the gynaecology clinic with a scan report of a bilateral ovarian mass. An MRI scan confirms a bilateral solid ovarian tumour. The blood test results show an increase in lactate dehydrogenase and placental alkaline phosphatase. She is referred to an oncology centre for further management, following which she undergoes staging for ovarian cancer and bilateral oophorectomy. Her final histology shows marked lymphocytic infiltration in the stroma surrounding the tumour cells.

7. A 20-year-old woman presents to the emergency department with abdominal distention and pain. Clinical examination reveals a palpable abdomino-pelvic mass and an ultrasound scan shows a unilateral solid ovarian mass on the right side. Her tumour marker alpha fetoprotein was 300 U/mL and CA 125 45 U/mL. She was then referred to the gynaecology oncology centre for further management. She had further imaging in the form of MRI and CT scans and underwent staging laparotomy and right-sided oophorectomy. The histology revealed a Schiller–Duval body.

8. An 18-year-old girl presents to her general practitioner with distention of the abdomen. An ultrasound scan reveals a unilateral solid/cystic mass on the left side. An MRI scan confirms that the ovarian tumour is confined to the left ovary and the right ovary looks normal. However, her tumour markers, beta human chorionic gonadotropin (beta hCG) and alpha fetoprotein, were normal. She is then referred to the gynaecology oncology centre for further management, following which she undergoes staging laparotomy and left-sided oophorectomy. One of the components of the histology shows elements of glial tissue.

9. A 55-year-old menopausal woman presents to the emergency department with irregular vaginal bleeding. An abdominal scan shows a large pelvic mass on the right side and a thickened endometrium (20 mm). An MRI scan reveals similar findings. The blood test shows a raised α subunit of inhibin and CA 125 48 U/mL. She gives a family history of breast cancer and is currently on tamoxifen.

10. A 58-year-old woman presents to the emergency department with abdominal bloating and a decreased appetite. She had opened her bowels 2 days ago. Clinical examination reveals a distended abdomen with signs of subacute bowel obstruction. A CT scan of the abdomen and pelvis revealed a large complex pelvic mass (size 15 × 12 × 12 cm) with raised CA 125 (1000 U/mL) and normal carcinoembryonic antigen (CEA) (2 U/mL).

Questions 11–15

Options for Questions 11–15

A	Cervical smear in 6 months	H	Punch biopsy of the cervical lesion
B	Cervical smear in 12 months	I	Refer to oncology centre
C	Cervical smear in 24 months	J	Repeat colposcopy in 3 months
D	Cervical random punch biopsy	K	Repeat colposcopy in 12 months
E	Knife cone biopsy	L	Repeat colposcopy in 24 months
F	Large loop excision of transformation zone (LLETZ)	M	Repeat colposcopy in 2 months
		N	Repeat colposcopy in 4 months
G	Needs discussion in the multidisciplinary team (MDT) meeting	O	Repeat colposcopy in 5 years

Instructions: For each scenario described below, choose the **single** most appropriate management from the list of options above. Each option may be used once, more than once, or not at all.

11. A 28-year-old nulliparous woman is referred to the colposcopy clinic by her general practitioner. She is up to date with smears and never had any previous abnormal smears other than the current cervical smear showing mild dyskaryosis. Colposcopy reveals a mild acetowhite area at the 11 o'clock position and is reported as satisfactory with no abnormal vessels.

12. A 41-year-old woman is referred to the colposcopy clinic with a cervical smear report of moderate dyskaryosis. She also gives a history of two borderline smears in the past. Colposcopy is satisfactory and reveals a severe acetowhite area with

coarse mosaicism at the 6 o'clock and 9 o'clock positions. She hates hospitals and did not attend her previous two appointments.

13. A 40-year-old woman is referred to the colposcopy clinic by her general practitioner with a referral cervical smear report of severe dyskaryosis. Colposcopy is unsatisfactory and reveals a severe acetowhite area at the 3 o'clock and 5 o'clock positions with abnormal vessels. She is a chain smoker and gives a family history of stroke.

14. A 30-year-old woman is referred to the colposcopy clinic by her general practitioner with a referral cervical smear report of moderate dyskaryosis. Colposcopy is satisfactory and normal. Medically she suffers from asthma and gives a family history of Huntington disease.

15. A 34-year-old woman is referred to the colposcopy clinic with a smear report of glandular neoplasia. Colposcopy is unsatisfactory and reveals high-grade abnormality intraepithelial neoplasia (CIN3) at the 5 o'clock and 10 o'clock positions and human papillomavirus (HPV) infection at the 6 o'clock position.

Questions 16–20

Options for Questions 16–20

A   Follow-up smear at 6 months
B   Follow-up smear at 8 months
C   Follow-up vault smear at 6 months
D   Follow-up vault smear at 6 and
      18 months
E   Follow-up vault smear at 24 months
F   Large loop excision of transformation
      zone
G   Knife cone biopsy
H   Needs to be seen in a colposcopy
      clinic within 1 week
I   Needs to be seen in a colposcopy
      clinic within 2 weeks

J   Needs to be seen in a colposcopy
      clinic within 3 weeks
K   Needs to be seen in a colposcopy
      clinic within 4 weeks
L   Needs to be seen in a colposcopy
      clinic within 8 weeks
M   Needs to be seen in a colposcopy
      clinic within 10 weeks
N   Needs to be seen in a colposcopy
      clinic within 14 weeks
O   Needs to be seen in a colposcopy
      clinic within 18 weeks

Instructions: For each scenario described below, choose the **single** most appropriate management from the list of options above. Each option may be used once, more than once, or not at all.

16. A 36-year-old woman, para 2, is referred to the colposcopy clinic after a routine smear showing mild dyskaryosis. She is up to date with her smears and gives a history of mild dyskaryosis on cytology 6 months ago. She is currently in a relationship and is using the progesterone only pill for contraception. She smokes 12 cigarettes per day.

17. A 38-year-old woman, para 4, is referred to the colposcopy clinic with a smear result of moderate dyskaryosis. She is generally up to date with her smears with no previous abnormal smears. She had a copper coil fitted 6 months

ago for contraception. She now suffers from heavy periods but does not have intermenstrual or postcoital bleeding. She is a social drinker and smokes five cigarettes per day. She also gives a strong family history of ovarian cancer

18. A 26-year-old woman is referred to the colposcopy clinic following a routine smear showing borderline abnormality in the endocervical cells. She is terrified that she has cancer. She has been on ethinylestradiol with drospirenone (Yasmin) for the last 2 years and complains of some headache and tiredness. She also smokes 10 cigarettes per day.

19. A 48-year-old woman, para 10, is referred to the colposcopy services with a clinical impression of suspicious cervix. She is up to date with her smears and has never had an abnormal smear. She has never had surgery before and is needle-phobic. She is social drinker and smokes 20 cigarettes per day. Recently, her mother died of breast cancer and her father has pancreatic cancer.

20. A 35-year-old woman is referred to the colposcopy clinic with a smear report of glandular neoplasia. Medically, she suffers from contact dermatitis and is allergic to peanut oil. She does not have any support at home.

Questions 21–25

Options for Questions 21–25

A	Follow-up cervical smear in 6 months	I	Vault smear in 6 months
B	Follow-up cervical smear in 10 months	J	Vault smear in 6 and 18 months
C	Follow-up cervical smear in 12 months	K	Vault smears and colposcopy as per protocols for follow-up of grade III cervical intraepithelial neoplasia (CIN3)
D	Follow-up cervical smear in 14 months	L	Vault smears and colposcopy as per protocol for follow-up for grade I cervical intraepithelial neoplasia (CIN 1)
E	Follow-up cervical smear in 6 months plus colposcopy		
F	May need hysteroscopy and endometrial biopsy	M	Vault smears at 1 year and 2 years
G	May need a knife cone biopsy	N	Vault smears at 1 year and 5 years
H	No need for a repeat cervical smear	O	Vault smear not indicated

Instructions: For each scenario described below, choose the **single** most appropriate management from the list of options above. Each option may be used once, more than once, or not at all.

21. A 46-year-old woman attends the general practitioner centre for her routine cervical smear. She is claustrophobic, but otherwise medically fit and well. She had a levonorgestrel IUS fitted 1 year ago for menorrhagia but it was removed 6 months ago due to missing threads. Since then, she has been having regular monthly periods and her last menstrual period was 3 weeks ago. The smear report shows normal squamous cells representative of transformation zone, endocervical cells and normal endometrial cells are seen on cytology.

22. A 36-year-old woman, para 3, presents to her general practitioner with an excessive white vaginal discharge. She has had three partners in the last year and is currently in a new relationship. She gives a history of an intrauterine copper device (IUCD) fitted 4 years ago. She drinks socially and smokes 20 cigarettes per day. Her cervical cytology a year ago was reported normal.

23. A 26-year-old woman had her first cervical smear recently which is reported as negative with some wart virus changes. She gives a history of childbirth 6 months ago.

24. A 25-year-old woman underwent a medical termination of pregnancy 3 months ago. She comes to the general practitioner centre today and has her first cervical smear, which is reported as borderline in squamous cells.

25. A 36-year-old woman presents to her general practitioner with vulval itching. Clinical examination reveals contact dermatitis. Her periods are generally regular and she is currently on her period. Her recent smear is normal but shows candida infection.

Questions 26–30

Options for Questions 26–30

A	CA 125	I	Repeat scan not necessary
B	Chemotherapy	J	Repeat the transabdominal ultrasound scan
C	Computed tomography (CT)		
D	Magnetic resonance imaging (MRI)	K	Repeat the transvaginal scan (TVS)
E	Ovarian cyst aspiration	L	Refer to the colposcopy clinic
F	Ovarian cystectomy	M	Refer to the cancer centre
G	Oophorectomy	N	Refer to the gynaecology clinic
H	Ovarian transposition	O	Staging laparotomy

Instructions: For each scenario described below, choose the **single** most appropriate management from the list of options above. Each option may be used once, more than once, or not at all.

26. A 20-year-old woman attends the emergency department with acute abdominal pain. The surgeon suspects appendicitis and performs a diagnostic laparoscopy. You are the on-call registrar for that night and the surgeon calls you to give an opinion on an incidentally found large solid ovarian mass in the right adnexa with papillary projections on the surface. There is some free fluid in the pelvis and the other ovary appears normal.

27. A 58-year-old woman presents to her general practitioner with gradual distension of the abdomen for the last 6 months. She is then referred to the gynaecology clinic for suspected ovarian cancer. An ultrasound scan of the pelvis reveals a large multilocular ovarian cyst on the right side. Her tumour markers are reported as: (a) CA 125 2000 U/mL, (b) CEA 1.2 ng/mL, and (c) CA 19.9 1 U/mL.

28. A 39-year-old woman is reviewed in the gynaecology clinic with symptoms of pelvic pain for the last 2 years. She was treated for endometriosis 5 years ago with laparoscopic laser ablation. Her ultrasound scan 2 months ago revealed a

left-sided ovarian cyst (5.8 cm) with diffuse low-level internal echoes with one thin internal septae. Her CA 125 level is raised (61 U/mL).

29. A 28-year-old woman is referred to the gynaecology clinic with symptoms of menorrhagia with no intermenstrual and postcoital bleeding. Her pelvic examination is normal. However, an ultrasound scan of the pelvis shows an incidental finding of a simple ovarian cyst (size 3 × 3 × 3 cm) on the right side. A serum CA 125 level is 15 U/mL. Her recent cervical smear was normal.

30. A 50-year-old woman is referred to the gynaecology clinic with two ultrasound scan reports: (a) a current one showing a simple left ovarian cyst of 3 × 4 cm in size, and (b) the previous one performed 4 months ago showing a simple left ovarian cyst of 5 × 4 cm in size. Her CA 125 is 6 U/mL. She is otherwise asymptomatic and well.

Questions 31–35

Options for Questions 31–35

A	Arrhenoblastoma	I	Mucinous cystadenoma
B	Brenner tumour	J	Mucinous cystadenocarcinoma
C	Borderline serous ovarian tumour	K	Papillary serous carcinoma
D	Clear cell carcinoma	L	Serous cystadenoma
E	Endometrioid carcinoma	M	Serous cystadenocarcinoma
F	Dermoid cyst	N	Struma ovarii
G	Granulosa cell tumour	O	Thecoma
H	Krukenberg tumour		

Instructions: For each of the pathological findings described below, choose the **single** most appropriate tumour diagnosis from the list of options above. Each option may be used once, more than once, or not at all.

31. Signet ring cells on histology.

32. Transitional epithelium from Wolffian remnants.

33. Low malignant potential with no stroma invasion.

34. Müllerian origin with poor prognosis.

35. Usually seen in postmenopausal women and is associated with fibroma (Meigs syndrome).

Questions 36–40

Options for Questions 36–40

A   Cervical biopsy
B   Cervical smear
C   Computed tomography (CT) scan
D   Hysteroscopy and endometrial biopsy
E   Diagnostic laparoscopy and proceed
F   Magnetic resonance imaging
     (MRI) scan
G   No further tests required

H   Transvaginal scan (TVS) for
     endometrial thickness
I   Thyroid function tests
J   Pregnancy test
K   Pelvic examination
L   Rectal examination
M   Renal function tests
N   Saline hysterosonography
O   Speculum examination of cervix

Instructions: For each case described below, choose the **single** most appropriate investigation in women with postmenopausal bleeding (PMB) from the above list of options. Each option may be used once, more than once, or not at all.

36. A 48-year-old Caucasian woman is referred to the rapid access gynaecology oncology clinic with PMB. Speculum examination reveals stenosed cervical os and two failed attempts at endometrial pipelle biopsy. A transvaginal ultrasound shows an endometrial thickness of 6 mm. She claims to be fit and well.

37. A 48-year-old Asian woman presents to her general practitioner with PMB. She had a left mastectomy and axillary node dissection for breast cancer 4 years ago. She is currently on two medications: tamoxifen and anastrozole. She has been up to date with her smears and all her previous smears including the current one are normal. A TVS performed in the clinic reveals 5 mm endometrial thickness and normal ovaries. A recent breast appointment shows no clinical evidence of recurrence of breast cancer.

38. A 48-year-old Caucasian woman visits the UK to see her daughter-in-law and her grandson. She is newly registered with a general practitioner and presents with PMB for the last 2 weeks. She is up to date with her smears and has never had any abnormal smears. Pelvic examination is normal.

39. A 48-year-old Asian woman is referred to the gynaecology oncology clinic for PMB which occurred 2 weeks ago. She did not have any further bleeding following that one episode. She is up to date with her smears which are normal, and a TVS reveals 3 mm endometrial thickness. Clinical examination reveals an atrophic cervix and vagina.

40. A 48-year-old Caucasian woman is referred to the gynaecology oncology clinic for ongoing PMB for the last 3 weeks. So far all her previous smears have been normal and her endometrial thickness measures 4 mm on recent TVS. Clinical examination is normal.

Answers

1. I Stage IIIC1

Endometrial cancer is surgico-pathologically staged. In this case the final histology shows pelvic node involvement. Therefore, this woman has stage IIIC1 endometrial cancer.

2. I Stage IIIC1

In this scenario, the preoperative MRI scan suggests serosal and pelvic lymph node involvement. The final histology confirms the MRI scan findings. Therefore, this woman has stage IIIC1 endometrial cancer.

3. G Stage IIIA

Do not be misled by findings of cervical involvement in this scenario. The final histology also reveals serosal involvement. Therefore, this woman has stage IIIA endometrial cancer.

4. D Stage II

According to the revised FIGO classification uterine cancer involving cervical stroma is described as stage II. The classification of II into IIa and IIb has been removed from the current classification. Glandular involvement of the cervix is no longer classified as stage II.

5. A Stage 1A

According to the new FIGO classification, the involvement of the endometrium and less than 50% of the myometrium is described as stage IA.

Positive peritoneal cytology no longer alters the stage of the disease according to the current FIGO classification.

The uterine tumours are surgico-pathologically staged.

The updated revised FIGO staging (2009) is as follows:

- **Stage I:** Tumour confined to the uterus
- **Stage IA:** Tumour confined to the endometrium or myometrial invasion of less than 50%
- **Stage IB:** Myometrial invasion of >50%
- **Stage II:** Invasion of the tumour into the cervical stroma but does not extend beyond the uterus
- **Stage III:** Local or regional spread of the tumour
- **Stage IIIA:** Tumour involves the serosa of the uterus, fallopian tubes or adnexae

- **Stage IIIB:** Vaginal or parametrial involvement
- **Stage IIIC:** Metastasis to pelvic or para-aortic lymph nodes
- **Stage IIIC1:** Metastasis to pelvic nodes
- **Stage IIIC2:** Metastasis to para-aortic nodes
- **Stage IV:** The tumour invades the bladder or bowel mucosa and/or distant metastasis
- **Stage IVA:** The tumour invades the bladder or bowel mucosa
- **Stage IVB:** Remote metastasis, including inguinal lymph nodes or intra-abdominal metastasis

Endocervical glandular involvement is no longer considered stage II.

Holland C. Endometrial cancer. Obstet Gynaecol Reprod Med 2010; 20:347–352.
Lewin SN. Revised FIGO staging system for endometrial cancer. Clin Obstet Gynecol 2011; 54:215–218.

6. C Dysgerminoma

Germ cell tumours

Germ cell tumours account for 10% of all ovarian tumours. They are derived from primitive germ cells of the embryonic gonad and usually occur in young women in their 20s. The major issue in managing these women is to be able to preserve fertility while not compromising the chances of a cure.

Dysgerminoma (the equivalent of seminomas in men) is the most common type of germ cell tumour. They are bilateral in 10% of the cases. The tumour cells resemble primordial germ cells and do not normally secrete hormones. However, raised βhCG is seen in 3% of these tumours. Lactate dehydrogenase and placental alkaline phosphatase can also be increased. Histologically, lymphocytic infiltration in the stroma is a hallmark of these tumours. The primary treatment is surgery followed by adjuvant chemotherapy in cases higher than stage IA. The overall survival rate is 90%.

7. D Endodermal sinus tumour

Germ cell tumours

The endodermal sinus tumour is the second most common tumour after dysgerminomas. They are usually large, fast-growing and unilateral in occurrence. Macroscopically, they are solid with areas of haemorrhage and necrosis. Microscopically, the characteristic feature is a Schiller–Duval body. The tumour marker alpha fetoprotein is increased.

8. K Malignant teratoma

Germ cell tumours

Mature teratomas are the same as dermoid cysts and are benign tumours. There is less than a 2% risk of developing cancer in a mature teratoma.

Immature teratoma is the same as malignant teratoma, it is usually unilateral and occurs before the 20s. They are derived from the ectoderm, endoderm and mesoderm. The degree of cellular immaturity decides the grade of the tumour and the element used is neural tissue. The treatment is surgery and chemotherapy.

Choriocarcinomas secrete βhCG while embryonal carcinomas secrete both βhCG and alpha fetoprotein.

9. G Granulosa cell tumour

Sex cord stromal tumours

The most common of these tumours is the granulosa cell tumour and it can occur at any age. They usually secrete oestrogens and this may cause endometrial hyperplasia and endometrial cancer. Women in menopause can present with vaginal bleeding and young women may present with precocious puberty. The tumour marker is inhibin, especially the α-subunit of inhibin. The main modality of treatment is surgery followed by chemotherapy in women with more than stage IA tumours. Long-term follow-up is necessary as these tumours have a tendency for late recurrence.

10. F Epithelial ovarian tumour

Epithelial cell tumours

The incidence of ovarian cancer is 15 in 100,000 women per year in the UK and about 90% of these tumours are epithelial in origin. These can be serous, mucinous and other tumours. Serous cystadenocarcinoma is three times more common (accounting for 50% of all epithelial ovarian cancers) than mucinous cystadenocarcinoma. Mucinous and endometrioid cancers are the next most common tumours accounting for 10–15% each. Undifferentiated and clear cell carcinomas are uncommon.

CA 125 is raised above the normal cut-off level (>35 U/mL) in about 80% of all women with epithelial ovarian cancers, while it is raised in only 50% of FIGO stage 1 ovarian cancer.

Sanusi FA, Carter P, Barton DPJ. Non Epithelial Ovarian Cancers. Personal assessment in continuing education. Reviews, questions and answers. Volume 3. London: RCOG Press, 2003: 38–39.
Kumar B and Davies-Humphreys J. Tumour Markers and Ovarian Cancer Screening. Personal assessment in continuing education. Reviews, questions and answers. Volume 3. RCOG Press, 2003: 51–53.

11. H Punch biopsy of the cervical lesion

Women with colposcopic findings of CIN should be followed up in the colposcopy clinic after 6 months. However, when adapting a surveillance policy for CIN1, a histological diagnosis should be obtained and therefore a punch biopsy of the cervical lesion should be performed in this case.

12. F Large loop excision of the transformation zone (LLETZ)

The chances of progression of moderate and severe dyskaryosis (amounting to CIN2 and CIN3) to invasive disease is much higher than mild dyskaryosis (amounting to CIN1), although it takes some time for progression. Therefore, the colposcopic finding of high grade abnormality warrants treatment. LLETZ can be performed at the same visit (see and treat) if the follow-up is going to be compromised.

13. E Knife cone biopsy

Unsatisfactory colposcopy and findings suggestive of invasive disease (abnormal vessels) are indications for a knife cone biopsy.

14. G Needs discussion in the multidisciplinary team (MDT) meeting

In this case there is a major disparity between cytology and colposcopic findings. Therefore, the woman's case should be discussed in the colposcopy MDT meeting with a review of her cytology slides before taking any further course of action.

15. E Knife cone biopsy

Glandular abnormality on cytology and positive colposcopy findings are an indication for knife cone biopsy.

The histology features analysed on colposcopy to make a colposcopic diagnosis are shown in **Table 23.1**.

Table 23.1 Histology features analysed on colposcopy			
	Low grade (CIN1)	**High grade (CIN2/CIN3)**	**Invasive**
Surface contour and edges	Smooth and irregular	Smooth, well demarcated	Smooth/rough/ulcerated/raised, well demarcated
Speed of uptake of acetowhite areas	Slow to appear and quick to disappear	Quick to appear and slow to disappear	Quick to appear and slow to disappear
Additional features on acetowhite areas	Plain or fine mosaicism and punctuation	Oyster white appearance, coarse mosaicism and punctuation	Oyster white appearance, coarse mosaicism and punctuation plus abnormal vessels
Iodine staining	Irregular or not distinct	Distinct and well demarcated	Distinct and well demarcated

NHS Cervical Screening Programme. Colposcopy and Programme Management. Guidelines for the NHS Cervical Screening Programme (2nd edn). Publication No 20. NHSCSP, 2010. http://www.bsccp.org.uk/docs/public/pdf/nhscsp20.pdf

International Agency for Research on Cancer (IARC). Modified Reid Colposcopy Index. http://screening.iarc.fr/colpoappendix5.php

16. L Needs to be seen in a colposcopy clinic within 8 weeks

Women can be referred to the colposcopy clinic following one test reported as mild dyskaryosis. It is not unreasonable to repeat the cytology in 6 months. Women should be referred to the colposcopy clinic after two tests reported as mild dyskaryosis without a return to routine recall. They should be seen in the colposcopy clinic within 8 weeks of referral.

17. K Needs to be seen in a colposcopy clinic within 4 weeks

Women with a referral smear result of moderate or severe dyskaryosis should be seen in a colposcopy clinic within 4 weeks of referral.

18. L Needs to be seen in a colposcopy clinic within 8 weeks

Women referred with a cytology report of borderline change should be seen in the colposcopy clinic within 8 weeks of referral. If the borderline change is shown in squamous cells, the smear can be repeated at six-monthly intervals. However, after three borderline smears, women need to be referred to colposcopy clinic.

In patients where borderline changes are seen in endocervical cells or where there is a suspicion of high grade disease, the cytopathologist should refer the woman immediately to the colposcopy clinic after one abnormal smear.

19. I Needs to be seen in a colposcopy clinic within 2 weeks

All women with an abnormal cervix or suspicious cervix for cancer should be referred to the colposcopy clinic immediately. It is recommended that they should be seen within 2 weeks of referral.

20. I Needs to be seen in a colposcopy clinic within 2 weeks

The cervical screening programme is not designed to pick up glandular abnormalities. These are rare but associated with an underlying malignancy (adenocarcinoma) in 40% of cases and cervical intraepithelial neoplasia in almost 50% of cases. All women with one report of glandular neoplasia should be seen in a colposcopy clinic within 2 weeks of referral to colposcopy services.

NHS Cervical Screening Programme. Colposcopy and Programme Management. Guidelines for the NHS Cervical Screening Programme (2nd edn). Publication No 20. NHSCSP, 2010. http://www.bsccp.org.uk/docs/public/pdf/nhscsp20.pdf

21. F May need hysteroscopy and endometrial biopsy

In women <40 years of age, the presence of benign endometrial cells has no significance and should not be reported. However, in women >40 years of age their significance varies with the menstrual cycle. During the secretory phase (after the 14th day of the menstrual cycle), the presence of benign endometrial cells in the cervical cytology sample may indicate endometrial pathology (the exceptions would be women using hormone replacement therapy (HRT) or tamoxifen and women fitted with an IUCD). It is important to report the presence of endometrial cells if the above history is unknown in a woman aged 40 years and over or during menopause. These women should be referred for a gynaecological opinion and should be seen in the clinic urgently, within 2 weeks of referral.

22. H No need for a repeat cervical smear

Supplementary cervical screening is not warranted in the following situations, provided the woman is in the cervical screening age and has undergone screening within the previous 3–5 years:

- women taking the combined oral contraceptive pill
- following insertion of an IUCD
- women taking or starting HRT
- following pregnancy, antenatal, postnatal or after termination unless a previous cytology is abnormal
- women presenting with vaginal discharge
- women who have multiple sexual partners
- women with pelvic infection or pelvic inflammatory disease
- women with genital warts
- women who smoke heavily

23. H No need for a repeat cervical smear

Wart virus infection in itself is not an indication for a repeat cervical smear. Most sexually active women will show these changes in the cervix when they are young, which eventually resolve themselves in 80% of cases.

24. A Follow-up cervical smear in 6 months

A borderline smear is a minor abnormality and most do resolve by themselves. A repeat smear is indicated in 6 months at the general practitioner centre and a referral to colposcopy should be made when three consecutive smears are reported as borderline in squamous cells. However, if the borderline abnormality is in the endocervical cells, a referral to colposcopy should be made after one abnormal smear.

25. H No need for a repeat cervical smear

Candida infection is not an indication for a repeat cervical smear.

NHS Cervical Screening Programme. Colposcopy and Programme Management. Guidelines for the NHS Cervical Screening Programme (2nd edn). Publication No 20. NHSCSP, 2010. http://www.bsccp.org.uk/docs/public/pdf/nhscsp20.pdf

26. M Refer to the cancer centre

This was an emergency surgery for acute appendicitis. The ovarian cyst was an unexpected finding and the intraoperative findings are suspicious of malignancy. She has not been consented for complete staging operation for suspected ovarian malignancy and this needs to be done in the gynaecology oncology centre following full investigation (MRI scan of pelvis, staging CT scan of pelvis, abdomen and chest plus tumour markers [CA 125, CEA, HCG and AFP]). She therefore needs urgent referral to the cancer centre.

27. M Refer to the cancer centre

The Risk of malignancy index (RMI) in this case is >250. RMI >250 is considered high risk and the risk of cancer is 75%. She therefore needs referral to the cancer centre.

RMI is calculated by multiplying three parameters:

- ultrasound (USG) features (U=0 for USG score of 0, U=1 for USG score of 1 and U=3 for USG score of 2–5)
- menopausal status (use 3 for postmenopausal women and 1 for premenopausal women)
- CA 125 levels (actual value from the blood test)

The final number acquired after multiplication of the above factors is regarded as the RMI. This number determines the risk of ovarian cancer, e.g. <25 is considered low risk and the risk of cancer is <3%, RMI 25–250 is considered moderate risk and the risk of cancer is 20%, and RMI >250 is considered high risk for malignancy and the risk of cancer is 75%.

28. D Magnetic resonance imaging (MRI)

CA 125 is non-specific and can be raised in benign conditions such as endometriosis, fibroids, pelvic inflammatory disease and anything that causes irritation to the pelvic peritoneum. In this case, the cyst is likely to be an endometrioma because it has the typical appearance of an endometrioma on the ultrasound scan (a cyst with diffuse low-level internal echoes). However, in women with an intermediate risk (RMI of 61) an MRI scan should be arranged and her case referred to an MDT before proceeding to surgery.

29. I Repeat scan not necessary

Around 10% of women will have surgery in some form during their lifetime for an ovarian mass. The majority are benign in premenopausal women. The overall incidence of a symptomatic ovarian cyst in a premenopausal woman being malignant is approximately 1 in 1000 increasing to 3 in 1000 at the age of 50 years.

In premenopausal women, functional or simple ovarian cysts (thin-walled cysts without internal structures) which are <50 mm in maximum diameter usually resolve over two to three menstrual cycles without the need for intervention. A serum CA 125 assay does not need to be undertaken in all premenopausal women when an ultrasonographic diagnosis of a simple ovarian cyst has been made.

Aspiration of ovarian cysts, both vaginally or laparoscopically, is less effective and is associated with a high rate of recurrence.

The RMI in this case is 15. RMI <25 is considered to be low risk for malignancy. The risk of malignancy in such ovarian cysts is <1% and more than 50% of cases will resolve spontaneously within 3 months. Therefore, it is reasonable to manage them conservatively. Asymptomatic premenopausal women with such cysts (<50 mm diameter) generally do not require a follow-up as these cysts are very likely to be physiological and almost always resolve within three menstrual cycles.

Women with simple ovarian cysts between 50 and 70 mm in diameter should have yearly ultrasound follow-ups and those with larger simple cysts should be considered for either further imaging (MRI) or surgical intervention.

Lactate dehydrogenase (LDH), alpha fetoprotein and βhCG should be measured in all women under the age of 40 years with a complex ovarian mass because of the possibility of germ cell tumours.

30. K Repeat the transvaginal scan (TVS)

The RMI in this case is 18 and is considered as low risk for malignancy. Hence, it can be followed by repeat scans and CA 125 levels every 3–4 months for 1 year when she can be discharged back to the general practitioner. Ovarian cyst aspiration is no longer recommended.

Royal College of Obstetricians and Gynaecologists. Green-top Guideline No. 34. Ovarian cysts in postmenopausal women. London: RCOG Press, 2003.
Royal College of Obstetricians and Gynaecologists. Green-top Guideline No. 62. Management of suspected ovarian masses in premenopausal women. London: RCOG Press, 2011.
National Institute for Health and Clinical Excellence. Guidelines on ovarian cancer: the recognition and initial management (CT122). NICE, 2011.

31. H Krukenberg tumour

It is a metastatic tumour of the ovary which accounts for 1–2% of ovarian cancers. The primary tumour is usually from the gastrointestinal tract and also from the breast.

Macroscopically, both ovaries are often (80%) involved and may be symmetrically enlarged, which is consistent with its metastatic nature.

Microscopically, it is characterised by mucin-secreting signet ring cells in the ovarian tissue.

Immunohistochemical studies are positive for CEA and cytokeratin 20 (CK20) and negative for cytokeratin 7 (CK7) if the primary is from the colon.

The management is to identify and treat the primary tumour. If the metastasis is confined to the primary tumour, surgical removal may improve survival. If the metastasis is extensive, the treatment is usually palliative. However, the optimum treatment for such tumours is unclear.

32. B Brenner tumour

Transitional epithelium is the epithelium of the ureter, bladder and urethra. It can be seen in Brenner tumour of the ovary.

33. C Borderline serious ovarian tumour

The hallmark of malignancy is stromal invasion. Ovarian tumours without stromal invasion and have malignant features rather than a benign appearance are referred to as borderline tumours.

34. D Clear cell carcinoma

Clear cell carcinoma is a poorly differentiated tumour and carries a poor prognosis.

35. O Thecoma

An ovarian mass (fibroma) when associated with right-sided pleural effusion is referred to as a fibroma (Meigs syndrome).

Pathological classification of ovarian tumours:

- epithelial cell tumours
- sex cord/stromal tumours
- germ cell tumours
- embryonic tumours
- miscellaneous
- metastatic

Epithelial tumours:

- eighty per cent of ovarian tumours
- ninety per cent of all primary malignant tumours

Types:

- serous cystadenoma
- serous cystadenocarcinoma
- serous borderline tumour
- mucinous cystadenoma

- mucinous cystadenocarcinoma
- mucinous borderline tumour
- Brenner tumour
- endometrioid tumour
- clear cell tumour

Serous tumours:

- most common epithelial tumour
- cystadenoma – usually uniocular or bilocular
- cystadenocarcinoma – partly cystic/solid
- increased CA 125

Mucinous tumours:

- cystadenoma – multilocular
- rupture may cause pseudomyxoma peritonei and small bowel obstruction
- cystadenocarcinoma – usually solid
- can be associated with appendicular cancer
- increased CEA and CA 125

Clear cell carcinoma:

- Müllerian origin
- poor prognosis
- ten per cent bilateral
- fifteen per cent associated with primary in the uterus
- highly malignant

Brenner tumours:

- transitional epithelium from Wolffian remnants
- fibrous elements
- usually benign (99%)
- if malignant, may be associated with bladder tumour

Borderline tumours:

- low malignant potential
- no stromal invasion
- may have extra ovarian spread in 20% of cases
- serous – 50% bilateral
- mucinous – 5% bilateral
- five-year survival: stage I = 97% and stage III = 85%

Endometrioid carcinoma:

- may be secondary from endometrial carcinoma
- can arise in endometriosis

Sex cord/stromal tumours:

- thecoma
- granulose cell tumour
- androblastoma

Thecoma:

- usually postmenopausal
- solid, yellow
- almost always benign
- fibroma (Meigs syndrome)

Granulosa cell tumours:

- solid and 75% have endocrine function
- usually occur in women >60 years of age but also can occur before puberty
- can present with PMB, irregular cycle and bleeding and precocious pseudo puberty
- juvenile – 5% are malignant and aggressive
- treatment is chemotherapy

Androblastoma (arrhenoblastoma):

- sertoli – most common, usually benign
- seventy per cent oestrogenic, 20% androgenic and 10% no secretion
- Leydig cell and mixed Sertoli–Leydig tumours – very rare

Germ cell tumours:

- most common type in woman aged <30 years
- malignant: 2–3%; 30% in women aged <20 years
- categorised by the degree of cellular differentiation

Dysgerminoma:

- fifty per cent of malignant germ cell tumours
- usually in women aged <30 years
- bilateral: 10–15%
- not associated with hirsutism
- secretes lactate dehydrogenase and placental alkaline phosphatase
- secretes βhCG in 3% of the cases
- has lymphoid infiltration of the stroma on histological examination
- radio and chemo sensitive
- chemotherapy preserves ovarian function

Embryonic tumours:

- mature cystic teratoma (dermoid) is a benign tumour and is usually seen in women of childbearing age. They are unilocular and bilateral in 10–15% of cases. In 1% of cases, malignant change can occur
- immature teratomas are common in the first two decades of life and are malignant. They are unilateral and frequently contain neural tissue. Occasionally, they may secrete thyroid hormones (struma ovarii) and serotonin (carcinoid)
- Embryonal carcinoma – secrete βhCG and alpha fetoprotein

Extra embryonic differentiation:

- yolk sac or endodermal sinus tumour – secrete alpha fetoprotein
- present at 14–20 years of age
- unilateral, chemosensitive

- malignant ovarian choriocarcinoma – secrete βhCG
- may present with precocious puberty
- poor prognosis and poor response to chemotherapy

Miscellaneous:

- gonadoblastoma – benign
- streak ovary or testis
- Leydig cell tumours
- small cell carcinoma

Metastatic tumours:

- constitute up to 10% of tumours
- most common from stomach, breast and colon
- Krukenberg tumour – mucin secreting tumour
- bilateral and solid
- signet ring cells on histology

Sanusi FA, Carter P, Barton DPJ. Non Epithelial Ovarian Cancers. Personal assessment in continuing education. Reviews, questions and answers. Volume 3. London: RCOG Press, 2003: 38–39.
Kumar B and Davies-Humphreys J. Tumour Markers and Ovarian Cancer Screening. Personal assessment in continuing education. Reviews, questions and answers. Volume 3. London: RCOG Press, 2003: 51–53.
Shafi MI, Luesley DM, Jordan JA. Handbook of Gynaecological Oncology. Edinburgh: Churchill Livingstone, 2001.

36. D Hysteroscopy and endometrial biopsy

Due to oestrogen deficiency the endometrial thickness in postmenopausal women is much thinner compared to premenopausal women. The probability of endometrial cancer increases with increasing endometrial thickness. A thickness of >5 mm increases the likelihood of endometrial cancer in postmenopausal women and thus warrants investigation in the form of endometrial pipelle sampling or hysteroscopy plus endometrial biopsy. A thickness of <5 mm has a negative predictive value of 98%. A meta-analysis also found that endometrial thickness of 5 mm or less reduced the risk of endometrial pathology by 84%.

The differential diagnosis of PMB includes:

- genital atrophy (88% of PMB)
- atrophic endometritis, atrophic vaginitis
- endometrial cancer (8% of PMB)
- endometrial hyperplasia (up to 10% of PMB)
- endometrial polyp (5–9% of PMB)
- cervical polyp and cervical cancer
- ovarian tumours (2% of PMB)

The majority (80%) of women with endometrial cancer present with PMB. The second most common malignancy is cervical cancer and the third most common is ovarian cancer. Malignancies arising from the vagina, vulva and fallopian tube are rare.

Extragenital causes of bleeding should be ruled out in women with recurrent PMB or PMB following hysterectomy (bleeding may be from bladder cancer or urethral polyps, caruncle or prolapsed urethral mucosa).

37. D Hysteroscopy and endometrial biopsy

PMB refers to any vaginal bleeding that occurs in menopausal women (absence of menstrual period for 1 year) other than the expected cyclical bleeding that occurs in women taking a sequential regimen of hormone replacement therapy. Until proven otherwise, this bleeding warrants investigation to rule out cancer and therefore needs referral to the gynaecology oncology clinic as a target patient. All patients should be seen in the clinic within 2 weeks of referral. However, the diagnosis can be made by 31 days once the patient is seen and if it is cancer the treatment should be initiated by 62 days from the time seen, or 30 days from the time of diagnosis.

Tamoxifen is an oestrogen antagonist in breast and an agonist in endometrial tissue. It is used in the treatment of breast cancer following surgery in women with receptor positive breast cancer. The duration used is usually 5 years as there is no evidence to show benefit after this period (risks outweigh benefits).

There is slightly increased risk of endometrial cancer in such women and there are no associated specific ultrasound findings. The only way forward is endometrial biopsy in women with abnormal vaginal bleeding. By agonist action, it causes endometrial thickening and it is difficult to define a cut-off value of endometrial thickness on ultrasonography for initiating investigation although some articles suggest 12 mm. However, women on tamoxifen presenting with PMB need urgent hysteroscopy and endometrial biopsy to rule out endometrial cancer.

38. H TVS for endometrial thickness

All women presenting with PMB need urgent TVS if clinical findings are normal. This helps the clinician to decide the necessity of an endometrial biopsy in such women. However, in women with normal endometrial thickness, one should take an individual approach in deciding the need for endometrial biopsy and this may depend on the risk factors in such women. If the endometrial thickness is >5 mm, an endometrial biopsy should be done in the form of an endometrial pipelle biopsy or hysteroscopy and endometrial biopsy.

39. G No further tests required

The most common cause of PMB is atrophic endometritis or vaginitis (88%). If the endometrial thickness is normal and the clinical findings are suggestive of atrophy, reassure women. However, if these women continue to bleed, they would need a hysteroscopy and endometrial biopsy.

40. D Hysteroscopy and endometrial biopsy

Any women with ongoing PMB will need an endometrial biopsy despite normal endometrial thickness on the TVS.

National Institute of Health and Clinical Excellence. Referral for suspected cancer (CG27). NICE, 2011. Rogerson L and Jones S. The investigation of women with postmenopausal bleeding. Pace review No. 98/07. London: RCOG Press, 2003: 10–13.

Gupta JK, Chien PF, Voit D, Clark TJ, Khan KS. Ultrasonographic endometrial thickness for diagnosing endometrial pathology in women with postmenopausal bleeding: a meta-analysis. Acta Obstet Gynecol Scand 2002; 81:799–816.

Franchi M, Ghezzi F, Donadello N, Zanaboni F, Beretta P, Bolis P. Endometrial thickness in tamoxifen-treated patients: an independent predictor of endometrial disease. Obstet Gynecol 1999; 93:1004–1008.

Smith-Bindman R, Weiss E, Feldstein V. How thick is too thick? When endometrial thickness should prompt biopsy in postmenopausal women without vaginal bleeding. Ultrasound Obstet Gynecol 2004; 24:558–565.

Sahdev A. Imaging the endometrium in postmenopausal bleeding. BMJ 2007; 334:635–636.

Chapter 24

Management of labour and delivery

Questions 1–5

Options for Questions 1–5

A   Break both the clavicles
B   Delivery of the posterior arm
C   Elective caesarean section
D   Emergency caesarean section
E   Episiotomy
F   Fundal pressure
G   Lovset manoeuvre
H   McRoberts position and suprapubic pressure

I   Rubin manoeuvre
J   Reverse Wood screw manoeuvre
K   Roll over onto all fours
L   Symphysiotomy
M   Suprapubic pressure
N   Wood screw manoeuvre
O   Zavanelli procedure

Instructions: For each clinical scenario described below, choose the **single** most appropriate management option from the list of options above. Each option may be used once, more than once, or not at all.

1. A 30-year-old woman, para 2, attends the antenatal clinic at 37 weeks of gestation to discuss mode of delivery. She had her last delivery two years ago and gives a history of a difficult forceps delivery following which her child developed Erb palsy.

2. A 30-year-old woman, para 1 (vaginal delivery), presents to the labour ward at 42 weeks of gestation with regular contractions. Clinically, the baby appears bigger than 4 kg (her previous child weighed 3.9 kg). She progresses quickly until 7 cm cervical dilatation but subsequently takes 8 hours to progress to full dilatation of cervix. Vaginal examination reveals an occipito-posterior position of the fetus with presenting part at +1 station. A turtle sign is noted following delivery of the head.

3. A 42-year-old primigravida presents to the labour ward with spontaneous labour at 38 weeks of gestation. She is a type 2 diabetic on insulin. Her last scan at 36 weeks of gestation revealed an estimated fetal weight of 3.7 kg. During labour she needed oxytocin augmentation to progress to full dilatation. Two hours after pushing, she had a spontaneous vaginal delivery with the head on the perineum. An emergency buzzer is pulled by the midwife. On entering the room, you notice the patient in McRoberts position and the midwife is giving traction to the fetal head.

4. A 30-year-old woman body mass index (BMI 41), para 1, presents to the labour ward at 40 weeks of gestation with a spontaneous onset of labour. Clinically, it is difficult to assess the size of the baby as she has a high body mass index (growth scan at 36 weeks of gestation revealed an estimated fetal weight of 3.8 kg). Ten hours later she has a vaginal delivery but the midwife puts out an obstetric crash call after noticing a turtle sign. The registrar attends and tries all the possible named rotational manoeuvres following McRoberts position but fails to deliver the impacted shoulders.

5. A 30-year-old Asian woman presents to the labour ward at 40 weeks of gestation with spontaneous onset of labour. She is unbooked (she has had no prior appointments, scans or blood tests) and clinically the baby appears big. Blood sugar levels are 10.1 mmol/L. She progresses slowly to full dilatation of the cervix after 18 hours. The registrar was called in anticipation of shoulder dystocia. The head is delivered and there is an obvious turtle sign. An obstetric crash call was put out. All the manoeuvres were tried including removal of the posterior arm but failed to deliver the impacted shoulder.

Questions 6–10

Options for Questions 6–10

A   Antenatal corticosteroids
B   Antenatal glucocorticoids and antibiotics
C   Antenatal corticosteroids plus antibiotics plus inpatient monitoring for 48–72 hours
D   Emergency cervical cerclage
E   Elective cervical cerclage
F   Immediate induction of labour with the aim of vaginal delivery plus intravenous antibiotics
G   Immediate delivery by caesarean section plus intravenous antibiotics
H   Prophylactic tocolysis and intravenous antibiotics
I   Prophylactic tocolysis plus antenatal corticosteroids plus intrauterine transfer
J   Reasonable to deliver at 34 weeks of gestation or after
K   Transabdominal amnioinfusion
L   Transvaginal amniocentesis
M   Tocolysis and antenatal corticosteroids
N   Tocolysis

Instructions: For each scenario described below, choose the **single** most appropriate initial management from the list of options above. Each option may be used once, more than once, or not at all.

6. A 34-year-old multiparous woman presents to the labour ward with a gush of fluid through the vagina at 26 weeks of gestation. A speculum examination by the on-call registrar confirms a spontaneous rupture of membranes. Abdominal examination reveals no uterine activity. Clinically, she feels well and vitals are normal.

7. A 40-year-old multiparous woman presents to the labour ward with a history of premature rupture of membranes (PROM) at 29 weeks of gestation. She complains of regular uterine contractions coming every 3 minutes. Speculum examination

confirms a rupture of membranes and her cervix appears to be 3 cm dilated. Clinically, there are no signs of chorioamnionitis.

8. A 38-year-old multiparous woman attends her antenatal clinic appointment at 35 weeks of gestation. She gives a history of PROM at 24 weeks of gestation. Abdominal examination reveals cephalic presentation with no signs of chorioamnionitis. An ultrasound scan reveals oligohydramnios. Her inflammatory markers are normal.

9. A 40-year-old multiparous woman attends the obstetric day assessment unit with reduced fetal movements at 32 weeks of gestation. A cardiotocograph (CTG) reveals a normal baseline, variable deceleration with reduced variability and no acceleration. Abdominal examination reveals a cephalic presentation and vaginal examination reveals a 2 cm cervical dilatation. An ultrasound scan confirms the cephalic presentation but also reveals severe oligohydramnios. She is tachypnoeic and tachycardic with spiking temperatures of 38°C. A review of her notes indicates that she had PROM at 28 weeks of gestation.

10. A 40-year-old multiparous woman attends the obstetric day assessment unit at 35 weeks of gestation. She gives a history of PROM at 30 weeks of gestation following which she received erythromycin for 10 days. She feels well in herself and her vitals are normal. However, her blood test results reveal a raised white blood cell count (19,000 per mm^3) and C-reactive protein (104 mg/L). An ultrasound examination reveals cephalic presentation with some liquor around the baby. A fetal cardiotocograph is normal.

Questions 11–15

Options for Questions 11–15

A	Artificial rupture of membranes	I	Forceps delivery
B	Augmentation with oxytocin	J	Fetal blood sampling (FBS)
C	Acyclovir – oral	K	Termination of pregnancy
D	Acyclovir – intravenous	L	Type specific herpes simplex virus
E	Acyclovir – intravenous followed		(HSV) antibody testing
	by oral	M	Symptomatic therapy
F	Consider vaginal delivery	N	Swabs for virology
G	Elective caesarean section at term	O	Screen for other sexually transmitted
H	Emergency caesarean section		infections (STIs) plus oral acyclovir

Instructions: For each clinical scenario described below, choose the **single** most appropriate initial management plan from the list of options above. Each option may be used once, more than once or not at all.

11. A 20-year-old pregnant woman presents at 35 weeks of gestation with a primary genital herpes infection. She is generally fit and well. She is worried about the implications for the baby as she has read about neonatal herpes on the internet.

12. A 30-year-old woman presents at 39 weeks of gestation with a primary active genital herpes infection. She gives a history of labour pains for the last 4 hours. Vaginal examination reveals a 2 cm cervical dilatation and intact membranes.

13. A 35-year-old pregnant woman presents with a history of recurrent herpes at term. She is contracting twice in 10 minutes on abdominal examination, and vaginal examination reveals a 6 cm cervical dilatation with intact membranes.

14. A 32-year-old pregnant woman presents to the labour ward at term with a primary genital herpes infection. She is contracting four times in 10 minutes and is currently 4 cm dilated. She declines caesarean section.

15. A 29-year-old woman comes to the day assessment unit with painful vesicles on the genital area. She is currently 16 weeks pregnant and clinical examination reveals a primary genital herpes infection.

Questions 16–20

Options for Questions 16–20

A   Apply a fetal scalp electrode
B   Facial oxygen therapy
C   Continue oxytocin
D   Continuous electronic fetal monitoring
E   Fetal scalp electrode application to monitor fetus
F   Fetal blood sampling (FBS) contraindicated
G   Forceps delivery
H   Intravenous 0.5 mg ergometrine
I   Intrauterine fetal blood transfusion
J   Intravenous fluids
K   Left lateral position
L   Perform FBS
M   Repeat FBS in 30 minutes
N   Reduce the rate of oxytocin
O   Subcutaneous 0.25 mg terbutaline

Instructions: For each scenario described below, choose the **single** most appropriate initial management from the list of options above. Each option may be used once, more than once, or not at all.

16. A 34-year-old woman, para 3, presents to the labour ward at 40 weeks of gestation with regular contractions. She makes good progress up to 8 cm cervical dilatation but does not progress further. Oxytocin was started at 2 mL/hour for augmentation. A CTG reveals a normal baseline heart rate, variability >5 beats/minute and typical variable decelerations for the last 40 minutes. The tocograph suggests that she is contracting seven times in 10 minutes. The midwife calls you to review the CTG as you are the on-call labour ward registrar for the night.

17. A 34-year-old primigravida is admitted to the antenatal ward for induction of labour at 41 weeks of gestation. She has first prostin at 0800 hours and was reassessed at 1400 hours for artificial rupture of membranes (ARM). A second prostin was inserted due to a poor Bishop score. She was put back on the CTG for fetal monitoring. One hour later CTG showed a fetal heart rate (FHR) of 160 beats/minute and atypical variable decelerations. A tocograph shows seven contractions in 10 minutes.

18. A 34-year-old, para 3, attends the labour ward at 40 weeks of gestation with regular contractions. Booking (her first midwife appointment) blood tests reveal she is positive for hepatitis B (low risk for fetal transmission). She was 4 cm at admission but did not progress further. ARM was performed but revealed thick

meconium-stained liquor. She was then augmented by oxytocin and 4 hours later, had progressed to 8 cm cervical dilatation. Currently, the CTG reveals a baseline of 170 beats/minute, variability <5 beats/minute, but no accelerations or decelerations.

19. A 34-year-old woman, para 5, attends the labour ward at 41 weeks of gestation with regular contractions and spontaneous rupture of membranes (SROM). She is admitted to the high-risk side on the labour ward for continuous fetal monitoring in view of high parity and meconium staining of liquor. Four hours later she has progressed to 9 cm cervical dilatation. FBS was performed at this stage as her CTG was pathological by the National Institute for Health and Clinical Excellence (NICE) criteria. The FBS results showed pH 7.26 and BE –0.3 mEq/L. Thirty minutes later the midwife informs you that the CTG has remained the same.

20. A 34-year-old woman, para 2, attends the labour ward at 40 weeks of gestation with SROM. She was discharged home to return in 24 hours for induction of labour. Twenty-four hours (0800 hours) later she returned contracting with a 4 cm cervical dilatation. She progressed to an 8 cm cervical dilatation at next vaginal examination (1200 hours). However, the CTG reveals a baseline FHR of 165 beats/minute, variability 5 beats/minute, occasional acceleration and typical variable decelerations for the last 60 minutes.

Answers

1. C Elective caesarean section

Shoulder dystocia

- **Definition:** failure to deliver the shoulders following delivery of the fetal head (>60 seconds)
- **Problem:** inlet
- **Incidence:** 0.5–2% of all vaginal deliveries
- **Prediction:** difficult to predict or prevent. One can only anticipate this in women with the risk factors mentioned below

Risk factors

- **D** – Diabetes
- **O** – Obesity, operative vaginal deliveries
- **P** – Prolonged labour (although labour progresses normally in 70% of cases)
- **E** – Estimated fetal weight >4 kg (although 50% occur in babies weighing <4 kg)
- **S** – Previous shoulder dystocia and prolonged second stage

Epidural analgesia is not associated with an increased risk of shoulder dystocia.

The incidence of recurrent shoulder dystocia is reported as being between 1 and 16%. A caesarean section may be considered for a previous history of severe shoulder dystocia with a poor outcome. The approach should be individualised and the decision should be made by the woman and her carers.

2. H McRoberts position and suprapubic pressure

Delivery is accomplished in 90% of cases by simple measures such as the McRoberts position and suprapubic pressure.

In this procedure the mother is placed in the supine position, the hips are abducted, and the hips and knees are flexed. This straightens the lumbosacral curvature and moves the symphysis superiorly, therefore releasing the anterior shoulder from behind the pubic symphysis. It increases the pelvic anteroposterior diameters by 1 cm.

3. M Suprapubic pressure

Suprapubic pressure should be tried following gentle traction and the McRobert position.

This is done with the flat of an assistant's hand behind the anterior shoulder (it is recommended to stand the side of the baby's back or fetal spine). This promotes adduction of the anterior shoulder and releases it from the symphysis pubis. It also reduces the bisacromial diameter. The initial pressure should be continuous and if there is no success after 30 seconds, a rocking motion should be tried. However, either of the two can be used.

4. B Delivery of the posterior arm

Rotational manoeuvres (Rubin, Wood screws and reverse Wood screws) promote the disimpaction of the shoulders from the pelvic inlet. These procedures normally push the shoulders into the oblique diameter of the pelvis (which is the larger diameter) and hence promotes the release of the anterior shoulder. It is recommended to use gentle neck traction and maternal pushing after every attempt of rotation. If the rotational manoeuvres fail, then go for the posterior arm without delay.

5. K Roll over onto all fours

Asking the mother to get on all fours may help with delivery. If this fails, Zavanelli procedure should be used.

Zavanelli procedure is rarely used in the management of shoulder dystocia. It is used as a last resort following failure of all other measures. The head is replaced with constant pressure (the palm of the hand is used) in order to flex the head and push it into the pelvis. Delivery of the head is then accomplished by caesarean section.

Royal College of Obstetricians and Gynaecologists. RCOG Green-top Guideline No. 42. Shoulder dystocia. London: RCOG Press, 2005.
Neill AC and Thornton S. Shoulder dystocia. Pace review No. 2/4 (B). Volume 3. London: RCOG Press, 2003: 55–57.

6. C Antenatal corticosteroids plus antibiotics plus inpatient monitoring for 48–72 hours

Women with PROM are at increased risk of going into labour within 24 hours. Hence, antenatal corticosteroids should be considered. The Royal College of Obstetricians and Gynaecologists (RCOG) recommends erythromycin (250 mg orally 6-hourly) for 10 days for women with a confirmed diagnosis of pre-term premature rupture of membranes (PPROM).

Women with PPROM should be monitored as outpatients only if facilities are available for rigorous monitoring. The risk of uterine infection is increased, especially in the first 3–7 days following PROM, hence the woman would need initial inpatient monitoring followed by outpatient monitoring once infection is ruled out. As part of outpatient monitoring, she should be observed for signs of chorioamnionitis. Also, weekly high vaginal swabs need not be performed. Maternal full blood counts and C-reactive protein have low sensitivity to detecting intrauterine infection and therefore need not be undertaken on a weekly basis. One should make sure that women are educated about the symptoms and signs of chorioamnionitis, so that they can report immediately if they are unwell.

A CTG should be performed as fetal tachycardia is used in the definition of clinical chorioamnionitis. A biophysical profile score and Doppler velocimetry can be carried out but women should be informed that these tests are of limited value in predicting fetal infection.

7. M Tocolysis and antenatal corticosteroids

The risk of respiratory distress syndrome (RDS) is increased at 29 weeks gestation and decreases with increasing gestational age. The neonatal admission rate is also increased during early gestation. The main aim is to decrease the risk of RDS and this can be achieved by giving antenatal corticosteroids. PPROM in itself is not a contraindication for administering antenatal corticosteroids. Tocolysis may be considered in women with PPROM who have uterine activity and would need either antenatal glucocorticoids or intrauterine transfer.

8. J Reasonable to deliver at 34 weeks of gestation or after

PPROM complicates 2% of pregnancies and is associated with 40% of pre-term deliveries. It can be associated with increased neonatal morbidity and mortality. The main causes of death associated with PPROM include prematurity, sepsis and pulmonary hypoplasia. For the mother, it carries risk of chorioamnionitis. In women with PPROM, about one third of pregnancies have positive amniotic fluid cultures. However, there is insufficient data to recommend amniocentesis as a modality for diagnosing infection.

Women with PPROM should receive erythromycin for 10 days and antenatal corticosteroids should be given to increase fetal lung maturity. Tocolysis is not routinely recommended in these women as this treatment does not significantly improve perinatal outcome.

In women with PPROM, delivery should be considered at 34 weeks of gestation as continuing pregnancy after this point may put women at risk of chorioamnionitis. If expectant management is considered beyond 34 weeks of gestation, one should balance the risk of uterine infection for the mother versus respiratory problems in the neonate, admission to neonatal intensive care and the increased risk of caesarean section.

9. G Immediate delivery by caesarean section plus intravenous antibiotics

If neonatal facilities are available the woman can be kept in the same hospital. However, if these facilities are not available she can be delivered and then transferred out to a different unit as the chances of survival at 32 weeks of gestation are high. The CTG findings (atypical variable decelerations) indicate fetal hypoxia and are categorised as pathological. Amnioinfusion is not recommended for such women with PPROM. This woman needs delivery in view of clinical findings of chorioamnionitis. The delivery should be expedited, hence delivery by caesarean section.

10. F Immediate induction of labour with the aim of vaginal delivery plus intravenous antibiotics

In this case the signs (inflammatory markers are raised) are suggestive of subclinical chorioamnionitis, hence delivery is indicated. If the cervix is favourable, induction of labour and vaginal delivery can be considered.

Royal College of Obstetricians and Gynaecologists. Green-top Guideline No. 44. Preterm prelabour rupture of membranes. London: RCOG Press, 2010.

11. O Screen for other sexually transmitted infections (STIs) plus oral acyclovir

Primary genital herpes infection during pregnancy

Genital herpes is caused by herpes simplex virus (HSV) type 1 and type 2 DNA virus, and is sexually transmitted. The incubation period is 7 days.

Women presenting with primary genital herpes should be referred to the genito-urinary clinic to screen for other STIs and should be treated with oral acyclovir for 5 days (200 mg five times a day) in order to reduce the severity and duration of symptoms and duration of viral shedding. However, it should be used with caution before 20 weeks.

One can also consider daily suppressive therapy with oral acyclovir from 36 weeks of gestation to reduce the likelihood of recurrent herpes simplex infection (evidence is lacking). Viral cultures can be offered at late gestation to predict the risk of viral shedding if the primary genital herpes infection was reported in the first and second trimesters.

If a woman presents with primary genital herpes within 6 weeks of the expected date of delivery, then maternal intravenous intrapartum acyclovir plus intravenous acyclovir to the newborn baby should be considered to reduce the risk of neonatal herpes.

All women presenting with primary herpes simplex infection within 6 weeks of the expected date of delivery or at delivery should be offered caesarean section (the highest risk to the fetus is within 6 weeks following primary genital herpes infection). However, there is no need for a caesarean section for women presenting with primary herpes simplex infection in the first and second trimesters.

Risk of transmission to fetus

- 30–60% if primary infection is within 6 weeks of delivery
- 3% in recurrent infection
- 1–3% if seropositive for HSV type 1 and HSV type 2
- less than 1% if no visible lesions

Investigation and diagnosis of primary genital herpes

- clinical: women characteristically present with painful vesicles or ulcerations on the genitalia and urinary retention
- laboratory: type specific HSV antibody testing with IgG is not recommended during pregnancy as it is not fully evaluated
- viral cultures: direct detection of genital HSV by swabs from the base of the ulcer, fluid sample following de-roofing the vesicle (PCR testing)

12. H Emergency caesarean section

Neonatal herpes

Neonatal herpes is caused both by HSV type 1 or type 2 and mostly occurs due to direct contact with maternal genital secretions when the baby is passing through the birth canal at delivery. It is a rare condition but is associated with high morbidity and mortality (30% if disseminated infection and 6% with local central nervous system infection). The prognosis is good if only the eyes, mouth and skin are involved.

The following factors influence fetal transmission from mother to baby:

- whether the infection is primary or recurrent
- the presence of maternal neutralising antibodies (antibody transfer to the baby before birth but does not prevent the neurogenic viral spread to the brain of the neonate)
- the duration of the rupture of membranes before delivery (deliver as soon as possible if PROM)
- the use of fetal scalp electrodes or fetal blood sampling; and mode of delivery

The risk to the fetus is high (neonatal infection) if the woman acquires primary genital herpes in the third trimester (<6 weeks of delivery, as viral shedding may persist and the baby is likely to be born before the transfer of passive immunity from the mother). Therefore, if the primary infection occurs at the time of labour, or within 6 weeks of the expected date of delivery, caesarean section is recommended for all women.

13. F Consider vaginal delivery

Recurrent genital herpes during pregnancy

The risk of transmission with recurrent genital herpes to the fetus is much lower compared to primary genital herpes and therefore caesarean section is not routinely recommended for such women (caesarean section is not indicated if episodes of recurrent herpes occur during the antenatal period). However, women should be counselled about the 3% risk of neonatal herpes with recurrent herpes during labour (caesarean section can be performed if the woman wishes after weighing the risks of caesarean section versus the risks of fetal transmission of infection). One may consider daily suppressive oral acyclovir from 36 weeks of gestation onwards in anticipation of reducing the recurrent herpetic lesions at term (especially in human immunodeficiency virus [HIV] patients but otherwise not routinely indicated).

There is no need for viral cultures or type-specific HSV antibody testing in women with recurrent herpes. Acyclovir is rarely indicated in the treatment of genital herpes. However, if the woman's partner has active genital herpes, she should be advised to avoid sexual intercourse (use of condoms is not fully protective against acquiring infection).

14. D Acyclovir – intravenous

Precautions during labour

For women wishing to deliver vaginally the following should be avoided: fetal blood sampling or fetal scalp electrode application during labour, delay or avoid artificial rupture of membranes and the neonatologist should be involved before delivery for neonatal care.

Intravenous administration of acyclovir to the mother during labour and the baby after birth should be considered to reduce the risk of neonatal herpes.

15. M Symptomatic therapy

Symptomatic and supportive therapy is the main form of treatment (analgesics and sitz baths). Acyclovir should be used with caution before 20 weeks of gestation. Admission to hospital and bladder catheterisation may be required in women presenting with severe pain and retention of urine. One should also be vigilant regarding the symptoms and signs of encephalitis and disseminated infection.

Royal College of Obstetricians and Gynaecologists. Green-top Guideline No. 30. Management of genital herpes during pregnancy. London: RCOG Press, 2007.

16. N Reduce the rate of oxytocin

In this case, the fetal heart rate (FHR) is suspicious and hyperstimulating on oxytocin. Only four or five contractions are expected for the labour to progress. Therefore, the dose of oxytocin should be reduced.

The NICE recommendations are:

- If the FHR trace is normal, oxytocin may be continued until the woman is experiencing four or five contractions every 10 minutes. Oxytocin should be reduced if contractions occur more frequently than five contractions in 10 minutes.
- If the FHR trace is classified as suspicious, this should be reviewed by an obstetrician and the oxytocin dose should only continue to increase to achieve four or five contractions every 10 minutes.
- If the FHR trace is classified as pathological, oxytocin should be stopped and a full assessment of the fetal condition undertaken by an obstetrician before oxytocin is recommenced.

17. O Subcutaneous 0.25 mg terbutaline

In the presence of abnormal FHR patterns and uterine hypercontractility not secondary to oxytocin infusion, tocolysis should be considered. A suggested regimen is subcutaneous terbutaline 0.25 mg which can be repeated every 15 minutes if necessary.

18. F Fetal blood sampling contraindicated

In this woman, the scenario describes the booking (her first midwife appointment) blood tests results as low risk for infection on hepatitis screening. This means she is negative for hepatitis 'e' antigen and positive for anti-e antibody. Women who are at high risk on hepatitis screening would be positive for e antigen and negative for anti-e antibody.

Contraindications to fetal blood sampling (FBS) include:

- maternal infection: HIV, hepatitis viruses and herpes simplex virus
- fetal bleeding disorders: haemophilia, low platelet disorders
- prematurity: less than 34 weeks

19. M Repeat FBS in 30 minutes

In this case the midwife informs you 30 minutes after FBS that the CTG has remained the same as before. Therefore, FBS needs to be repeated in 30 minutes and this will be 1 hour from the previous normal FBS.

The NICE recommends the results of FBS should be interpreted carefully, taking into account previous pH measurements, the rate of progress in labour and the clinical features of the woman and baby.

Interpretation of a FBS result (pH):

- ≥7.25 – normal FBS result
- 7.21–7.24 – borderline FBS result
- ≤7.20 – abnormal FBS result

FBS should be performed when fetal compromise is suspected (which is interpreted on CTG as pathological):

- After a normal FBS result, sampling should be repeated no more than 1 hour later if the FHR trace remains pathological, or sooner if there are further abnormalities.
- After a borderline FBS result, sampling should be repeated no more than 30 minutes later if the FHR trace remains pathological, or sooner if there are further abnormalities. The time taken to take a fetal blood sample needs to be considered when planning repeat samples.
- If the FHR trace remains unchanged and the FBS result is stable after the second test, a third/further sample may be deferred unless additional abnormalities develop on the trace.
- Where a third FBS is considered necessary, a consultant obstetrician's opinion should be sought.

20. L Perform FBS

In this case the CTG shows two non-reassuring features (which is by definition considered to be a pathological CTG). Therefore, FBS should be performed.

The NICE definitions of normal, suspicious and pathological FHR traces

- Normal – an FHR trace in which all four features are classified as reassuring
- Suspicious – an FHR trace with one feature classified as non-reassuring and the remaining features classified as reassuring
- Pathological – an FHR trace with two or more features classified as non-reassuring or one or more classified as abnormal

National Institute of Health and Clinical Excellence. Chapter 13: Complicated labour: monitoring babies in labour. Intrapartum care. Care of healthy women and their babies during childbirth. (CG55). NICE, 2008: 47–50.

Chapter 25

Menopause

Questions 1–5

Options for Questions 1–5

A   Continuous oestrogens and progestogens (oral) hormone replacement therapy (HRT)
B   Desogestrel
C   HRT not recommended
D   Levonorgestrel IUS (Mirena)
E   Norgestimate
F   Oestrogens plus progestogens plus testosterone (oral)
G   Testosterone only (oral) HRT
H   Oestrogens only (oral) HRT
I   Oestrogen transdermal patch and vaginal progesterone cream HRT
J   Oestrogen transdermal patch only HRT
K   Oestrogen cream or pessaries vaginally HRT
L   Oestrogen cream for vaginal application and oral progestogens HRT
M   Progestogens only (oral) HRT
N   Sequential oestrogens and progestogens (oral) HRT
O   Cyproterone acetate

Instructions: For each scenario described below, choose the **single** most appropriate hormonal drug therapy from the list of options above. Each option may be used once, more than once, or not at all.

1. A 50-year-old Asian woman presents to her general practitioner with one episode of postmenopausal minimal vaginal bleeding which lasted for 2 days but has now stopped. Clinical examination reveals atrophic vagina and cervix. A transvaginal scan shows an endometrial thickness of 4 mm. She gives a history of breast cancer in her first cousin who is 69 years old.

2. A 50-year-old Caucasian woman presents to her general practitioner with severe menopausal symptoms (hot flushes and night sweats). She gives a past history of total abdominal hysterectomy and bilateral salpingo-oophorectomy 10 years ago for menorrhagia. Currently, she is on citalopram and levothyroxine for depression and hypothyroidism respectively. She is receiving dermatological treatment for psoriasis.

3. A 50-year-old Asian woman presents with severe hot flushes and night sweats. Her periods have been very irregular for the last 8 months and she has not had any periods for the last 4 months. Her follicle-stimulating hormone (FSH) level is 45 IU/mL. She is very religious and wishes to have regular menstrual periods every month. She is happy to take tablets.

4. A 50-year-old Afro-Caribbean woman presents to her general practitioner with severe menopausal symptoms. She gives a past history of menorrhagia and myomectomy 5 years ago. A recent cervical smear is negative. She does not like to have cyclical vaginal bleeding.

5. A 50-year-old Caucasian woman presents to her general practitioner with severe menopausal symptoms (hot flushes and night sweats). She had a vaginal hysterectomy for genital organ prolapse 2 years ago. However, she is a known epileptic who is taking 600 mg carbamazepine twice a day.

Answers

1. K Oestrogen cream or pessaries vaginally HRT

Oestrogen deficiency during the menopause causes atrophy of the genital organs. This makes the tissues in the genital organs fragile (especially the epithelium of the vagina and the cervix) and thus can result in bleeding with minimal trauma (e.g. sexual intercourse) or even without. The treatment is local oestrogens (oestrogen vaginal cream or tablets). This may be required in the long term to revert the symptoms of urogenital atrophy (late manifestation of oestrogen deficiency). It appears to be more effective than systemic therapy.

Low dose vaginal oestrogens can be used in the management of recurrent urinary tract infection in postmenopausal women once underlying pathology has been excluded. There is no evidence that local vaginal oestrogen is associated with any significant risks.

2. H Oestrogens only (oral) HRT

HRT is beneficial in relieving symptoms for women with severe menopausal symptoms that adversely affect quality of life. The standard preparation contains oestrogen and progestogen. In women with a uterus, progestogens are given along with oestrogens for endometrial protection as only unopposed oestrogens can cause endometrial hyperplasia which can even lead to endometrial cancer. In women who have undergone a hysterectomy, only oestrogens can be used as there is no uterus.

The minimum effective dose should to be used for the shortest duration of time and then should be reviewed on a yearly basis. An individualised approach is necessary and HRT should be started with the informed consent of the woman after appropriate counselling of the risks (breast cancer, thromboembolism and stroke) and benefits. If symptoms return after stopping HRT, it can be restarted.

A short duration of HRT can be used for up to 5 years for symptom relief in menopausal woman in their early 50s.

Younger women with premature menopause can be treated with HRT for their menopausal symptoms and for preventing osteoporosis until the age of normal menopause, following which the therapy should be reviewed.

HRT can be used as an 'add-back' therapy to avoid menopausal symptoms in women on gonadotrophin-releasing hormone (GnRH) agonist therapy.

3. N Sequential oestrogens and progestogens (oral) HRT

Sequential oestrogens and progestogens cause cyclical monthly bleeding. Women who wish to have a monthly withdrawal bleed should be prescribed a sequential regimen of HRT. However, they should be warned about the slightly increased risk of endometrial cancer.

4. A Continuous oestrogens and progestogens (oral) HRT

Women who do not like to have cyclical bleeding should be prescribed a continuous regimen of oestrogen and progestogen.

5. J Oestrogen transdermal patch only HRT

This woman needs only oestrogens since she has had a hysterectomy in the past. She is on a liver enzyme inducing drug (carbamazepine) and therefore would benefit from a transdermal oestrogen patch rather than oral oestrogens to avoid first bypass metabolism.

Royal College of Obstetricians and Gynaecologists. Menopause and Hormone Replacement: study group statement. Consensus views arising from the 47th Study Group: Menopause and Hormone Replacement Clinical Practice. http://www.rcog.org.uk/womens-health/clinical-guidance/menopause-and-hormone-replacement-study-group-statement

Royal College of Obstetricians and Gynaecologists. Scientific Advisory Committee Opinion Paper 6 (2nd edn). Alternatives to HRT for the Management of Symptoms of the Menopause. London: RCOG Press, 2010.

StratOG.net. Managing menopausal symptoms. http://www.rcog.org.uk/stratog/page/managing-menopausal-symptoms

RCOG and hormone replacement therapy debate. http://www.rcog.org.uk/what-we-do/campaigning-and-opinions/briefings-and-qas-/rcog-and-hrt-debate

Chapter 26

Puerperium

Questions 1–5

Options for Questions 1–5

A   Assess for mental capacity
B   Admit to the antenatal ward
C   Admit to the high dependency unit
D   Admit to the gynaecology ward
E   Admit to the surgical ward
F   Admit to the mother and baby unit and drug therapy
G   Antidepressant drug therapy
H   Cognitive behavioural therapy
I   Counselling
J   Referral to a bereavement midwife
K   Referral to a general physician
L   Referral to a neurologist
M   Referral to a cardiologist
N   Referral to the perinatal mental health team
O   Section under Mental Health Act

Instructions: For each clinical scenario described below, choose the **single** most appropriate initial management option from the list above. Each option may be used once, more than once, or not at all.

1.   A 20-year-old woman presents to the emergency department on the fourth postnatal day following a caesarean section. She is tearful and has not felt like breastfeeding her baby for the last couple of days. She has good family support and has not had depression or any other psychiatric problems in the past.

2.   A 20-year-old woman, para 1, is brought to the emergency department by her mother. She had a vaginal delivery 2 weeks ago which she considered quite traumatic as she suffered a massive postpartum haemorrhage. She feels listless, depressed and shows no interest in her child or in things she enjoyed before. She has had thoughts of harming herself for the last few days.

3.   A 20-year-old woman is brought to the emergency department by her partner. She tried harming herself with a knife and does not seem to have any insight into it. She does not show any interest in her 3-week-old child or want to breastfeed the baby. Her history suggests she has been on treatment for schizophrenia in the past and had stopped taking tablets. She refuses to have any treatment or be admitted to the hospital.

4.   A 20-year-old woman presents to her general practitioner with mild vaginal spotting. She thinks she is 10 weeks pregnant in the light of a positive pregnancy test 4 weeks ago. She gives a history of depression and is currently taking citalopram.

5.   A 20-year-old woman presents to the obstetric day assessment unit for symptoms of depression. She is currently 28 weeks pregnant and is under the care of

a perinatal mental health team. However, she does not have any psychotic symptoms or suicidal tendencies. As she was free of symptoms, antidepressant medications were stopped prior to pregnancy.

Questions 6–10

Options to Questions 6–10

A	Aspirin	I	Isoniazid
B	Bromocriptine	J	Lithium
C	Chloramphenicol	K	Nitrofurantoin
D	Cabergoline	L	Nalidixic acid
E	Combined oral contraceptive pill	M	Propylthiouracil
F	Diazepam	N	Sulphonamides
G	Ergotamine	O	Tetracycline
H	Iodine		

Instructions: For each side effect in neonates described below during breastfeeding or the neonatal period, choose the **single** most appropriate drug received by the mother in the antenatal or postnatal period from the list of options above. Each option may be used once, more than once, or not at all.

6. A 40-year-old Asian woman had a vaginal delivery 2 days ago. She is para 5 with all previous vaginal deliveries. She had a stroke 2 years ago from which she has recovered. She was restarted on her previous medication following delivery. She comes to the paediatric emergency department with her child who has suddenly become lethargic, started vomiting and developed a rash on the palms of his hands and feet. The registrar makes a differential diagnosis of Reye syndrome.

7. A 40-year-old woman had an emergency caesarean section 2 days ago under an epidural top-up. She has now developed meningitis and is on treatment with antibiotics. She is breastfeeding and the baby suddenly shows signs of vomiting and becomes lethargic. The blood tests show aplastic anaemia and a differential diagnosis of grey baby syndrome is made. The mother is asked to stop breastfeeding.

8. A 40-year-old woman attends for the growth scan of her fetus at 32 weeks of gestation. She has been told that the fetus has developed a swelling in front of her neck which looks like a thyroid goitre. She has recently been diagnosed with Graves' disease and is under treatment with drugs. However, her levels of thyroid stimulating antibodies, thyroid stimulating hormone (TSH) and thyroxine (T4) are within normal range.

9. A 40-year-old woman had a forceps delivery 2 days ago. She was diagnosed with malaria 1 week ago and was started on anti-malarial medication. The paediatricians notice severe worsening jaundice in the baby.

10. A 40-year-old woman had a ventouse delivery 24 hours ago. She suffered from a recurrent urinary tract infection during pregnancy and was on long-term antibiotic prophylaxis which she stopped only 1 week ago. The paediatricians have diagnosed her baby as having severe anaemia due to haemolysis.

Answers

---

1. I Counselling

The diagnosis in this case is postpartum blues. This woman has insight into her symptoms and is seeking advice. Postpartum blues are mild and temporary mood symptoms seen in up to 80% of women during the postpartum period. They typically last for a few hours to several days. The symptoms include tearfulness, sleeplessness, irritability, anxiety, low mood, feelings of isolation and disinterest in her child.

At 10–14 days after birth, women should be asked about the resolution of symptoms of baby blues. If symptoms have not resolved, the woman should be assessed for postnatal depression, and if symptoms persist, evaluated further (urgent action).

---

2. N Referral to the perinatal mental health team

Perinatal mental health disorders

Mental diseases have been identified as the second leading indirect cause of maternal morbidity and mortality in the UK (according to The Confidential Enquiry into Maternal and Child Health [CEMACH] Report of 2003–2005, there were 42 psychiatric deaths and of these 68% were from suicide).

During pregnancy and the postnatal period, perinatal mental health problems can have serious consequences for the mother, her infant and other family members. The mother and baby unit provides specialist inpatient care to women suffering from such problems including postnatal depression, related postnatal illnesses or a recurrence of pre-existing mental health diseases. The aim is to keep the woman and the baby together to promote bonding whenever possible.

The diagnosis in this case is severe depression with suicidal tendencies. She should be referred urgently to the perinatal mental health team, followed by admission to the mother and baby unit before initiating treatment.

---

3. N Referral to the perinatal mental health team

Patients with mental health problems have the right to accept or decline life-threatening treatment while people without capacity cannot make such decisions, and therefore the Mental Health Act (2005) allows someone else (a professional) to make decisions for them. This patient does not have insight or capacity and is refusing treatment. Therefore, she needs to be urgently referred to the perinatal mental health team before sectioning under the Mental Health Act to initiate treatment.

---

4. N Referral to the perinatal mental health team

Women with a history of depression should be referred to the perinatal mental health team for assessment at their first antenatal visit during pregnancy.

To identify possible depression, all women should be asked at least two questions during the first contact with primary care during pregnancy, at her booking visit (her first midwife appointment) and postnatally (usually at 4–6 weeks and 3–4 months) by healthcare professionals (midwives, obstetricians, health visitors and general practitioners). For example:

- during the past month, have you often been bothered by feeling down, depressed or hopeless?
- during the past month, have you often been bothered by having little interest or pleasure in doing things?

A third question should be considered if the woman answers 'yes' to either of the initial questions:

- is this something you feel you need or want help with?

Also, at first contact all women should be asked about:

- past and present severe mental illness including schizophrenia, bipolar disorder, psychosis in the postnatal period and severe depression
- previous treatment by a psychiatrist/specialist mental health team including inpatient care
- a family history of perinatal mental illness

5. G Antidepressant drug therapy

This woman has insight as she is seeking medical advice. As she does not have any psychotic symptoms or suicidal tendencies, admission to hospital is not required. She is depressed and therefore needs antidepressant therapy.

Antidepressant drugs

While choosing an antidepressant medication for pregnant and breastfeeding women, one should bear in mind that the safety of these drugs is not well understood:

- Tricyclic antidepressants (amitriptyline, imipramine and nortriptyline) have fewer known risks during pregnancy than other antidepressants.
- Fluoxetine (a selective serotonin reuptake inhibitor [SSRI]) has the least known risk during pregnancy.
- Imipramine, nortriptyline and sertraline are present at relatively low levels in breast milk.
- Citalopram and fluoxetine are present in at relatively high levels in breast milk.
- SSRIs taken after 20 weeks of gestation may be associated with an increased risk of persistent pulmonary hypertension in the neonate.
- Paroxetine taken in the first trimester may be associated with fetal heart defects.
- Venlafaxine may be associated with an increased risk of high blood pressure at high doses, higher toxicity in overdose than SSRIs and some tricyclic antidepressants, and increased difficulty in withdrawal.
- All antidepressants carry the risk of withdrawal or toxicity in neonates; in most cases the effects are mild and self-limiting.

National Institute of Health and Clinical Excellence. NICE guideline on antenatal and postnatal mental health: clinical management and service management (CG45). NICE, 2007 (revised 2010).
Nicholas N and Nicholas S. Understanding the Mental Capacity Act 2005: a guide to clinicians. The Obstetrician & Gynaecologist 2010; 12:29–34.

6. A Aspirin

Aspirin is secreted in breast milk and Reye syndrome is a side effect of aspirin use.

Reye syndrome is a fatal disease which mainly affects the brain and liver but can affect any organ in the body. It is commonly seen in children following consumption of aspirin with viral illness. Its use is therefore not recommended in the UK for children under 16 years of age unless really indicated (Committee on Safety of Medicines). The Food and Drug Administration (FDA) does not approve its use in children under the age of 19 years.

The disease itself can cause a fatty liver and severe encephalopathy. Jaundice is not a feature of Reye syndrome. Most children will recover with conservative supportive therapy. Brain injury and death are potential complications.

http://www.mhra.gov.uk/committees/medicinesadvisorybodies/committeeonsafetyofmedicines/index.htm

7. C Chloramphenicol

Chloramphenicol is an antimicrobial drug effective against gram-positive and gram-negative bacteria, including most anaerobic organisms. It is no longer a first line treatment due to the development of resistance and safety issues. The most common and serious side effect is bone marrow suppression which is usually reversible. The less common side effect is aplastic anaemia which is idiosyncratic and generally fatal (unpredictable and unrelated to the dose).

Oral chloramphenicol crosses the placenta and is also excreted in the breast milk. When used in late pregnancy or during puerperium it is known to cause grey baby syndrome in the neonate. Therefore, its use near term and during breastfeeding is not recommended.

8. M Propylthiouracil

Hyperthyroidism (50% of affected women have a family history of autoimmune thyroid disease) is more common in women than men and 95% of these in pregnancy are due to Graves disease. Such women are usually treated with antithyroid drugs: carbimazole and propylthiouracil are the most commonly used drugs in the UK. Both of these drugs cross the placenta, propylthiouracil less easily than carbimazole, and are generally safe to use in pregnancy using the minimum effective dose to maximise the therapeutic effect. However, reports of aplasia cutis (scalp defect) have been noted with the use of carbimazole and fetal hypothyroidism and goitre have been noted with both drugs when used in high doses.

Propylthiouracil is preferred during puerperium as very little is excreted in the breast milk (0.07% of the dose taken by the mother).

Fetal hypothyroidism may be caused by placental passage of maternal thyroid stimulating hormone (TSH) inhibitory immunoglobulins or high doses of propylthiouracil, more often the latter. The risk can be minimised by using vigorous antithyroid treatment before conception and by the use of lower doses of these drugs during pregnancy. However, fetal hyperthyroidism can be caused by transplacental passage of thyroid stimulating antibodies and is reported in 1% of the babies born to mothers with a past or current history of Graves' disease. If it develops *in utero* and is left untreated the mortality is 50%, while if it develops at birth and is left untreated the mortality is 15%. *In utero*, the fetus may present with fetal tachycardia, fetal growth restriction and fetal goitre. The risk of the fetus being affected with hyperthyroidism is higher if the TSH-binding inhibiting immunoglobulin (TBI) index is >30% (predictive) and increases further if the TBI index is >70% (strongly predictive).

9. N Sulphonamides

Long acting sulphonamides should be avoided in the last few weeks of pregnancy because they increase the risk of neonatal kernicterus (bilirubin binds with albumin but sulphonamides interfere with bilirubin binding with albumin by competitively binding to albumin).

10. K Nitrofurantoin

Urinary tract infection (UTI): the antibiotic choice depends on the sensitivity of the organism. Three days of antibiotics are sufficient to treat asymptomatic bacteriuria. It is recommended that regular urine cultures are done to ensure eradication of the organism as 15% of women will have recurrent bacteriuria during their pregnancy, thus needing a second course of antibiotics.

Amoxicillin, ampicillin and cephalosporins are safe to use in pregnancy. Nitrofurantoin (50–100 mg four times daily for 7 days, if using a long-acting preparation, the dose would be 100 mg twice daily) is a safe alternative to treat UTI but should be avoided in the third trimester as it can precipitate neonatal haemolytic anaemia. Trimethoprim should be avoided in the first trimester due to its antifolate action.

Nelson-Piercy C. Handbook of Obstetric Medicine (4th edn). London: Informa Healthcare, 2010.

Chapter 27

Reproductive medicine

Questions 1–5

Options for Questions 1–5

A	Androgen insensitivity syndrome	I	Hypogonadotrophic hypogonadism
B	Androgen secreting tumour	J	Granulosa cell tumour of the ovary
C	Adenomyosis	K	Ovarian remnant syndrome
D	Autoimmune disease	L	Ovarian resistant syndrome
E	Cushing syndrome	M	Residual ovary syndrome
F	Endometriosis	N	Parovarian cyst
G	Fibroid uterus	O	Premature ovarian failure
H	Fitz–Hugh–Curtis syndrome	P	Unexplained infertility

Instructions: For each clinical scenario described below, choose the **single** most appropriate diagnosis from the list of options above. Each option may be used once, more than once, or not at all.

1. A 38-year-old Asian woman attends the infertility clinic with her partner. She has been trying to conceive for the last 3 years without success. She gives a history of regular periods associated with dysmenorrhoea which outlasts the periods. She is 5 feet tall and is a normal weight for her height. Pelvic examination reveals thickened, tender uterosacral ligaments. Hormonal tests reveal normal luteinising hormone (LH), follicle-stimulating hormone (FSH), testosterone, prolactin and ovulatory day 21 progesterone. Her partner's semen analysis is normal.

2. A 20-year-old Asian woman attends the infertility clinic with her husband. She has been trying to conceive for the last 2 years without any success. She is very anxious as her mother-in-law is pressuring her and abusing her for not conceiving. Clinically, she has a blind vagina with small breasts and scant pubic hair. Investigations reveal grossly elevated testosterone levels above the normal range and relatively elevated oestrogen levels.

3. A 38-year-old Caucasian woman attends the infertility clinic with her partner. She has been trying to conceive for the last 2.5 years. She has a normal body mass index (BMI) and gives a history of regular menstrual cycles. Hormonal tests reveal normal FSH, LH, testosterone, prolactin and ovulatory day 21 progesterone. Her partner's semen analysis is normal. A hysterosalpingogram (HSG) confirms bilateral patent fallopian tubes.

4. A 40-year-old Caucasian woman attends the infertility clinic. She has been trying to conceive for the last year and had noticed very scant periods over the last

6 months. She gives a history of rapid hair growth on the face, chin and chest in the last 4 months. Her voice has deepened and she has noticed an increase in muscle bulk. The rest of the physical examination is normal. Her partner's semen analysis is normal.

5. A 30-year-old Caucasian woman attends the day surgery unit for a diagnostic laparoscopy. She has been trying to conceive for the last 3 years and has some pelvic pain on the right side. She is a normal weight and gives a history of regular menstrual cycles. Hormonal tests reveal normal LH, FSH, prolactin, thyroid function tests (TFTs) and ovulatory day 21 progesterone. Laparoscopy reveals absence of spill in both fallopian tubes and perihepatic adhesions. Her partner's semen analysis is normal.

Questions 6–10

Options for Questions 6–10

A	Admit to the ward	I	Laparotomy and salpingectomy
B	Arrange *in vitro* fertilisation (IVF)	J	Laparoscopy and ovarian cystectomy
C	Bilateral ovarian drilling	K	Offer medical termination of pregnancy
D	Counsel and offer support		
E	Do serial beta human chorionic gonadotropin blood tests	L	Perform suction evacuation
		M	Perform laparoscopy and dye test
F	Explain and offer laparoscopic salpingectomy	N	Refer to the recurrent miscarriage clinic
G	Intramuscular methotrexate	O	Repeat scan in 1 week
H	Intramuscular tranexamic acid		

Instructions: For each clinical scenario described below, choose the **single** most appropriate management from the list of options above. Each option may be used once, more than once, or not at all.

6. A 36-year-old Asian woman attends the early pregnancy assessment unit with mild vaginal bleeding. She gives a history of an embryo transfer 2.5 weeks ago at a fertility centre, hence she is anxious. She is under a lot of family pressure to have children. A pregnancy test performed today is negative.

7. A 36-year-old Caucasian woman attends the early pregnancy assessment unit with abdominal pain. She had an embryo transfer 5 weeks ago at a fertility centre and has come for a routine scan. A transvaginal scan reveals a single viable intrauterine pregnancy and a 3.5-cm echogenic mass seen adjacent to the left ovary suggestive of an ectopic pregnancy. There is no free fluid in the pouch of Douglas and both ovaries appear normal.

8. A 36-year-old Asian woman attends the infertility clinic with her husband. She has been trying to conceive for the last 2 years. She is overweight and gives a history of irregular periods over the last 2 years. Her history and investigations are suggestive of polycystic ovary syndrome (PCOS). She has been using clomiphene citrate for the last 6 months with day 21 progesterone of 30 nmol/L. Her husband's semen analysis is normal.

9. A 36-year-old Caucasian woman attends the infertility clinic with her partner. She is a normal weight and gives a history of regular menstrual cycles. However, her periods are heavy and are associated with severe pain that outlasts her periods. Hormonal tests reveal normal LH, FSH, prolactin and ovulatory day 21 progesterone levels. She recently had a laparoscopy and a dye test that showed pelvic adhesions with an absence of dye spill in both fallopian tubes. Her partner's semen analysis is normal.

10. A 36-year-old Caucasian woman attends the infertility clinic with her husband. She has been trying to conceive for the last 2 years. She is overweight and gives a history of irregular cycles for the last 2 years. Her history and investigations are suggestive of PCOS. She has been using clomiphene citrate for the last 8 months. Hysterosalpingogram reveals patent fallopian tubes. Her husband's semen analysis is normal.

Answers

1. F Endometriosis

Endometriosis

Endometriosis can cause symptoms which include deep dyspareunia, severe dysmenorrhoea, chronic pelvic pain, ovulation pain, cyclical or premenstrual bowel or bladder symptoms, infertility and dyschezia (painful defaecation).

Clinical examination may reveal deeply infiltrating nodules when performed during menstruation. The gold standard for diagnosing endometriosis is by visual inspection of the pelvis at laparoscopy. However, ultrasonography is a useful tool to diagnose ovarian endometrioma.

Serum CA 125 may be elevated in this condition but has no value as a diagnostic tool compared to laparoscopy.

Medical therapy

A therapeutic trial of hormone drug therapy to reduce menstrual flow is appropriate if the woman has symptoms suggestive of endometriosis and wants treatment. It has been shown that suppression of ovarian function can reduce endometriosis-associated pain. Levonorgestrel IUS use is also known to reduce endometriosis-related pain. However, recurrence of symptoms is common following medical treatment of endometriosis. The duration of therapy depends on the drug choice, response to therapy and side effect profile.

There is not enough evidence to suggest non-steroidal anti-inflammatory drugs (NSAIDs) are effective in reducing endometriosis-associated pain.

A gonadotropin-releasing hormone (GnRH) agonist with 'add back' therapy with oestrogen and progesterone can be used for treatment. 'Add back' therapy protects against bone mineral density loss during GnRH therapy and for a further 6 months after.

Surgical treatment

Endometriosis-related pain can be reduced by removing the entire lesions in severe deeply infiltrating lesions. However, before undertaking such extensive surgery planning is important and this should be done in a multidisciplinary context.

The involvement of the bladder, bowel and ureters should be assessed to plan the extent of surgery. Therefore, consider performing an MRI scan or ultrasound (transrectal or renal) scan with or without intravenous urogram and barium enema studies to map the disease.

The ideal treatment is removal of endometriosis. However, ablation of endometriotic lesions has been shown to reduce endometriosis-related pain compared to diagnostic laparoscopy alone.

Laparoscopic uterine nerve ablation has not been shown to reduce endometriosis-associated pain.

There is not sufficient evidence to justify the use of hormonal therapy prior to or after surgical treatment.

Infertility treatment

Ovarian hormone suppression to improve fertility in minimal to mild endometriosis is not effective and there is no evidence that it is effective in more severe disease. However, ablation of endometriotic spots with adhesiolysis is effective for improving fertility in minimal−mild endometriosis compared to diagnostic laparoscopy alone. Also, in women with endometriosis-related infertility, tubal flushing appears to improve pregnancy rates while treatment with intrauterine insemination also improves fertility. One should offer IVF treatment especially if there is a contributing tubal factor or male factor, or if other treatments have failed.

GnRH agonist use for 3−6 months before IVF in women with endometriosis increases the rate of clinical pregnancy.

The role of surgery in improving pregnancy rates in moderate to severe endometriosis is not certain.

Laparoscopic ovarian cystectomy for ovarian endometrioma is better than drainage and coagulation. It is recommended for lesions ≥4 cm.

Hormonal therapy following surgery does not improve pregnancy rates.

The role of complementary therapies is uncertain.

2. A Androgen insensitivity syndrome

Androgen insensitivity syndrome (46XY) is an X-linked recessive condition where testicular function is normal but cell receptors are unable to respond to androgens. This can impair or prevent the masculinisation of male genitalia in a developing fetus and also the development of male secondary sexual characteristics at puberty. Most women present at puberty with primary amenorrhoea.

The defect may be due to 5α-reductase enzyme deficiency or partial or complete androgen insensitivity (**Table 27.1**).

3. P Unexplained infertility

The chance of conceiving following 1 year of regular unprotected intercourse is 80% and after 18 months is 90%. In a couple seeking help to conceive, investigations should be performed only if there is at least a 1-year history of infertility.

Couples are said to have unexplained infertility when there is failure to conceive when basic infertility investigations are normal. It is reported in 10−20% of cases and the chances of conception depend on the age of the female partner, duration of the infertility and whether the infertility is primary or secondary. The pregnancy

Table 27.1 Androgen insensitivity syndrome

5α-reductase enzyme deficiency

- autosomal recessive trait
- normal levels of testosterone
- low dihydrotestosterone
- internal genitalia male
- external genitalia ambiguous or female
- male phenotype at puberty

Complete androgen insensitivity

- X-linked recessive disorder
- normal female external genitalia
- male internal genitalia
- blind vaginal pouch
- absent uterus and ovaries
- absent Wolffian structures
- breast growth at puberty
- sparse pubic and axillary hair
- testes are found in the labial folds, inguinal canal or intra-abdominal
- gonads should be removed at puberty because of risk of malignancy
- elevated testosterone levels
- relatively elevated oestradiol levels which are testicular in origin and are also derived from peripheral conversion of testosterone to oestradiol

Partial androgen insensitivity

- X-linked recessive disorder
- mainly caused due to the reduced binding affinity of dihydrotestosterone or a receptor defect in the transcription of the nucleus
- most common presentation is hypospadias during infancy
- ambiguous genitalia
- male internal genitalia
- blind vaginal pouch
- phallic enlargement
- absent uterus and ovaries
- rudimentary or normal Wolffian ducts
- testes are azoospermic
- poor development of secondary sexual characters at puberty
- breast development at puberty
- gonadectomy and hormone replacement therapy is indicated if assigned as a female

rate within 3 years of follow-up is reported to be 60–70% with no specific treatment. Counselling is an important aspect of management but may be frustrating to couples.

4. B Androgen secreting tumour

Androgen secreting tumours may arise in the adrenal gland or the ovary.

Adrenal adenomas and late onset congenital adrenal hyperplasia can give rise to such symptoms. The onset is usually sudden and of a short duration. The symptoms are that of virilisation. If the woman is pregnant, it may cause masculinisation of the fetus.

One should differentiate this from Cushing syndrome.

Cushing syndrome

Cushing syndrome is due to an excess of glucocorticoids in the blood (glucocorticoid therapy and tumours that produce cortisol or adrenocorticotropic hormone [ACTH]). In this condition, there will be other symptoms in addition to hirsutism. These include typical weight gain in the trunk and face, buffalo hump, excessive sweating, telangiectasia and easy bruising due to thinning of the skin, purple skin stria, hyperpigmentation, insulin resistance and diabetes, proximal muscle weakness, baldness, hirsutism, hypertension, hypercalcaemia, osteoporosis, euphoria or psychosis, amenorrhoea and infertility.

ACTH-induced Cushing syndrome causes hypokalaemic alkalosis and hypertension together with glucose intolerance, while there is no hypokalaemia with increased glucocorticoid excess due to a pituitary cause.

Types

- Pituitary Cushing or Cushing disease: it is responsible for 70% of endogenous Cushing syndrome and is caused by increased ACTH secretion from a benign pituitary adenoma.
- Adrenal Cushing: it is caused by excessive cortisol secretion by adrenal gland tumours or hyperplasia.
- Ectopic or paraneoplastic Cushing disease: ectopic secretion of ACTH can have an influence on the adrenal gland, e.g. ACTH production from small cell lung cancer.

Diagnosis

- 24-hour urinary cortisol measurement will be high
- Dexamethasone suppression test (normally the administration of dexamethasone would suppress the ACTH production by negative feedback and thereby reduce cortisol secretion. If cortisol levels are high, it would be indicative of Cushing syndrome because there is an ectopic source of cortisol or ACTH that is not inhibited by dexamethasone)

Ovarian tumours which are androgen secreting include arrhenoblastoma, luteoma, Leydig cell tumour and gynandroblastoma.

5. H Fitz–Hugh–Curtis syndrome

The presence of perihepatic adhesions in women with previous pelvic inflammatory disease is known as Fitz–Hugh–Curtis syndrome.

Royal College of Obstetricians and Gynaecologists. Green-top Guideline No. 24. The investigation and management of endometriosis. London: RCOG Press, 2008.
Keith Edmonds D. Chapter 13: Sexual differentiation – normal and abnormal. In: Shaw RW, Luesley D, Monga A (eds). Gynaecology (4th edn). Edinburgh: Churchill Livingstone, 2011.

6. D Counsel and offer support

A pregnancy test is usually positive at 2 weeks after an embryo transfer. If the pregnancy test is negative it means that the IVF cycle has failed. Hence, this woman needs counsel and support.

7. F Explain and offer laparoscopic salpingectomy

This woman has heterotopic pregnancy (the incidence is 1 in 30,000 pregnancies). She will need a laparoscopic salpingectomy for removal of the ectopic pregnancy (these days most ectopic pregnancies are managed laparoscopically in the UK). She cannot be offered medical management with methotrexate as she also has a viable intrauterine pregnancy.

The small risk of miscarriage with surgery and anaesthesia performed in early pregnancy should be explained to her.

8. M Perform laparoscopy and dye test

Midluteal progesterone levels of >30 nmol/L is suggestive of ovulation.

This woman is responding to clomiphene citrate with serum progesterone levels showing ovulation, hence her tubes should be checked for patency before offering other forms of fertility treatment.

9. B Arrange IVF

This woman has endometriosis and both tubes are damaged. Hence, one should offer IVF treatment especially if there is a contributing tubal factor or male factor or if other treatments have failed.

10. C Bilateral ovarian drilling

Ovarian drilling should be offered to women with clomiphene resistant PCOS.

Hamilton M. Chapter 20: Disorders and investigation of female reproduction. In: Shaw RW, Luesley D, Monga A (eds). Gynaecology (4th edn). Edinburgh: Churchill Livingstone, 2011.
Vogiatzi M and Shaw RW. Chapter 17: Ovulation induction. Gynaecology (4th edn). In: Shaw RW, Luesley D, Monga A (eds). Gynaecology (4th edn). Edinburgh: Churchill Livingstone, 2011.

Chapter 28

Research, ethics, consent and risk management

Questions 1–5

Options for Questions 1–5

A Abortion Act 1967
B The case should be individualised and registered as a stillbirth in case of doubt
C England and Wales: Stillbirth Definition Act 1992
D Female Genital Mutilation Act 2003
E Female Genital Mutilation Act March 2004
F Northern Ireland: Stillbirth Definition Northern Ireland Order 1992
G Registration under the Stillbirth Act not required

H Registration under the Abortion Act not required
I Scotland: Stillbirth Definition Act 1992
J Human Fertilisation and Embryology Act 1990
K Human Fertilisation and Embryology Authority's Code of Practice
L Human Rights Act
M Human and Animal Rights Act
N Human Tissue Act
O Human Organ Donation Act

Instructions: For each of the scenarios described below, select the **single** most appropriate Act from the list of options above. Each option may be used once, more than once, or not at all.

1. A 39-year-old woman, para 3, presents to the labour ward at 32 weeks of gestation with pre-term labour. She progresses very quickly and proceeds to have a normal vaginal delivery. The baby is admitted to the special care unit for prematurity. Following delivery a fetus papyraceus is found coincidentally.

2. A 25-year-old woman, para 1, presents to the labour ward at 23 weeks of gestation with abdominal pain and reduced fetal movements. Clinical examination reveals a soft abdomen and closed cervical os. An ultrasound scan reveals no fetal heart activity. She is in denial and refuses to accept the death of the baby. She goes home and returns 8 days later with abdominal pain and vaginal bleeding. The fetus and the placenta are expelled and the patient is discharged home the following day.

3. A 39-year-old woman, para 2, presents to the labour ward at 28 weeks of gestation with multiple pregnancies. Clinically, she is contracting four times every 10 minutes with a 4 cm cervical dilatation. An ultrasound scan reveals twin 1 and twin 2 are in breech presentation. Therefore, an emergency caesarean section is

performed. The babies are admitted to the special care baby unit due to extreme prematurity. The woman had triplets and had selective feticide of one baby at 20 weeks of gestation for fetal abnormality.

4.   A 28-year-old woman, para 3, presents to the labour ward. She is unbooked (She has had no prior appintments, scans or blood tests) and is unsure of the first day of her last period. Clinically, the contractions are strong and uterine fundal height measures 25 cm. An ultrasound scan reveals no fetal heart activity. On questioning she gives a history of recent travel to Africa and was treated for malaria.

5.   A 29-year-old woman, para 1, comes to the UK for the summer holidays with her 5-year-old child. She is brought to a hospital in an ambulance straight from the airport as she is pregnant and complains of abdominal pain. Clinically, her fundal height measures 39 cm and the midwife calls you as she cannot locate a fetal heartbeat. An ultrasound scan by an obstetric registrar reveals the absence of fetal heart activity. The woman is in denial as she felt fetal movements the previous morning. She is induced the next day followed by delivery of a macerated fetus 16 hours later.

Questions 6–10

Options for Questions 6–10

A	1–2%		I	30–40%
B	2–3%		J	56%
C	5%		K	77%
D	6–10%		L	88%
E	12%		M	85%
F	10–20%		N	99%
G	30%		O	100%
H	32%			

Instructions: For each scenario described below, choose the **single** most appropriate percentage for the events described from the list of options above. Each option may be used once, more than once, or not at all.

6.   A 24-year-old primigravida presents to the labour ward at 25 weeks of gestation with contractions. She does not give any history of rupture of membranes. Clinical examination reveals palpable contractions (two to three contractions in 10 minutes) and a cervical dilatation of 2 cm. An ultrasound scan reveals breech presentation. A diagnosis of pre-term labour is made and intravenous atosiban commenced with steroids as per local protocol to improve survival.

7.   A 24-year-old woman presents to the labour ward at 28 weeks of gestation with labour pains. Clinical examination reveals palpable contractions (one to two contractions in 10 minutes) and closed cervical os with minimal effacement. She does not give any history of rupture of membranes. A vaginal fibronectin test is positive. It is explained to the patient that this gives a positive predictive value (PPV) for pre-term labour (chance of going into labour).

8. A 24-year-old primigravida presents to the labour ward at 28 weeks of gestation with labour pains. Clinical examinations reveal palpable contractions (one to two in 10 minutes) and open cervical os. She does not give any history of rupture of membranes. Her C-reactive protein (CRP) is 55 mg/L. It has been explained to her that CRP may predict amniotic fluid infection if a sample is taken for culture.

9. A 24-year-old multiparous woman presents to the labour ward at 28 weeks of gestation with labour pains. Clinical examination reveals palpable contractions (two to three in 10 minutes) and a 3 cm cervical dilatation. She gives a strong history of rupture of membranes. A discussion is undertaken with the patient as to the chance (percentage) of going into premature labour in women with rupture of membranes at this gestation.

10. A 24-year-old primigravida presents to the labour ward at 28 weeks of gestation with labour pains. Clinical examination reveals palpable contractions (two to three in 10 minutes) and a 2 cm cervical dilatation. She does not give any history of rupture of membranes. A diagnosis of pre-term labour is made and intravenous atosiban is commenced to buy time for the administration of corticosteroids. Her risk of amniotic infection at this stage is discussed.

Questions 11–15

Options for Questions 11–15

A Abandon surgery and discuss with the patient	H Perform a laparotomy to remove the ovary
B Ask the patient to sign a new consent form	I Perform a laparotomy to remove the endometriosis
C Ask the hospital solicitor	J Perform a laparotomy to do an internal iliac artery ligation
D Abandon the surgery and arrange a clinic follow-up in 3 months	K Do nothing
E Abandon the surgery and contact the partner	L Discharge to the general practitioner
F Call consultant for second opinion	M Perform a laparoscopic ovarian cystectomy
G Check the consent form	N Perform a laparoscopic oophorectomy
	O Repeat the scan in 4 months

Instructions: For each scenario described below, choose the **single** most appropriate course of action from the list of options above. Each option may be used once, more than once, or not at all.

11. A 32-year-old woman with 5 years of infertility is booked for a laparoscopic dye test with or without treatment of endometriosis on a registrar list. While doing the laparoscopy, you are alarmed to see a 4 cm haematoma in the right infundibulopelvic ligament which is expanding and starts bleeding while you are manipulating the uterus.

12. A 40-year-old woman gives consent for laparoscopic sterilisation. You have finished the sterilisation procedure and notice a 3 cm cyst on the left side. Her scan report from 8 months ago showed an incidental finding of a dermoid cyst.

13. A 19-year-old woman presents with pain in the right iliac fossa (RIF). The on-call surgical team performs a diagnostic laparoscopy for suspected appendicitis. On examination the appendix looks normal with few omental adhesions to the anterior abdominal wall. The surgical team also find a small 3 cm simple left ovarian cyst which is mobile with a smooth surface and looks benign. The surgeons request the removal of the left ovary.

14. A 65-year-old woman presents with postmenopausal bleeding. The ultrasound scan shows endometrial thickness of 2 mm and also a 4 cm simple cyst on the right side. A review of the notes reveals the same findings 1 year ago with normal CA 125 levels and a risk of malignancy index (RMI) of 22.

15. A 50-year-old postmenopausal woman is referred to the fast track gynaecology oncology clinic for an incidental finding of a 4.5 cm right-sided simple ovarian cyst with CA 125 levels 8 U/mL. She is quite anxious.

Answers

---

1. G Registration under the Stillbirth Act not required

In the case of a fetus papyraceus, it is known that the fetus must have died before 24 weeks of gestation and thus it would be incorrect to register it as a stillbirth. Also, when a fetus papyraceus is present at the birth of a live baby born after 24 weeks of gestation, it would be clear from its stage of development that the fetus papyraceus had died in the womb at a stage prior to the 24 weeks of gestation. Thus, the woman can be taken not to have been pregnant with that fetus on giving birth to the surviving child or for the purpose of the legislation after 24 weeks of gestation.

---

2. G Registration under the Stillbirth Act not required

Fetuses which have died prior to 24 weeks of gestation would not be registered as stillbirths.

---

3. G Registration under the Stillbirth Act not required

Fetuses known to have died prior to the 24 weeks of gestation (e.g. where there has been a delay between a diagnosed intrauterine death and delivery, vanishing twins or selective or multifetal pregnancy reduction in multiple pregnancies) would not be registered as stillbirths.

---

4. B The case should be individualised and registered as a stillbirth in case of doubt

In cases where one or more fetuses have been born dead after 24 weeks of gestation but it was not known prior to their birth that they had died, and it is not known precisely when they died, it may be appropriate to use the stage of development of the fetus as an indicator of when death occurred and as a basis for determining when that particular pregnancy ended relative to the 24-week limit. This would need to be agreed on a case-by-case basis by the medical professionals involved; this responsibility should not be left to the attending midwife. The decision and the basis on which it was made would need to be clearly detailed in the mother's notes in case any queries arise at a later date.

Where there is any doubt about the gestational age at which the fetus died, the default position would be for medical professionals to register the birth as a stillbirth.

---

5. C England and Wales: Stillbirth Definition Act 1992

The current law on stillbirth registration as set out in the Births and Deaths Registration Act 1953 (as amended by the Still-Birth (Definition) Act 1992), Section 41, is as follows:

'a child which has issued forth from its mother after the twenty-fourth week of pregnancy and which did not at any time after being completely expelled from its mother breathe or show any other signs of life, the expression "still-birth" shall be construed accordingly'

The law in England and Wales (Section 41 of the Births and Deaths Registration Act 1953 as amended by the Stillbirth Definition Act 1992), Scotland (Section 56(1) of the Registration of Births, Deaths and Marriages (Scotland) Act 1965 as amended by the Stillbirth Definition Act 1992) and Northern Ireland (Births and Deaths Registration Order 1976 as amended by the Stillbirth Definition Northern Ireland Order 1992), requires that any 'child' expelled or issued forth from its mother after the 24th week of pregnancy that did not breathe or show any other signs of life be registered as a stillbirth.

Royal College of Obstetricians and Gynaecologists. Good Practice Guideline No. 4. Registration of stillbirth and certification for pregnancy loss before 24 weeks of gestation. London: RCOG Press, 2005.

6. B 2–3%

The incidence of pre-term labour is between 6% and 10% of all pregnancies. About 30% of these would be due to medical intervention. A 2–3% of improvement in survival is noted by postponing delivery for 24 hours around the period of viability. However, survival of infants is not much different at 32 weeks compared to term babies.

7. K 77%

A fibronectin test is performed in women suspected of being in pre-term labour. It has a PPV of 77% in predicting pre-term labour. On the other hand, less than 3% of women with a negative test will go into labour in the next 3 weeks.

8. J 56%

Inflammatory markers are poor predictors of infection. The sensitivity of the white blood count and CRP for predicting amniotic fluid infection is 32% and 56%, respectively.

9. I 30–40%

The majority of pre-term labour is preceded by premature rupture of membranes (30–40%). The aetiological factors for pre-term labour include infection, multiple pregnancy, low socioeconomic status, smoking, low prepregnancy weight, young maternal age (<18 years), previous pre-term labour, incompetent cervix, Müllerian duct anomalies and early pregnancy bleeding.

10. E 12%

Infection is one of the most common causes of pre-term labour. Twelve per cent of cases of preterm labour with intact membranes and 34% of cases with premature rupture of membranes are associated with intraamniotic infection when amniocentesis is performed.

Howe DC and Calder AA. Preterm labour. Pace review. Volume 3. London: RCOG Press 2003: 14–15.

11. F Call the consultant for second opinion

The broad ligament is a potential space which can expand with blood. The ureter runs closely at the base of the broad ligament before entering into the bladder laterally in front of the uterus.

As the haematoma is expanding, the bleeding will need to be stopped and you will need the help of a consultant.

12. K Do nothing

She is asymptomatic and has not consented to a cystectomy. A conservative approach with a follow-up appointment in the gynaecology clinic to discuss further management is important.

Small asymptomatic dermoid cysts can be managed conservatively with follow-up ultrasound scans following a discussion of the complications (cyst accidents such as torsion and rupture). If the cyst is significantly growing in size or if the patient develops symptoms, she would need a surgical approach to treat. However, both options (conservative as well as surgical) should be discussed with the patient to make an informed choice.

13. K Do nothing

This woman has RIF pain and the ovarian cyst is on the left side which is totally unrelated to the pain. This woman has not consented to any ovarian procedure, which is unnecessary considering the intraoperative findings. However, if the ovarian cyst was twisted or bleeding due a haemorrhagic cyst, it would have been dealt with at the same time in the patient's best interests.

14. L Discharge to the general practitioner

A RMI of 22 indicates a low risk of ovarian malignancy. In asymptomatic women, ovarian cysts can be managed conservatively with follow-up scans and repeated tests for CA 125 levels every 3–4 months for 1 year before they can be discharged back to their general practitioner.

Since this woman already had a scan 1 year ago with similar findings she can be discharged back to the general practitioner.

Protocol for triaging women:

- Low risk – RMI <25 = <3% risk of cancer
- Moderate risk – RMI 25–250 = 20% risk of cancer
- High risk – RMI >250 = 75% risk of cancer

RMI = menopausal status × results of ultrasound scan findings × absolute CA 125

15. O Repeat the scan in 4 months

A RMI of 24 indicates low risk of malignancy. This patient is asymptomatic and the ultrasound scan features indicate a benign appearance (simple unilocular cyst). She needs follow-up repeat scans and tests for CA 125 levels for 1 year and then if the clinical situation remains the same she can be discharged to her general practitioner.

Royal College of Obstetricians and Gynaecologists. Green-top Guideline No. 34. Ovarian cysts in postmenopausal women. London: RCOG Press, 2003.
Royal College of Obstetricians and Gynaecologists. Green-top Guideline No. 62. Management of suspected ovarian masses in premenopausal women. London: RCOG Press, 2011.
National Institute of Health and Clinical Excellence. Guidelines on ovarian cancer: the recognition and initial management (CG122). NICE, 2011.

Chapter 29

Urogynaecology

Questions 1–5

Options for Questions 1–5

A	Amitryptyline	I	Trospium chloride
B	Botulinum toxin	J	Propiverine HCl
C	Darifenacin	K	Dobutamine
D	Desmopressin	L	Drospirenone
E	Duloxetine	M	Desogestrel
F	Fesoterodine	N	Digoxin
G	Oxybutynin	O	Fexofenadine
H	Tolterodine		

Instructions: For each mechanism of action described below, choose the **single** most appropriate drug from the list of options above. Each option may be used once, more than once, or not at all.

1. Selective serotonin and noradrenergic reuptake inhibitor.

2. Anticholinergic plus musculotrophic plus local anaesthetic.

3. Anticholinergic plus calcium channel blocker.

4. Competitive muscarinic receptor antagonist which is a prodrug.

5. Uroselective, M3 muscarinic acetylcholine receptor antagonist.

Answers

1. E Duloxetine

Duloxetine is a selective serotonin and noradrenergic reuptake inhibitor, which increases the contraction of the rhabdosphincter. It is used in the treatment of stress incontinence. The dose is 40 mg twice daily and can be reduced to 20 mg daily after reassessment in 2 weeks. The side effects include nausea, vomiting, constipation, diarrhoea, dry mouth, insomnia, drowsiness, headache, dizziness, anorexia and blurred vision. The contraindications to its use include liver disease, pregnancy and breastfeeding.

2. G Oxybutynin

Oxybutynin is anticholinergic, musculotropic and also has local anaesthetic effect. The dose is 2.5 mg three times daily to 5 mg four times daily. It causes more dryness of mouth than selective anticholinergic drugs and is used in the treatment of detrusor instability.

3. J Propiverine HCl

Propiverine HCl is an anticholinergic plus a calcium channel blocker. It antagonises muscarinic receptors and directly relaxes the muscle. The side effects are dry mouth and blurring of vision. The dose is 15–30 mg twice daily.

4. F Fesoterodine

Fesoterodine is a newer anticholinergic drug used in the treatment of detrusor instability. It is a competitive, non-uroselective muscarinic receptor antagonist and is a prodrug. The dose is 4–8 mg once daily. The side effects include insomnia, less often nasal dryness, pharyngo-laryngeal pain, cough and vertigo.

5. C Darifenacin

Darifenacin is a M3 muscarinic acetylcholine receptor antagonist and is uroselective. The daily dose is 7.5–15 mg once daily. It is not recommended for women with severe hepatic impairment.

Solifenacin has similar actions to darifenacin and is not recommended in women a with severe hepatic impairment.

Other drugs

Trospium chloride is a non-selective, anticholinergic drug and a competitive muscarinic receptor antagonist. The dose is 20 mg twice daily. It causes less dry mouth compared to oxybutynin. It is used in the treatment of detrusor instability.

Tolterodine is a competitive, non-uroselective muscarinic antagonist (M1, 2, 3, 4 and 5), which causes less dryness of the mouth than oxybutynin. The dose is 2–4 mg once daily.

Desmopressin enhances the reabsorption of water in the kidneys by increasing cellular permeability of the collecting ducts and is highly effective for women with nocturia. The dose is 200–400 µg once daily at night-time.

Abboudi H, Fynes MF, Doumouchtsis SK. Contemporary therapy for the overactive bladder. The Obstetrician and Gynaecologist 2011; 13:98–105.

Chapter 30

Women's sexual and reproductive health

Questions 1–5

Options for Questions 1–5

A   Condoms
B   Copper intrauterine device (IUD)
C   Danazol
D   Medroxyprogesterone acetate
E   Co-cyprindiol (Dianette)
F   Levonorgestrel 1.5 mg
G   Ethinylestradiol/drospirenone (Yasmin)

H   Ethinylestradiol/levonorgestrel (Microgynon)
I   Mifepristone
J   Levonorgestrel IUS
K   Norethisterone
L   Progestogen only pill
M   Sterilisation
N   Gestrinone
O   GnRH analogues

Instructions: For each scenario described below, select the **single** most appropriate method of contraception from the list of options above. Each option may be used once, more than once, or not at all.

1. A 42-year-old woman presents to the labour ward at 34 weeks of gestation in pre-term labour. She progress very quickly and proceeds to have an emergency caesarean section for fetal distress. She was discharged home after 1 week as her baby was admitted to the special care baby unit. Two weeks later, she attends the general practitioner centre seeking contraception. She wants to continue to breastfeed her baby.

2. A 20-year-old woman presents to the emergency gynaecology services at a hospital at midnight for advice. She gives a history of condom rupture while having sexual intercourse 3 hours ago. She is worried that she will get pregnant and her parents will abandon her.

3. A 28-year-old happily married woman presents to the family planning clinic for advice. She gives a history of unprotected intercourse 3 days ago and does not want to get pregnant. She is also looking for long-term contraception. She has two children who are primary school age.

4. A 20-year-old young Asian woman is about to start a new relationship. She had previously used progestogen only pills for contraception but became pregnant after the delayed intake of two consecutive pills. The pregnancy had to be

terminated as it was unwanted. She is still keen to take pills. She has suffered from acne for the last 6 months and is worried that her boyfriend will leave her because of this problem.

5. A 28-year-old woman, para 2, attends the family planning centre for contraceptive advice. She is keen to take long-term contraception. However, she suffers from menorrhagia for which she is currently taking tranexamic acid.

Answers

1. L Progestogen only pill

In women who are willing to breastfeed, the progestogen only pill is recommended as it does not affect lactation. It can be started as early as 3 weeks post delivery in such women. The combined oral contraceptive pill should not be used if women are continuing to breastfeed as this can affect both quantity and quality of the breast milk.

2. F Levonorgestrel 1.5 mg

Levonorgestrel 1.5 mg (Levonelle) can be taken up to 72 hours after unprotected intercourse, although the efficacy decreases with time. Women should be advised to take a further dose if vomiting occurs within 2 hours.

3. B Copper intrauterine device (IUD)

The levonorgestrel IUS is not recommended or licensed for emergency contraception. A copper intrauterine device can be inserted up to 5 days after unprotected intercourse or from ovulation. It is important to consider antibacterial prophylaxis and infection screening (for possible sexullay transmitted infections) at the same time.

4. G Ethinylestradiol/drospirenone (Yasmin)

Yasmin is a new monophasic combined oral contraceptive pill which contains 30 µg of ethinyl oestradiol and 3 mg of drospirenone. Its anti-mineralocorticoid properties help to counteract the salt and fluid retaining properties of oestrogen and helps women who have symptoms of bloating, while its anti-androgenic properties make it useful to prescribe for women with acne and polycystic ovary syndrome. It can be used as an alternative to co-cyprindiol in the latter condition.

5. J Levonorgestrel IUS

Either levonorgestrel IUS or endometrial ablation should be offered before discussing hysterectomy.

Guillebaud J. Your Questions Answered: Contraception (5th edn). Edinburgh: Churchill Livingstone, 2008.

Section C

SAQs

Chapter 31

Gynaecology

31.1 BRCA1 mutation

A 22-year-old nulliparous woman is known to carry the BRCA1 mutation. She has two sisters and the eldest of them died recently at the age of 35 years with ovarian cancer.

1. What risks of developing ovarian cancer should she be aware of? Marks (6)

2. How can those risks be reduced? Marks (8)

3. How should she be managed? Marks (6)

Key points

- 22 years
- nulliparous
- BRCA1 mutation
- sister died of ovarian cancer
- associated risks
- reduce risks
- implications to family members

Essay plan

1.

- autosomal dominant
- genetic predisposition: seen in 10% of women with the disease
- seven per cent of patients give family history of ovarian cancer
- lifetime risk of developing ovarian cancer if positive for BRCA1 is 40–60%
- associated with Lynch-type II variant of hereditary non-polyposis colorectal cancer (HNPCC)
- lifetime risk of endometrial cancer if positive for HNPCC is 30%

2.

- lifestyle modification
- combined oral contraceptive pill (COCP)
- planning of pregnancies
- prophylactic bilateral oophorectomy
- oophorectomy does not eliminate the risk of primary peritoneal cancer
- screening and detection

3.

- confirm her sister had the BRCA1 mutation
- screening for ovarian, breast, endometrial cancer and HNPCC
- complete family early
- prophylactic oophorectomy once family complete
- implications to other family members to be screened

31.1 Suggested answer

1.

Predisposition (genetic) to ovarian cancer occurs in 10% of patients with the disease while only 7% report a family history of ovarian cancer. The BRCA1 gene is found on chromosome 17 and has an autosomal dominant inheritance. Women positive for the BRCA1 mutation have a 40–60% lifetime risk of developing ovarian cancer.

There can be an association with Lynch-type II variant of HNPCC. When positive for this condition, there is a 5–10% chance of developing ovarian cancer and a 30% lifetime risk of developing endometrial cancer.

It can affect other family members as they may be carrying the BRCA1 mutation.

2.

The lifestyle factors that can modify the risk include parity, breastfeeding and avoiding ovulation induction drugs and *in vitro* fertilisation (IVF)-related treatments.

There is also evidence that the COCP may offer protection to these patients' ovaries (with a 40% risk reduction in developing ovarian cancer).

Ovarian cancer in women with such mutation has a tendency to occur at an earlier age than is found for sporadic cases. Therefore one should offer prophylactic oophorectomy following completion of the family as this has shown benefit. However, one should be aware when counselling such women that this does not eliminate the risk of primary peritoneal cancer.

In the meantime, regular screening with transvaginal scan and CA 125 should be offered.

3.

One should first confirm that her sister had an ovarian cancer and the BRCA1 mutation (index case).

She should be advised to complete her family early as the risk of developing ovarian cancer is high and has future fertility implications. Once the family is complete, she should be offered prophylactic oophorectomy. If she does undergo a surgical oophorectomy, she should be appropriately counselled about its disadvantages (osteoporosis and cardiac disease) and hormone replacement therapy (HRT) implications (increased risk of thromboembolism and breast cancer).

One should screen her for other cancers (e.g. breast, endometrial and HNPCC) as these conditions have an association in these women.

Other family members should be screened for the BRCA1 mutation and treated accordingly if positive.

Acheson N and Chan KK. Chapter 12: Epithelial ovarian cancer. In: Shafi MI, Luesley DM, Jordan JJ (eds). Handbook of Gynaecological Oncology. Edinburgh: Churchill Livingstone, 2001.

31.2 Complications during laparoscopy

A 20-year-old woman is the first case on the list for a diagnostic laparoscopy due to pelvic pain. After entering the abdomen with the scope, blood is found in the entry field which starts filling up slowly.

1. What is the immediate course of action? Marks (7)

2. After some time it is noticed that there is continuing bleeding from a retroperitoneal vessel. What is the next course of action and why? Marks (9)

3. How should she be managed postoperatively? Marks (4)

Key points
- diagnostic laparoscopy
- 20 years old
- blood on entry

Essay plan

1.

- look all around
- identify the source of bleeding
- inform the anaesthetist
- inform the on-call gynaecology consultant if a consultant is not in the theatre
- inform the theatre scrub nurse
- blood group and save (should have been done)

2.

- cross-match four units of blood
- central venous or arterial line
- get vascular surgeons
- midline laparotomy
- pressure on the aorta above the bifurcation
- suturing of the vessel by vascular surgeons
- intraperitoneal drain
- Foley's catheter with an hourly bag
- prophylactic antibiotics

3.

- intensive therapy unit (ITU)

- close monitoring
- assess for need for further blood and blood products (check clotting profile, depending on blood loss)
- assess for any further bleeding
- antibiotics and thromboprophylaxis
- debrief the woman
- follow-up in clinic
- incident/risk management form

31.2 Suggested answer

1.

It is important to identify the source of bleeding. The most common site for the source of a trickle of blood is the port site itself. However, if there is no port site bleeding, one should consider the bleeding to be due to a vascular injury. If the bleeding persists, one should inform the anaesthetist and theatre scrub nurse and contact the on-call consultant to come for a review. A group and save should have been undertaken preoperatively; if not then one should be sent off immediately as an urgent sample. The blood transfusion department should be informed about the urgency, the location and the person to contact. It is important to cross-match blood. The theatre sister should be informed that the laparotomy trolley is to be available in case it is needed.

2.

If the bleeding is persistent one should cross-match blood and ask for blood products (fresh frozen plasma). By this time the on-call gynaecology consultant should have arrived. The anaesthetist and theatre nurse should be informed again about the conversion to laparotomy. The vascular surgeons may be urgently called to the theatre for help. In the meantime, a midline laparotomy should be performed and another senior gynaecology consultant may be called for help (two brains are better than one). Following this, the bleeding source should be identified and pressure applied on the abdominal aorta above the bifurcation to reduce the bleeding while awaiting the vascular surgeons.

The vascular injury should be sutured to achieve haemostasis and a Robinson intraperitoneal drain used. Blood and blood products should be given as necessary. Intravenous antibiotics for prophylaxis and low molecular weight heparin (LMWH) for thromboprophylaxis should be given once there are no signs of bleeding.

The rectus sheath should be closed with Loop ethilon (No. 1) or polydioxanone. Skin should be closed with staples.

3.

The woman should be transferred and closely monitored in the ITU or high dependency unit (HDU). Antibiotics should be continued and thromboprophylaxis initiated once she is clinically stable. She should be debriefed along with her family and the need for further follow-up in the gynaecology clinic for a detailed discussion of her pelvic pain explained.

As in all adverse/unexpected incidents, especially with transfer to ITU, a risk incident form should be completed.

Royal College of Obstetricians and Gynaecologists. Green-top Guideline No. 2. Diagnostic laparoscopy. London: RCOG Press, 2008.

31.3 Delayed puberty

A 16-year-old Asian girl attends the gynaecology clinic with her mother. The general practitioner letter reveals that she has not attained menarche. She and her mother seek reassurance.

1. What are the causes of delayed puberty and how would one classify them?   Marks (8)

2. How should she be investigated and why? How should she be managed?   Marks (12)

Key points

- 16 years old
- delayed menarche
- anxious parent

Essay plan

1.

- constitutional
- hypothalamic causes
- medical illness
- Müllerian development abnormalities
- abnormal karyotype
- endocrinological disorders
- others

2.

- history
- examination
- investigation
- diagnosis
- treatment

31.3 Suggested answer

1.

Constitutional delay

This is the most common cause of delayed menarche.

Hypothalamic causes

These are excessive exercise (athlete), weight loss (body mass index <18) and stress.

Endocrinological causes

Endocrinological causes are hyperprolactinaemia, hyperthyroidism and polycystic ovary syndrome (PCOS).

Medical illnesses

These include tuberculosis, cystic fibrosis, chronic renal disease, malabsorption syndromes and inflammatory bowel disease.

Müllerian abnormalities

Müllerian abnormalities are Mayer–Rokitansky–Küster–Hauser syndrome, imperforated hymen, transverse vaginal septum and vaginal agenesis.

Abnormal karyotype

These include Turner syndrome and testicular feminisation syndrome.

Other causes

Other causes could be skull trauma, history of radiotherapy, chemotherapy and prolactinoma of the pituitary.

2.

The management consists of taking an appropriate history, examination, investigations, coming to a diagnosis and treatment of the causative factor.

A detailed history including constitutional delay in the family, family history of PCOS, past history of medical illnesses, personal history of eating disorders and excessive weight loss is important. A past history of childhood cancers, radiotherapy and chemotherapy is important as these may lead to permanent destruction of pituitary or ovarian hormone production.

One should enquire about the physical development and secondary sexual characters including the breast, axillary hair, pubic hair and height.

In the presence of normal secondary sexual characters one should suspect Müllerian abnormalities such as Mayer–Rokitansky–Küster–Hauser syndrome, imperforate hymen and transverse vaginal septum. The ovarian function and the karyotype are normal (46XX). An imperforate hymen needs a cruciate incision under general anaesthetic to let the collected blood out and open up the passage. With Mayer–Rokitansky–Küster–Hauser syndrome one should offer vaginal dilators to attain the maximum length of the vagina for sexual intercourse and the need for *in vitro* fertilisation (IVF) to conceive in the future should be discussed.

The presence of good breast development in testicular feminisation syndrome can be misleading. However, there is scanty axillary and pubic hair, tall stature, absent uterus and a blind-ending vagina. One should suspect the presence of the

Y chromosome in the absence of a uterus. Gender assignment is a major concern at this stage as she has been brought up as female and she should be appropriately counselled by a specialist. The use of vaginal dilators should be encouraged to maintain the vaginal length or increase the vaginal length if sexually active. Future fertility issues should be discussed (e.g. adoption, egg donation and surrogacy).

In the absence of secondary sexual characters and the presence of features such as short stature, webbed neck, wide-spaced nipples, wide-carrying angles and coarctation of aorta, one should strongly suspect Turner syndrome. A karyotype will reveal 45XO. She will need hormonal therapy for growth and secondary sexual characteristic development (e.g. growth hormone, oestrogen and progesterone). Also the need for IVF to conceive in the future may need to be discussed.

A hormonal profile including serum follicle-stimulating hormone (FSH), luteinising hormone (LH), oestradiol, testosterone, prolactin and thyroid function tests are important to exclude hypothalamic, pituitary and thyroid causes. Normal or slightly low FSH and LH levels are seen in hypothalamic causes while high levels are seen in ovarian failure. An extremely low level of FSH and LH implies pituitary failure. One should (appropriately) treat these conditions with supplementation if necessary.

A systematic examination (general and genital organs) will give a clue to the cause of primary amenorrhoea. A pelvic ultrasound scan will reveal the presence (imperforate hymen, transverse vaginal septum) or absence of a uterus (testicular feminisation syndrome and Mayer–Rokitansky–Küster–Hauser syndrome). The uterus is small in size in Turner syndrome due to streak gonads.

Balen A. Chapter 14: Disorders of puberty. In: Shaw RW, Luesley D, Monga A (eds). Gynaecology (4th edn). Edinburgh: Churchill Livingstone, 2011.
Critchley HOD, Horne A, Munro K. Chapter 16: Amenorrhoea and oligomenorrhoea, and hypothalamic–pituitary dysfunction. In: Shaw RW, Luesley D, Monga A (eds). Gynaecology (4th edn). Edinburgh: Churchill Livingstone, 2011.

31.4 Ectopic pregnancy

A 20-year-old woman presents to the early pregnancy assessment unit with a small amount of vaginal spotting but no pain. One week later she attends for an ultrasound scan which reveals an ectopic pregnancy in the left fallopian tube (size 20×15 mm). Her serum beta human chorionic gonadotropin (βhCG) level is 999 IU/mL.

1. What is the incidence and what are the risk factors for developing an ectopic pregnancy?   Marks (2)

2. She is scared of surgery and requests expectant management. What are the criteria for expectant management and how should they be followed?   Marks (4)

3. The patient is reviewed 1 week later in the early pregnancy assessment unit. A repeat blood test shows her βhCG level to be 1400 IU/mL. She is clinically stable and asymptomatic except for minimal vaginal bleeding. She is not keen for surgery as she is asymptomatic but agrees to have medical management. What are the criteria for medical

management of her ectopic pregnancy and what should one warn this
woman regarding adverse affects and further management?   Marks (8)

4. One week later this woman presents to the emergency department with
    severe abdominal pain and dizziness. How should she be managed?   Marks (6)

Key points

*   20 years old
*   absence of pain
*   tubal pregnancy <3 cm
*   βhCG <1000
*   incidence
*   risk factors
*   management

Essay plan

1.

*   incidence
*   may not have risk factors
*   previous pelvic inflammatory disease (PID)
*   previous tubal surgery/pelvic surgery
*   progestogen only contraception (POP)
*   *in vitro* fertilisation

2.

*   criteria for expectant management
*   haemodynamically stable
*   small adnexal mass
*   βhCG <1000
*   absence of free fluid in the pelvis
*   facilities for close follow-up with βhCG and transvaginal scan (TVS)
*   decreasing βhCG levels and size of adnexal mass
*   compliance of the patient

3.

*   criteria for medical management
*   haemodynamically stable
*   adnexal mass <3 cm
*   βhCG <3000
*   facilities for follow-up
*   compliance of the patient
*   adverse effects of methotrexate
*   need for further dose of methotrexate
*   need for surgical management if clinical situation changes

4.

*   ruptured ectopic pregnancy
*   laparoscopy

- laparotomy
- salpingectomy
- salpingotomy
- anti-D immunoglobulin
- future advice

31.4 Suggested answer

1.

The incidence is approximately 1 in 100 pregnancies (11 in 1000 or approximately 1% from the Triennial Report on Maternal Mortality 2003–2005).

The risk factors include previous ectopic pregnancy, past history of PID, tubal surgery (including sterilisation), previous pelvic surgery, POP and *in vitro* fertilisation. However, 50% of ectopic pregnancies occur in women with no obvious history of risk factors.

2.

Expectant management should be used only for asymptomatic, clinically stable women with an ultrasound diagnosis of ectopic pregnancy, with no evidence or minimal fluid in the pouch of Douglas and decreasing βhCG levels that are less than 1000 IU/L at initial presentation.

If women are managed expectantly, serial serum βhCG measurements should be performed until βhCG levels are less than 20 IU/L. They should be followed twice weekly with serial βhCG measurements and weekly by transvaginal scans to ensure rapidly decreasing βhCG levels (ideally they should fall to less than 50% of their pretreatment levels within 7 days) and a reduction in the size of the adnexal mass by day 7. This approach is important as there are reports of tubal rupture caused by low levels of βhCG.

3.

Methotrexate is the drug of choice for medical management of ectopic pregnancies. It is used as an intramuscular injection and is given as a single dose with dose calculation related to the patient's body surface area (50 mg/m^2).

Medical therapy should be offered only to women who are clinically stable and asymptomatic.

The size of the ectopic pregnancy should be less than 3 cm as in this case (data concerning the effect of ectopic pregnancy size on outcome are less clear but women with large adnexal masses are more likely to have already ruptured).

The absence of cardiac activity on ultrasound scan is important as its presence is associated with a reduced chance of success following medical therapy and should be considered a contraindication to medical therapy.

Women most suitable for methotrexate therapy are those with a serum βhCG below 3000 IU/L (the βhCG level in this case is 1400 IU/L). However, one should bear in mind that women with βhCG >1500 IU/L may need further treatment and prolonged follow-up.

The woman should be free of any liver and haematological disorders.

Early pregnancy assessment units which offer medical management should have strict protocols for the treatment and follow-up of ectopic pregnancies. The woman should be given clear information (preferably written) about the possible need for further treatment and adverse effects following treatment. Women should be able to return easily for assessment at any time during follow-up.

Nearly 75% will experience abdominal pain following treatment. Occasionally, women will also experience conjunctivitis, stomatitis and gastrointestinal upset. A repeat treatment (more than one dose of methotrexate) may be needed in at least 15% of medically treated women. Women should be advised to attend the emergency department immediately in the case of severe abdominal pain and other symptoms (e.g. dizziness, fainting and shoulder tip pain) as this may indicate tubal rupture (there is a 7% risk of tubal rupture during follow-up) and may need immediate surgery.

4.

The above symptoms are likely to indicate tubal rupture and should be managed surgically.

A laparoscopic approach to the surgical management of tubal pregnancy, in the haemodynamically stable patient, is preferable to an open approach.

Management of tubal pregnancy in the presence of haemodynamic instability should be by the most expedient method. In most cases this will be laparotomy.

In the presence of a healthy contralateral tube, salpingectomy should be used instead of salpingotomy. This approach is associated with a lower rate of persistent trophoblast and subsequent tubal ectopic pregnancies while achieving similar intrauterine pregnancy rates.

Laparoscopic salpingotomy should be considered as the primary treatment when managing tubal pregnancy in the presence of contralateral tubal disease and the desire for future fertility. The woman should be warned about the risk of persistent trophoblast and the 20% risk of ectopic pregnancy with salpingostomy.

Non-sensitised women who are Rhesus negative with a confirmed or suspected ectopic pregnancy, managed medically or surgically, should receive anti-D immunoglobulin.

An increased risk of recurrence in future pregnancies (10%) should be explained and the need for an early scan (at 6 weeks) in future pregnancies should be emphasised.

Royal College of Obstetricians and Gynaecologists. Green-top Guideline No. 21. Management of tubal pregnancy. London: RCOG Press, 2004.

Magowan B. Churchill's Pocketbook of Obstetrics and Gynaecology (3rd edn). Edinburgh: Churchill Livingston, 2005.

Stovall TG, Ling FW, Carson SA, Buster JE. Nonsurgical management of unruptured ectopic pregnancy: an extended trial. Am J Obstet Gynecol 1993; 168:1759–1765.

31.5 Endometrial cancer

A 52-year-old menopausal woman presents to the rapid referral clinic with postmenopausal bleeding (PMB). Following a hysteroscopy and endometrial biopsy she is diagnosed with endometrial cancer.

1. What investigations should be performed for this patient prior to surgery and why? Marks (6)

2. What is the sub-classification of stage 1 endometrial cancer? Marks (2)

3. Following imaging and a multidisciplinary team (MDT) meeting she is diagnosed to have stage 1 endometrial carcinoma. Critically discuss her management. Marks (12)

Key points

- 52 years old
- menopausal
- PMB
- endometrial cancer

Essay plan

1.

- chest X-ray/electrocardiogram (ECG)
- magentic resonance imaging (MRI) scan of pelvis and abdomen with contrast
- blood tests (full blood count [FBC], liver function tests [LFTs], renal function tests [RFTs])
- histological type may alter recommended surgery

2.

- stages 1a and 1b (previously stages 1a, 1b and 1c)

3.

- discussion with a multidisciplinary team (MDT)
- standard treatment – total abdominal hysterectomy (TAH) and bilateral salpingo-oophorectomy (BSO)
- laparoscopy or laparotomy
- role of vaginal hysterectomy
- with or without pelvic lymphadenectomy
- postoperative radiotherapy

31.5 Suggested answer

1.

A chest X-ray is organised as part of her routine preoperative workup and also to rule out lung metastasis which is very uncommon. An ECG may be requested by the anaesthetist depending on any co-morbidities.

Further imaging in the form of an MRI of the pelvis and abdomen to identify metastatic disease, depth of myometrial invasion and cervical involvement is important. This helps when deciding on treatment options. An MRI scan is more sensitive in predicting the depth of myometrial invasion and cervical stromal invasion in 92% of cases compared to transvaginal scans (TVS) and computed tomography (CT) scans. In cases of uterine sarcomas, a chest CT scan may be necessary due to high-risk metastasis. A baseline FBC, RFT and LFT are performed.

Following investigation, her case should be discussed at a specialist gynaecological oncology cancer MDT meeting and the histology wll also be reviewed.

2.

According to the International Federation of Gynecology and Obstetrics (FIGO) classification for endometrial cancer (2009), stage 1 is classified as follows: 1a – no or less than 50% myometrial invasion; 1b – more than 50% of myometrial invasion.

3.

Surgery is important for FIGO staging using intraoperative findings and histological assessment. The mainstay of treatment is TAH and BSO in a woman with endometrial cancer confined to the uterus (stage 1). The argument for removing the ovaries is that they may be involved with metastatic disease, or as a precaution as they can be an abnormal source of oestrogen (e.g. granulose cell tumour).

Surgery (TAH and BSO) is therapeutic in low grade stage 1a and stage 1b endometrial cancer and lymphadenectomy is not required as the risk of metastasis to lymph nodes is low. In stage 1b and grade 3 endometrial cancer controversy exists with regards to lymphadenectomy despite two randomised controlled trials (RCTs) showing no survival advantage in the lymphadenectomy group. The argument is that these factors are considered high risk for lymph node metastasis.

The rarer types including clear cell and malignant mixed Müllerian tumours (MMMT) may warrant lymphadenectomy.

Traditionally an abdominal approach with midline vertical incision was undertaken to have good visual access to the upper abdomen and to perform lymphadenectomy. A Pfannenstiel approach helped in the quicker recovery of the patients.

Women with co-morbidities pose a significant challenge to surgery and anaesthesia. A laparoscopic approach is increasingly used in such women. It has recently been shown that laparoscopically assisted vaginal hysterectomy or total laparoscopic hysterectomy with BSO is associated with reduced operative morbidity and mortality. Also lymphadenectomy can be performed with a laparoscopic approach and has been shown to give equally good lymph node yield when compared to open surgery and has been found to be feasible in both elderly and obese women. There is no difference between the overall or disease-free survival in women with open or laparoscopic surgery. The risk of port site metastasis with laparoscopy should not be overlooked.

A regional anaesthesia and vaginal approach may be used in women with severe co-morbidities where general anaesthesia is contraindicated.

Postoperative radiotherapy is associated with a reduced rate of pelvic recurrence in women with stage 1 endometrial cancer. However, it does not show any survival advantage and in fact increases treatment-related morbidity (bowel and bladder dysfunction). Radiotherapy is recommended in women with grade 3 and stage 1b endometrial cancer and beyond (considered as a high-risk disease) to improve survival.

Primary radiotherapy is rarely used in a situation where a patient is unfit for surgery for medical reasons.

Close follow-up for 5 years following treatment is necessary (the new cancer guidelines recommend 6-monthly follow-ups for 3 years in the UK). Recurrence is most common in the first 3 years; the overall survival for this type of cancer is good.

Holland C. Endometrial cancer. Obstet Gynaecol Reprod Med 2010; 20:347–352.
Edey K and Murdoch J. FIGO staging in vulval and endometrial cancer. The Obstetrician and Gynaecologist 2010; 12:245–249.

31.6 Endometrial hyperplasia

A 48-year-old woman presents with continuous vaginal bleeding for the previous 2 months. A hysteroscopy and endometrial biopsy reveals endometrial hyperplasia.

1. What should one ask in her history?   Marks (5)

2. What further investigations should be arranged for her and why?   Marks (5)

3. Critically evaluate her management regarding endometrial hyperplasia.   Marks (10)

Key points

- 48 years old
- continuous bleeding
- endometrial hyperplasia
- history
- investigation and why
- management of endometrial hyperplasia (critically evaluate)

Essay plan

1.

- menstrual history (regularity, intermenstrual bleeding, postcoital bleeding)
- cervical smear history
- premenopausal or menopausal
- gynaecological history (polycystic ovary syndrome [PCOS])
- drugs, e.g. tamoxifen, hormone replacement therapy (HRT)
- family history of cancer
- past history of breast cancer
- medical history (hypertension and diabetes)
- body mass index

2.

- calculate body mass index
- examination to rule out any pelvic masses
- full blood count (FBC) to rule out anaemia and the need for blood transfusion
- transvaginal scan (TVS) to rule out an ovarian tumour
- serum oestradiol in the presence of solid ovarian tumour
- magnetic resonance imaging (MRI) if it is atypical endometrial hyperplasia (25–50% of cases with atypical hyperplasia have coexistent endometrial cancer which is missed on endometrial biopsy)

3.

- simple hyperplasia
- complex hyperplasia
- atypia or no atypia
- fertility wishes if young
- lose weight with high body mass index
- remove ovarian tumour in case of oestrogen-producing tumours
- stop tamoxifen
- surgery versus medical treatment

31.6 Suggested answer

1.

One should ask about ongoing vaginal bleeding, cervical smear history, menopausal status, history of PCOS (risk of endometrial hyperplasia and cancer), history of tamoxifen or HRT usage (increases the risk of endometrial hyperplasia and cancer), family history of ovarian, breast or endometrial cancer, heriditary non-polyposis colorectal cancer, weight gain and also medical history regarding diabetes and hypertension.

2.

Endometrial hyperplasia results from unopposed oestrogenic action on the endometrium. Therefore any further investigation should aim to identify the source and remove the oestrogen which is responsible for endometrial hyperplasia.

Calculate body mass index and if high help to inform the woman how to lose weight (including bariatric surgery) to reduce the production of peripheral hormones.

Examine the woman to ascertain the size of the uterus, mobility and also to rule out any pelvic masses (especially ovarian tumours).

A FBC is important in a woman with ongoing vaginal bleeding as this will help to rule out anaemia and the need for iron tablets and blood transfusion.

A TVS is necessary to exclude any ovarian tumours (these may be a source of excessive oestrogen hormones).

If the histology is atypical endometrial hyperplasia, it is important to arrange an MRI scan due to the increased incidence of coexistent (25–50%) endometrial carcinoma (to rule out any metastasis).

3.

Endometrial hyperplasia is a precursor of endometrial carcinoma.

Management depends on fertility wishes, associated co-morbidities, type of hyperplasia (simple or complex hyperplasia without or with atypia), presence or absence of oestrogen-producing ovarian tumours (granulose cell tumours) and current drug therapy.

This woman is already 48 years old and fertility should not be an issue in her case.

If she is taking medication such as tamoxifen or HRT, then it should be discontinued.

Simple hyperplasia without atypia has a low malignant potential (<1%). Therefore conservative management may be appropriate. Medical therapy in the form of long-term or cyclical progestogen for symptom control as well as resolution of hyperplasia can be given. If there is a recurrence of symptoms, the patient should be investigated further and a hysterectomy offered.

Complex hyperplasia without atypia has a slightly higher malignant potential (10–25%). Either medical treatment or a hysterectomy can be offered at this age. Medical treatment is not unreasonable if the woman does not wish to have a hysterectomy. However, a repeat endometrial biopsy (3 months later) should be offered to such women following progestogen therapy (e.g. oral medroxyprogesterone or levonorgestrel IUS insertion) to check for resolution or progression of endometrial pathology. In any case close follow-up in the gynaecology clinic should be offered and hysterectomy offered if there is a recurrence of symptoms.

Atypical endometrial hyperplasia has a greater potential for the development of endometrial cancer (25–50%). There is also a 25–50% chance of coexistent carcinoma in association with complex atypical hyperplasia. Therefore hysterectomy plus bilateral salpingo-oophorectomy (BSO) should be offered to such women.

If the woman is unfit for surgery, alternative options should be discussed, for example levonorgestrel IUS or long-term high dose oral progestogens, with follow-up arrangements in the gynaecology clinic.

In cases of isolated unilateral solid oestrogen-producing ovarian tumour, they should be removed.

Women with a high body mass index should be advised to lose weight to reduce the peripheral source of oestrogen which is a culprit for endometrial hyperplasia.

Fritz MA and Speroff L. Clinical Gynaecologic Endocrinology and Infertility (8th edn), Philadelphia: Lippincott Williams and Wilkins, 2011.
Teale G and Jordan J. Chapter 7: Lower genital tract intraepithelial neoplasia. In: Shafi MI, Luesley DM, Jordan JJ (eds). Handbook of Gynaecological Oncology. Edinburgh: Churchill Livingstone, 2001.

31.7 Glandular neoplasia 1

A 35-year-old woman presents to her general practitioner with postcoital bleeding (PCB). A cervical smear taken 2 weeks ago is reported as having atypical glandular cells suggestive of cervical glandular intraepithelial neoplasia (CGIN).

1. What are the factors affecting her treatment? Marks (7)

2. What are the principles of the treatment of CGIN? Marks (6)

3. What will be the indications for hysterectomy while managing the woman? Marks (7)

Key points

- 35 years old
- PCB
- cervical smear
- CGIN

Essay plan

1.

- fertility wishes
- age
- colposcopic findings
- location of lesion
- visibility of upper extent of lesion
- excision margins
- type of treatment

2.

- cone biopsy
- appropriate depth
- clear margins
- close surveillance
- good compliance
- endocervix brush for cytology
- with or without hysteroscopy and endometrial biopsy
- hysterectomy once family complete

3.

Simple hysterectomy

- completed family
- women declines conservative management
- positive margins
- absence of invasive disease
- an adequate cytological follow-up not possible
- high grade cytological abnormality at follow-up

Radical hysterectomy
- early invasive disease

31.7 Suggested answer

1.

- age and desire for fertility
- the location (ectocervical or endocervical) of the lesion on colposcopy
- satisfactory or unsatisfactory colposcopy, i.e. can the full extent of the lesion be visualised
- associated cervical intraepithelial neoplasia (CIN) may be present
- no abnormality may be detected on colposcopy
- whether upper limit of the lesion is seen
- whether excision margins are clear or not clear of disease
- type of previous treatment received – large loop excision of transformation zone (LLETZ), laser or knife cone
- high risk of malignancy with glandular abnormality on cytology

2.

- laser or knife cone preferred as easier to achieve depth and cleaner endocervical margin
- margins should be clear of disease
- cone depth should be at least 20 mm
- close surveillance in the colposcopy clinic following treatment with good compliance of the woman is required due to a high recurrence rate. The cytology should include endocervical brush
- once the family is complete offer a hysterectomy
- if the colposcopy is normal, look for lesions higher up in the reproductive organs (perform hysteroscopy and endometrial biopsy and also arrange transvaginal pelvic ultrasound)

3.

Simple hysterectomy, preferably vaginally, can be done in the following situations:

- the woman does not wish to preserve her fertility
- a positive margin despite adequate excision
- invasive disease has been excluded.
- an adequate cytological follow-up is not possible following treatment
- women declines conservative management
- high grade cytological abnormality on smear following excision treatment for CGIN

Radical hysterectomy is undertaken if there is an early stage underlying cervical malignancy on histology.

NHS Cervical Screening Programme. Colposcopy and Programme Management. Guidelines for the NHS Cervical Screening Programme (2nd edn). Publication No 20. NHSCSP, 2010. http://www.bsccp.org.uk/docs/public/pdf/nhscsp20.pdf

31.8 Glandular neoplasia 2

A 40-year-old woman presents to her general practitioner with postcoital bleeding (PCB). A cervical smear taken 2 weeks ago is reported as having atypical glandular cells suggestive of cervical glandular intraepithelial neoplasia (CGIN).

1. What is CGIN? What is its incidence on cytology?   Marks (2)

2. Enumerate the differences between CGIN and cervical intraepithelial neoplasia (CIN).   Marks (9)

3. Critically discuss the initial investigation and management plan.   Marks (9)

Key points
- 40 years old
- cervical smear
- CGIN
- differences between CGIN and CIN
- investigation
- management
- indications for hysterectomy

Essay plan
1.
- premalignant disease in the columnar cells of the endocervix
- incidence

2.
- natural history unknown and unpredictable
- age at presentation is different
- low incidence on cytology
- underlying malignancy high with glandular abnormality on cytology
- difficulty in diagnosis at colposcopy
- difficulty in treatment as the disease may be multifocal
- difficulty in follow-up due to possible skip lesions higher up in the canal

3.
- urgent colposcopy – target wait <2 weeks
- experienced person performing colposcopy
- cone biopsy
- with or without transvaginal scan (TVS)
- with or without hysteroscopy and endometrial biopsy
- multidisciplinary team (MDT) review if any concerns
- repeat cone biopsy if margins are positive
- hysterectomy offered where fertility is not an issue
- follow-up in the colposcopy clinic at the discretion of the clinician
- cervical cytology using endocervical brush

31.8 Suggested answer

1.

CGIN is a premalignant glandular cervical lesion and affects the columnar cells in the endocervical canal. It coexists with cervical intraepithelial lesions (squamous) in 50% of cases and therefore pure disease is uncommon.

Glandular abnormalities of the cervix are relatively rare and account for only 0.05% (1 in 2000) of cytological abnormalities.

2.

Natural history and difficulty in diagnosis on cytology

CGIN has an uncertain natural history unlike squamous lesions and the screening programme mainly aims to detect squamous and not glandular lesions.

Age at presentation

Women present a decade earlier than CIN (mean age 36 years).

Low incidence on cytology but associated with underlying malignancy

The incidence of CGIN:CIN is 1:50 and is usually associated with high grade CIN in 40–50% of cases. It can be associated with underlying adenocarcinoma in the cervix, endometrium and very rarely in the ovary.

Difficulty in colposcopic diagnosis and treatment

There is unfamiliarity with CGIN in view of the low incidence and no definitive identifying patterns on colposcopy. Small lesions are difficult to visualise and a lesion in the endocervical canal can be missed.

CGIN is multifocal in 15% of cases (skip lesions) and this has implications for diagnosis (unsatisfactory colposcopy) and treatment. Even with presumed adequate treatment with clear margins the risk of recurrence is high (15% with CGIN and 5% with CIN).

Usually CGIN is human papillomavirus (HPV) 18 positive whereas CIN (high grade) is usually HPV 16 positive.

Histological interpretation in differentiating CGIN and micro invasive disease can be difficult.

3.

The NHS Cervical Screening Programme publication recommends urgent colposcopy referral after one test is reported as possible glandular neoplasia (100%) as the natural history of this condition is unclear. All women should be seen in the colposcopy clinic within 2 weeks of receipt of referral as there is an increased risk of an underlying (cervical) malignancy (40%).

Colposcopy should be undertaken by an experienced colposcopist

Almost 50% of CGIN is associated with high grade CIN. The presence of squamous lesions should be taken into account in managing these cases. Ninety-five per cent of the CGIN extends within 25 mm of the anatomical external cervical os. Despite originating from the columnar cells, 85% of the CGIN is found in the transformation zone (TZ) and deep clefts up to 5 mm from the margin of the canal can be involved.

A relationship between age and proximal linear extent of disease suggests more limited excision of the endocervix (a cylindrical-shaped cervical excision including the whole TZ and at least 1 cm of the endocervix) above the squamo-columnar junction (SCJ) in younger women and/or women who desire to preserve fertility. However, glandular lesions tend to be more aggressive and these women are more likely to have an unsatisfactory colposcopy. Hence, a cylindrical biopsy should be undertaken that includes all the visible TZ and 20–25 mm of the endocervical canal.

If all investigations are normal (colposcopy, hysteroscopy and transvaginal scan), the smear should be reviewed by a MDT and a knife or laser cone biopsy is suggested.

One needs to counsel the women regarding the multifocal nature of this condition, high recurrence rate (15% within 4 years) and need for further treatment in 21.5% of the cases. Also, one needs to explain the high false-positive rate of glandular abnormality in cervical cytology and consequent negative biopsy on histology.

If the margins of the first cone biopsy are not clear, it is reasonable to offer a repeat cone biopsy in order to exclude invasion and obtain negative margins. A hysterectomy (preferably vaginally) should be offered if the woman has completed her family or does not wish to conceive in the future.

Close surveillance for 10 years of conservatively treated women should consist of cytology (with an endocervical brush) and may best be managed in a colposcopy clinic.

NHS Cervical Screening Programme. Colposcopy and Programme Management. Guidelines for the NHS Cervical Screening Programme (2nd edn). Publication No 20. NHSCSP, 2010. http://www.bsccp.org.uk/docs/public/pdf/nhscsp20.pdf

31.9 Incontinence

A 52-year-old woman is referred to the gynaecology clinic by her general practitioner. She complains of incontinence for the last 5 years.

1. What are the relevant aspects one should ask in her history? Marks (7)

2. She suffers from some frequency and incontinence following coughing and weighs 98 kg. She is also a smoker. However, she is embarrassed to socialise with her friends due to the smell of urine and incontinence problems. What investigations should be requested following this consultation? Marks (5)

3. Describe the initial plan of management for her. Marks (8)

Key points

- 52 years old
- incontinence
- weight 98 kg
- smoking
- relevant history and investigations
- management

Essay plan

1.

- a detailed history of incontinence
- basic gynaecology and obstetric history
- previous gynaecological surgeries, e.g. hysterectomy and pelvic floor repair
- fluid type, amount and timing of intake of beverages especially caffeine and alcohol
- smoking
- chronic cough
- constipation – needing to strain
- weight gain or obesity
- menopausal status

2.

- mid-stream specimen of urine (MSU)
- blood sugar
- three-day bladder diary
- may need urodynamics at a later date
- important to examine patient

3.

- general measures: lifestyle modifications, weight reduction
- specific measures: pelvic floor exercises
- treat any urinary tract infection (UTI)

31.9 Suggested answer

1.

One needs to ask more about her incontinence symptoms. This includes frequency, urgency, urge incontinence (suggestive of an overactive bladder), incontinence following coughing, sneezing or straining (suggestive of stress incontinence), or problems with voiding and dribbling (outflow obstruction).

The amount and type of fluid (tea, caffeine, alcohol, soft drinks) intake during the day and night is important to assess if her symptoms are due to excessive fluid intake and bladder irritants. Also important is her history of smoking which can act as an irritant to the bladder and lead to chronic cough which may also affect intra-abdominal pressure.

High body mass index is associated with an increased risk of incontinence problems and women should be routinely weighed and asked about recent weight gain.

A basic gynaecology history including her last period and last cervical smear test, and a basic obstetric history about parity, difficult labours and weight of previous babies are important. Information regarding any previous gynaecological surgeries (e.g. hysterectomy and pelvic floor repair) and menopausal status should also be sought.

2.

A baseline urine dipstick and MSU are performed to check for UTI and a random blood glucose to exclude diabetes. A bladder diary should be kept for 3 days to record fluid balance measurements (input, output, frequency, urge incontinence, stress incontinence and nocturia) is crucial in making the diagnosis as well as to see improvement during follow-up.

Urodynamics may be necessary at a later date if there is no improvement in the symptoms following initial therapy.

It is always important to examine the woman to exclude any anatomical problems.

3.

The management should be individualised and can be divided into two categories: general and specific.

General management is mainly to do with lifestyle modifications, which include weight loss, cessation of smoking, reduction of fluid intake in the evening, reduction of the amount of tea and avoidance of caffeine. If the investigations reveal a UTI or diabetes, they should be treated.

The National Institute for Health and Clinical Excellence (NICE) recommends referral to physiotherapy and pelvic floor exercises for 3 months as a first step in management. A follow-up should be arranged in the gynaecology clinic to review whether her symptoms have improved.

If the symptoms do not improve, however, one may need to consider continence surgery (transvaginal tape, TVT) following urodynamic studies if genuine stress incontinence is diagnosed.

National Institute of Health and Clinical Excellence. Guideline on urinary incontinence (CG40). NICE, 2006.

31.10 Laparoscopy

A 29-year-old woman attends the gynaecology clinic with complaints of chronic pelvic pain. She has a body mass index of 40 and previous midline laparotomy for a torted ovarian cyst. Her name is placed on the waiting list for a diagnostic laparoscopy.

1. What questions should one ask in her history?   Marks (4)

2. What risks and additional procedures should be discussed with her regarding laparoscopy?   Marks (8)

3. How could the risks of laparoscopy be minimised for this woman?   Marks (8)

Key points

- 29 years old
- chronic pelvic pain
- history
- risks of laparoscopy
- specific risks to her
- minimise risks, both medical and surgical

Essay plan

1.

- details of pain – menstrual history and any associated dyspareunia
- parity and mode of delivery
- fertility wishes
- medical history
- surgical history
- allergy
- family history
- social history

2.

- serious risks
- frequent risks
- additional procedures
- anaesthetic risk

3.

- reduce body mass index before surgery
- medical: prevention of thromboembolism
- surgical: use of Palmer's point entry to avoid midline adhesions
- intraoperative: use of appropriate length (e.g. 100 mm) of trocars
- postoperative: good pain relief and promote early mobilisation and discharge

31.10 Suggested answer

1.

One should ask details about the pain. If she is currently asymptomatic, surgery is not indicated.

If she remains symptomatic, then she should be asked about her fertility wishes, weight, diet, previous medical and surgical history, history of allergy, family history, social history and any menstrual upset or pain with intercourse.

2.

The overall risk of serious complications (2 in 1000 women) include damage to the bowel, bladder, ureter and major blood vessels which may need laparotomy to repair the damage. However, 15% of the bowel injuries are not recognised at the time of surgery and may present at a later date.

It may not be possible to gain entry into the abdominal cavity (especially in women with a high body mass index) and complete the intended procedure laparoscopically due to extensive adhesions.

There is risk of hernia at the port sites. Therefore, a lateral port more than 7 mm in size and central ports >10 mm should be closed with a J-shaped needle.

The risk of death is 8 in 100,000 as a result of complications and is not routinely discussed by doctors when obtaining consent.

The risk of frequent complications include shoulder tip pain (due to left over gas in the abdomen irritating the diaphragm), wound bruising, gaping and infection.

The additional procedures one should discuss include laparotomy, the rectification of serious complications (e.g. repair of damage to bowel, bladder, ureter and vessels) and blood transfusion.

3.

Methods to minimise risks

Medically, she should have anti-embolism stockings and flowtrons if the duration of surgery is going to be more than 1 hour.

One can possibly postpone the surgery if her body mass index is high (reduce body mass index before surgery).

Use Palmer's entry instead of umbilical entry as there is risk of midline adhesions and damage to the bowel. The length of the trocars can be 100 mm instead of 75 mm so the length is appropriate for the depth of the abdominal wall.

The woman should be clearly warned about failure to gain entry into the abdomen due to high her body mass index and therefore failure to complete the procedure laparoscopically. Laparotomy is associated with increased morbidity in women with a high body mass index. The documentation should therefore be clear about proceeding to laparotomy or abandoning the operation.

Postoperatively, good pain relief is important as it will promote early mobilisation and discharge from the hospital.

Royal College of Obstetricians and Gynaecologists. Green-top Guideline No. 2. Diagnostic laparoscopy. London: RCOG Press, 2008.

31.11 Medical management of missed miscarriage

A woman presents to the early pregnancy assessment unit at 8 weeks of gestation with mild vaginal bleeding. An ultrasound on the same day shows a missed miscarriage. Following counselling and discussion of options, she wants to have medical management only because she is scared of surgery.

1. What are the drugs used in the medical management of missed miscarriage and what is their success rate?   Marks (4)

2. What are the common side effects and complications of medical management?   Marks (8)

3. What are the absolute contraindications to the use of medical management?   Marks (4)

4. What should one tell this woman when using misoprostol vaginally?   Marks (4)

Key points

- 8 weeks of gestation
- missed miscarriage
- medical management
- side effects
- complications
- absolute contraindications

Essay plan

1.

- medical management
- drugs used for medical management
- success rate

2.

- medical management
- side effects
- complications

3.

- medical management
- contraindications

4.

- misoprostol
- vaginal route – unlicensed

31.11 Suggested answer

1.

The drugs used in the medical management of missed miscarriage include mifepristone (antiprogestogen) and prostaglandin analogues gemeprost and misoprostol.

The earlier the use of this method during pregnancy, the higher the success rate and the fewer associated complications. At 6–7 weeks, it has shown to be effective in 97.5% of women whereas at 7–9 weeks the success rate is 93% and 89% for gemeprost and misoprostol, respectively.

2.

Common side effects include headache, dizziness, nausea, vomiting, diarrhoea, abdominal pain (in 28–35% of cases) and tiredness. There is a risk of excessive bleeding and blood transfusion may even be required in 0.7–1% of cases.

The woman needs to be appropriately counselled and warned that there is a 5% risk of needing surgical treatment (which can be done under general anaesthesia), and a risk of continuation of the pregnancy with the use of gemeprost (0.3%) and misoprostol (7%). An association between misoprostol and defective formation of the temporal and frontal bones has been described. Therefore surgical evacuation is recommended if medical management or treatment fails.

Anti-D immunoglobulin should be given to all women who are Rhesus negative as there is risk of sensitisation.

3.

Mifepristone is contraindicated in the following conditions:

- porphyrias
- smokers >35 years of age
- known allergy to mifepristone
- anaemia
- women on long-term glucocorticoid therapy
- women with known major haemoglobinopathies
- women on anticoagulant therapy
- adrenal insufficiency
- suspected ectopic pregnancy

The relative contraindications include hypertension and severe asthma.

Misoprostol is contraindicated in women with a known allergy.

Medical management is also less suitable in women with excessive vaginal bleeding, with low haemoglobin, with signs of infection and with medical contraindications as above.

4.

The vaginal use of misoprostol is unlicensed. When used with mifepristone, the vaginal route (95%) is more successful than the oral route (87%). The incidence of adverse side effects is also reduced with vaginal use of misoprostol.

Amis S. Medical management of first trimester induced abortion and miscarriage. Personal assessment in continuing education. Reviews, questions and answers. Volume 3. London: RCOG Press, 2003: 67–68.

31.12 Ovarian hyperstimulation syndrome

A slim 35-year-old woman presents to the emergency department with abdominal distension and mild pain. She had an intrauterine embryo transfer 3 weeks previously at an infertility centre in the private sector. Clinical examination reveals gross ascites causing her discomfort and pain. Her urine output is reported to be less than 100 mL in the last 4 hours. Her urine test reveals a positive pregnancy test and the haematology result reveals haematocrit of 48%.

1. What is the definition of ovarian hyperstimulation syndrome (OHSS) and explain its pathophysiology.   Marks (4)

2. What are the risk factors for OHSS? What measures should one take to prevent it?   Marks (8)

3. Critically discuss her management. Marks (8)

Key points

- embryo transfer
- pregnant
- distension and pain abdomen
- ovarian hyperstimulation syndrome (OHSS) – definition/pathophysiology
- risk factors

Essay plan

1.

- OHSS
- iatrogenic complications of *in vitro* fertilisation (IVF) – graded mild/moderate/severe
- pathophysiology – raised vascular permeability due to the release of vasoactive substances

2.

- risk factors – young age, slim women, previous OHSS, polycystic ovary syndrome (PCOS) and gonadotropin-releasing hormone (GnRH) use for ovulation induction
- prevention – use simple forms of ovulation induction (clomiphene citrate), use purified follicle-stimulating hormone (FSH) instead of GnRH analogues, monitor follicles by transvaginal scan (TVS) and cancel the cycle in the case of excessive response, withhold human chorionic gonadotrophin (hCG) in cases of excessive response, and cryopreserve the embryos to be replaced at a later date

3.

- admission to the gynaecology unit – baseline blood tests
- symptomatic treatment
- pain relief – use of paracetamol and opioids but avoid non-steroidal anti-inflammatory drugs (NSAIDs)
- correction of the intravascular volume and electrolytes
- thromboprophylaxis due to increased risk of thrombosis
- close input and output chart as risk of renal shut down
- drainage of ascites if symptomatic or renal compromise despite correction of intravascular volume
- drainage of pleural fluid if symptomatic

31.12 Suggested answer

1.

The incidence of mild OHSS is around 33%, while moderate or severe OHSS occurs in 3–8% of IVF cycles.

OHSS is an iatrogenic complication of ovarian stimulation, especially following the use of gonadotrophins for numerous follicular growths preceding assisted reproduction.

The systemic symptoms and signs are a result of vasoactive substances released from enlarged ovaries. This results in increased capillary permeability, leading to loss of protein-rich fluid into the third space or serous cavities (e.g. ascites, pleural and rarely pericardial effusion). As a result, it causes depletion of the intravascular volume, haemoconcentration and an increased predisposition to develop thrombosis. Furthermore, renal and liver dysfunction and adult respiratory distress syndrome can result.

2.

Risk factors

Early OHSS is usually caused by excessive ovarian hyperstimulation (increased oestradiol levels, number of ovarian follicles) and late OHSS is related to pregnancy.

The risk factors include slim body structure, young age, PCOS, past history of OHSS and the use of GnRH analogues in the ovarian stimulation regime.

Women who get pregnant or use hCG for luteal support are more likely to develop OHSS compared to women who do not get pregnant and use progesterone for luteal support.

Prevention

Simple forms of ovulation induction such as clomiphene citrate should be used where possible. If the ovaries are resistant, then laparoscopic ovarian drilling should be considered as it carries less risk of OHSS than gonadotrophins.

It is suggested that purified FSH by a low dose incremental regime is less likely to lead to OHSS than GnRH analogue plus human menopausal gonadotrophin.

Follicular monitoring by using ultrasound is important, so that one can cancel the cycle in the case of an excessive response and very high oestradiol levels.

The triggering factor is usually the administration of βhCG or luteinising hormone (LH). Withholding an HCG injection or cancellation of the cycle in women with excessive ovarian response will prevent OHSS provided that an endogenous LH surge does not occur. Gonadotrophin administration can be discontinued and HCG administration delayed to also reduce the risk in women with an excessive response awaiting a decrease in serum oestradiol levels.

It is advisable to cryopreserve all the embryos and put them back at a later date when the ovaries do not need to be stimulated, thus reducing the risk of severe OHSS.

Intravenous albumin administration at the time of oocyte collection has been shown to reduce the incidence of OHSS in women with excessive ovarian response. Its value in preventing late OHSS is unclear.

3.

OHSS tends to be more severe in women who are pregnant compared to those who are not. It is a self-limiting condition and therefore management is mainly supportive with analgesia, fluid balance and thromboprophylaxis.

This woman has severe OHSS. She should be admitted to the gynaecology ward and managed as an inpatient until the symptoms have resolved. Close supervision and assessment on a day-to-day basis is necessary to detect improvement or worsening of the condition.

The following are key steps in the management of OHSS:

- She should be managed by somebody senior who has experience in managing OHSS.
- Pain relief: opiates should be used liberally for pain relief after paracetamol and codeine. NSAIDs should be avoided as they may precipitate renal failure due to their anti-prostaglandin activity. If the abdominal pain is severe, cyst accident (torsion, rupture or haemorrhage) should be excluded.
- Correction of intravascular volume: due to loss of protein-rich fluid in the third space, there is depletion of intravascular volume in OHSS. Fluids should be replaced with crystalloids and clinically assessed by correction of dehydration, decreasing haematocrit and normalising electrolyte levels. Intravenous colloids should be considered in women who have large volumes of ascitic fluid drained.
- Oliguria: correction of the intravascular depletion alone should improve her urine output. If it does not improve, she may need invasive monitoring (a central venous line). The other clinical scenario where urine output can be low is when there is compression of the inferior vena cava (it reduces venous return and thereby cardiac output) by massive ascites. In such cases, an ultrasound-guided ascitic tap may be necessary along with infusion of albumin to replace protein and maintain intravascular volume. It should be ultrasound-guided because of the risk of inadvertently rupturing the enlarged ovaries.
- She is at risk of thrombosis due to the depletion of her intravascular volume and haemoconcentration. She should be encouraged to mobilise and wear thrombo-embolic stockings. She should receive prophylactic enoxaparin sodium injection to prevent thrombosis.
- Caution: diuretics (which will further deplete intravascular volume) and NSAIDs (which will precipitate renal failure) should be avoided in this woman.
- Others: Strenuous exercise and sexual intercourse should be avoided as there is a theoretical risk of injury or torsion of grossly enlarged fragile ovaries. Women on luteal support with progesterone can continue it using while women on HCG luteal support should stop HCG.
- She should be reassured that the pregnancy may continue normally and there is no increase in the risk of miscarriage or the development of congenital abnormalities.

Royal College of Obstetricians and Gynaecologists. Green-top Guideline No. 5. Management of ovarian hyperstimulation syndrome. London: RCOG Press, 2006.
Jenkins J and Mathur R. Ovarian hyperstimulation syndrome. Personal assessment in continuing education. Reviews, Questions and Answers. Volume 3. London: RCOG Press, 2003.

31.13 Ovarian cyst

A 48-year-old postmenopausal Asian woman is referred to the gynaecology clinic with a scan report of an ovarian cyst. The features on the pelvic scan show a unilateral complex pelvic mass 7 cm in size (multilocular with no solid areas or free fluid) arising from her right ovary. She has some vague dull abdominal pain which is tolerable and does not require any analgesics. Medically, she suffers from asthma and hypertension and does not have any allergies. The serum CA 125 level is 60 U/mL (normal 0–34 U/mL).

1. What should one ask in her history?   Marks (4)

2. How is the risk of malignancy index (RMI) calculated and what is its significance? What is the value of RMI in the assessment of her case?   Marks (10)

3. How should her case be managed?   Marks (6)

Key points

- 48 years old
- Asian
- postmenopausal
- ovarian cyst
- abdominal pain
- CA 125 60 U/mL
- RMI

Essay plan

1.

- more details about pain
- bowel and bladder symptoms
- appetite and weight loss
- gynaecological and obstetric history
- family history
- any past history of pelvic infection

2.

- RMI is calculated by the multiplication of three factors (ultrasound features [U] × menopausal status [M] × CA 125 level)
- significance of RMI
- differential diagnosis

3.

- a complex mass in a postmenopausal woman needs further investigation in the form of higher imaging
- malignancy needs to be excluded
- referral to an oncology multidisciplinary team (MDT) meeting to review her case and plan further management

31.13 Suggested answer

1.

One needs to ask more details about the nature and severity of the pain, any medical co-morbidities to assess fitness for surgery, the kind of support she has from family and friends, past cervical smear history, parity, family history of cancer and past history of pelvic inflammatory disease (PID). No history is complete without bowel and bladder symptoms (the ovarian cyst may cause pressure symptoms or rule out any bowel pathology).

2.

RMI = U × M × CA 125 concentration

- U = 0 (for ultrasound score of 0); U = 1 (for ultrasound score of 1); U = 3 (for ultrasound score of 2–5).Ultrasound scans are scored 1 point for each of the following characteristics: multilocular cyst, evidence of solid areas, evidence of metastases, presence of ascites, bilateral lesions
- M = 3 for all postmenopausal women dealt with by this guideline (1 if premenopausal)
- CA 125 measurement in U/mL

RMI is categorised as:

- RMI <25 (low risk)
- RMI 25–250 (moderate risk)
- RMI >250 (high risk)

It gives an indication for the risk of malignancy (low [3%], moderate [20%] and high [75%]).

In her case the RMI is: U = 1, M = 3 and CA 125 = 60 (1 × 3 × 60) = 180 (moderate risk).

CA 125 is a very non-specific marker and can be mildly raised in benign pelvic pathology. The differential diagnosis includes:

- PID
- tuberculosis
- endometriosis
- fibroids
- borderline ovarian tumour or ovarian malignancy

3.

She is at a moderate risk of an underlying malignancy (RMI = 180). Further imaging with a computed tomography (CT) scan and possibly a magnetic resonance imaging (MRI) scan is appropriate.

A referral to an oncology MDT is recommended for a decision about the diagnosis, the extent of her surgery, place of her surgery (gynaecological oncology unit or oncology centre) and operating surgeon (oncologist or person with a special interest in gynaecological oncology).

In either case she will need surgery for removal of the ovary to know the exact pathology. In a case of suspected malignancy, she will need to be put in touch with a clinical specialist nurse in an oncology clinic for counselling and support. A staging laparotomy will be arranged at the oncology centre. She also needs to be warned that she may need further therapy in the form of chemotherapy but this will depend on the histopathological finding. A long-term follow-up in the clinic to assess for wellbeing and recurrence would be necessary if the cyst is malignant. If the cyst is benign an oophorectomy may be indicated.

Royal College of Obstetricians and Gynaecologists. Green-top Guideline No. 34. Management of ovarian cysts in postmenopausal women. London: RCOG Press, 2003.
Royal College of Obstetricians and Gynaecologists. Green-top Guideline No. 62. Management of suspected ovarian masses in premenopausal women. London: RCOG Press, 2011.
National Institute of Health and Clinical Excellence. Guidelines on ovarian cancer: the recognition and initial management (CG122). NICE, 2011.

31.14 Ovarian torsion

A 31-year-old woman attends the emergency department with a history of right-sided severe abdominal pain for the last 24 hours. A clinical diagnosis of suspected ovarian torsion is made as there is marked tenderness as well as guarding on abdominal palpation. An ultrasound scan reveals a large ovarian cyst on the right side ($8 \times 7 \times 6$ cm) with absent blood flow.

1. Enumerate ovarian cyst accidents and describe the pathophysiology of ovarian cyst accidents. Marks (8)

2. Critically evaluate the approach to managing ovarian cyst accidents. Marks (8)

3. How should one manage this woman? Marks (6)

Key points
- 31 years old
- ovarian cyst accidents
- severe abdominal pain
- approach to management
- ovarian torsion
- ovarian cyst accidents
- absent blood flow on scan

Essay plan

1.

- ovarian cyst rupture, haemorrhage and torsion
- pathophysiology
- age
- possible theories for torsion
- histopathology of the ovarian tumours

2.

- conservative
- surgical
- critically evaluate each method

3.

- counselling
- surgical approach

- different surgical approaches
- debrief
- follow-up
- future

31.14 Suggested answer

1.

Ovarian accidents include ovarian cyst rupture, ovarian cyst torsion and haemorrhage into the ovarian cyst.

Ovarian cyst rupture and haemorrhage usually occur in association with physiological functional cysts and are generally self-limiting.

Ovarian torsion is defined as partial or complete rotation of the ovarian vascular pedicle. The majority of ovarian cyst torsion occurs in the reproductive age but about one quarter of cases occur in children.

An ovarian mass has been found in 64–82% of cases of confirmed torsion. The size of the cyst is usually 6 cm or more (moderate size) with long pedicles. Cysts of this size are usually lifted over the confines of the pelvis and become more freely mobile. It is postulated that a heavy ovary allows the ovary to swing on its pedicle. The tube and ovary usually undergo torsion as a single unit, rotating around the broad ligament as an axis. Commonly, the ovary twists alone, around the mesovarium. In the absence of an ovarian cyst, the torsion occurs where there is an unusually long pedicle. This causes occlusion of the venous return followed later by occlusion of the arterial inflow to the ovarian tumour. An ultrasound scan shows an oedematous ovary with peripheral displacement of the follicles.

Ovarian torsions occur twice as often with the right adnexa than with the left adnexa suggesting anatomic differences such as the presence of the sigmoid colon (it restricts the mobility of the left ovary). In accordance with Kushner's rule, the right ovary twists in a clockwise manner and the left counterclockwise.

Mature cystic teratomas are common tumours leading to torsion (3.5–10% of them undergo torsion), followed by cystadenomas, dysfunctional cysts, ovarian hyperstimulation, polycystic ovaries and paraovarian cysts. It is less common in women with endometriosis, previous pelvic inflammatory disease (PID) or malignancy (2% of the ovarian malignancies undergo torsion) as these are relatively fixed in the pelvis and therefore less mobile.

2.

The approach can be conservative or surgical.

Conservative

Ovarian cyst rupture and haemorrhage are usually generally self-limiting. More than 20% of patients with haemorrhagic ovarian cysts can be managed conservatively. Laparoscopy is indicated if there is haemodynamic compromise or if there is doubt.

Most cases of ovarian torsion require surgical intervention except in mild and early cases where there is the possibility of untwisting naturally.

Surgical

Surgery can be completed laparoscopically or by laparotomy.

The surgery itself depends on the findings at operation. It can be in the form of a cystectomy where the ovary is viable or unilateral oophorectomy if the ovary appears non-viable and gangrenous. Women should therefore be counselled appropriately.

Conventionally, laparotomy was performed to manage cases of ovarian cyst torsion, rupture, haemorrhage or infection with acute or subacute symptoms. This results in a less mobile patient, prolonged hospital stay, more time for healing, a bigger scar on the abdomen and a higher possibility of developing adhesions.

Today with more and more people being trained in laparoscopy, most cases can be managed laparoscopically. However, this should not be at the expense of a patient's wellbeing.

The advantages of laparoscopic surgery include reduced postoperative pain, shorter hospital stay, shorter healing time and a quicker return to normal activities. It may also result in less adhesion formation than an open procedure, although the evidence is not convincing. The disadvantages include spillage of cyst contents, incomplete excision of the cyst wall and an unexpected histological diagnosis of malignancy. Up to 83% of malignant ovarian tumours at a laparoscopic operation for a 'cyst' are treated inadequately. These operations require considerable skill in laparoscopic manipulation and should not be attempted without appropriate training, especially in acute emergencies.

3.

The role of counselling cannot be overemphasised.

This woman should be managed surgically and the approach can be laparotomy or laparoscopy. This depends on the availability of expertise.

The aim should be fertility-sparing surgery where possible in young women. If the ovarian tissue can be preserved, an ovarian cystectomy should be performed, while unilateral oophorectomy is considered in the worst case scenario where the ovary is non-viable.

The other approach described in the literature includes detorsion at first-look laparoscopy to restore the blood supply to the ovary and ovarian cystectomy at second-look laparoscopy to treat the pathology. This approach preserves the ovarian tissue and also proves that detorsion helps to resolve the oedema and ischaemia caused by torsion.

Following surgery, debriefing is very important. This woman should be followed up in the clinic to discuss the histology results.

She should be informed that her fertility is unlikely to be affected.

Bottomley C and Bourne T. Diagnosis and management of ovarian cyst accidents. Best Pract Res Clin Obstet Gynaecol 2009; 23:711–724.

31.15 Premenstrual syndrome

A 35-year-old has been suffering from premenstrual syndrome (PMS) for the last 12 months. Her symptoms have become worse over a period of time leading to disharmony with her partner and an inability to cope with her personal, social and work life.

1. What is PMS and how is it graded?   Marks (4)

2. What is its aetiology and how is PMS diagnosed in this woman?   Marks (4)

3. Critically discuss her management.   Marks (12)

Key points

- PMS
- affecting quality of life

Essay plan

1.

- definition of PMS
- grading of PMS in terms of severity

2.

- aetiology unclear
- criteria for diagnosis of PMS

3.

- general advice regarding diet, exercise and stress
- specific therapy – medical (first, second and third line drugs) or surgical

31.15 Suggested answer

1.

PMS, also known as premenstrual dysphoric disorder, is a condition manifesting with distressing physical, behavioural and psychological symptoms in the absence of organic or underlying psychiatric disease. This regularly repeats during the luteal phase (second half) of each menstrual cycle and disappears by the end of menstruation.

Symptoms can be mild, moderate or severe:

- mild: it does not interfere with personal, social or professional life
- moderate: interferes with personal, social or professional life but still able to interact and function
- severe: unable to interact personally, socially and professionally

Underlying psychopathology should be ruled out.

2.

The exact cause for PMS is unknown. Recurrence of symptoms with cyclical ovarian activity points to the effect of oestradiol and progesterone on the neurotransmitter serotonin and gamma-aminobutyric acid (GABA). This is further supported by the absence of cyclical ovarian activity in women who are pregnant, menopausal and prepubertal. It is also less common in women using hormonal contraception. Although these findings point to a hormonal effect, measuring hormonal levels are not helpful as studies have shown no relationship with PMS symptom severity.

PMS is known to be common in women who are obese and exercise less often.

The diagnosis of PMS is based on history: the woman should be assessed prospectively with a symptom diary over her next two menstrual cycles. Symptoms appear 1–2 weeks before the period and disappear following menstruation.

3.

Her symptoms point to severe PMS. She should be managed in a multidisciplinary setting involving a gynaecologist, a psychologist and a counsellor.

Once underlying psychopathology is ruled out, the treatment can be started. The effect of symptom improvement with treatment should be assessed with a symptom diary.

The initial step is general advice regarding diet, exercise and decreasing stress levels. Non-randomised trials have shown that exercise improves PMS symptoms.

The Royal College of Obstetricians and Gynaecologists (RCOG) provides an algorithm to manage women with severe PMS symptoms.

The first line is exercise, cognitive behavioural therapy and vitamin B6, the combined new-generation pill (such as ethinylestradiol with drospirenone [Yasmin], ethinylestradiol with norgestimate [Cilest] – cyclically or continuously) and continuous or luteal phase (days 15–28) low-dose selective serotonin reuptake inhibitors (SSRIs).

Cognitive behavioural therapy and exercise have been shown to be helpful and should be considered in all women. SSRIs (either during the luteal phase or continuously throughout the cycle) should be considered first line drug therapy in the treatment of severe PMS in view of proven efficacy and safety.

The combined oral contraceptive pill (COCP) (second generation) has not shown any benefit. In fact its progestogen content worsens the symptoms of PMS. This is well-handled with the new generation COCP (Yasmin) and has been shown to improve PMS symptoms due to its anti-mineralocorticoid and anti-androgenic progestogen, drospirenone.

Vitamin B6 has not been shown to be of benefit.

The second line is estradiol patches plus oral progestogen or levonorgestrel and high dose SSRIs continuously or during the luteal phase only.

Various hormonal combinations (oestrogen alone, oestrogen plus progestogen and progestogen) have been tried to treat PMS. However, randomised controlled trials (RCTs) have shown only a placebo effect with these hormonal therapies. Oestrogens may be helpful in women with the migraine component of PMS, but they may need progestogens for endometrial protection if the uterus is present. Oral or parenteral use of progestogens may be limited by adverse effects. However, with the advent of medical technology, this can be overcome with the newer device levonorgestrel IUS which acts more locally.

Due to the underlying aetiology as mentioned above, SSRIs have been tried and found useful in alleviating both physical and psychological symptoms. They should be withdrawn gradually to avoid withdrawal effects.

The third line is GnRH analogues with hormone replacement therapy (HRT) add back treatment (continuous combined oestrogen plus progestogen or tibolone). GnRH analogues have been shown to reduce or totally abolish the physical symptoms. If the above measures fail, the third line of therapy can be tried (it is also useful earlier on in making a diagnosis of PMS). However, its long-term use is limited by adverse effects such as trabecular bone loss. Therefore it is recommended that add back HRT should be used alongside to limit its adverse effects.

The fourth line is total abdominal hysterectomy and bilateral oophorectomy. This has been shown to be of benefit as it suppresses ovulation permanently and removes cyclical ovarian activity. It should only be used for severe PMS when all other treatments have failed and following thorough counselling. It is advised that GnRH analogues should be used as a test of cure before undertaking this major step. It is also important to ensure that women tolerate HRT.

Others

The use of danazol is limited due its virilising side effects. If it is used for treatment, then women should be advised to use contraception.

Evening primrose oil has shown to be beneficial only in women with cyclical mastalgia and has not been shown to improve PMS symptoms.

Various complementary therapies such as homeopathy, acupuncture and reflexology have been tried but not proven to be effective.

Royal College of Obstetricians and Gynaecologists. Green-top Guideline No. 48. Management of premenstrual syndrome. London: RCOG Press, 2007.

31.16 Puberty menorrhagia

A 16-year-old girl comes to the emergency department with a heavy period which has lasted for 3 weeks. Her haemoglobin is 8 g/dL.

1. What should one ask in her history? Marks (2)

2. What are the possible causes of menorrhagia in this young girl and how should she be investigated? Marks (6)

3. What are the medical implications of diagnosing inherited bleeding disorders? Marks (4)

4. Justify the management of this girl.   Marks (8)

Key points
- 16 years old
- heavy period
- haemoglobin 8 g/dL
- history
- investigations
- management

Essay plan

1.

- detailed menstrual history/could she be pregnant
- anovulatory bleeding
- family history of polycystic ovary syndrome (PCOS)
- thyroid disorders
- haemophilia A and B
- von Willebrand's disease
- immune idiopathic thrombocytopenic purpura
- leukaemia

2.

Investigations
- full blood count
- blood film
- platelet count
- von Willebrand's factor
- factor VIII and IX levels
- thyroid function tests
- pregnancy test with or without ultrasound scan

3.

Medical implication
- effective medical therapy
- preoperative preparation
- prophylactic treatment before surgery
- genetic implications

4.

- management depends on cause

31.16 Suggested answer

1.

A detailed menstrual history (e.g. age at menarche, regularity, duration of periods, protection used), history of menorrhagia since menarche, history of bleeding after tooth extraction, history of postoperative bleeding, history of postpartum haemorrhage, drug history (any hormonal treatment), family history of PCOS and inherited bleeding disorders. In all women of reproductive age with irregular bleeding, pregnancy needs to be considered, with a high index of suspicion for an ectopic pregnancy.

2.

Anovulatory bleeding is common in extremes of age and also with PCOS, and is probably the most likely cause in this case.

Blood clotting disorder should be ruled out if there is intractable menorrhagia in the young woman. These include von Willebrand's disease; factor V, VII, VIII, IX, X and XI deficiency; idiopathic thrombocytopenic purpura; and platelet dysfunction.

Hypothyroidism should be excluded. Acquired von Willebrand's disease is associated with hypothyroidism and is seen mainly in women.

The investigations include a pregnancy test, full blood count (FBC), platelet count, clotting profile, blood film (leukaemia) and also the above clotting factors if indicated. Enzyme-linked immunoassay is the most sensitive assay for the screening of von Willebrand's disease. Bleeding time and activated partial thromboplastin time (APTT) is prolonged in women with severe haemophilia. Also, genetic diagnosis is possible in this condition.

The Royal College of Obstetricians and Gynaecologists (RCOG) guidelines for the management of menorrhagia recommend testing for bleeding disorders only when there are features in the history and examination of bleeding disorders.

However, the American College of Obstetricians and Gynecologists (ACOG) guidelines recommend screening for von Willebrand's disease in all adolescents with menorrhagia.

3.

There will be an alteration to the medical therapy if the girl is diagnosed to have inherited bleeding disorders (e.g. ↑ factor VIII levels in women with haemophilia A). These women also need to be investigated for clotting factor levels and if the levels are low, they need to be replaced before surgery.

Finally, other members of the family need to be screened in view of the genetic implications.

4.

The first line of treatment is medical. The most commonly used first line options include tranexamic acid, combined oral contraceptive pill (COCP) and progestogens. Also desmopressin (DDAVP) is administered by intranasal spray or subcutaneous injection in women with von Willebrand's disease.

Anovulatory bleeding is common in this age group. Oral progestogens 5 mg three times daily from days 5–26 of the cycle cyclically can be given. This reduces menstrual blood loss by up to 30%. It can be used back to back for 3 months to build up the haemoglobin level. Progestogens are advisable in patients with irregular and unpredictable cycles. They are also used as a second line in therapy for treatment of inherited bleeding disorders not responding to the other treatments or when these other treatments are contraindicated.

The COCP is commonly used in the treatment of menorrhagia. It causes endometrial atrophy and decreases endometrial prostaglandins and fibrinolysis. Menstrual loss is decreased by 50%. This can be used back to back for 3 months to build up the haemoglobin level. COCPs are especially useful in the presence of an irregular menstrual cycle and where there is a need for contraception.

Desmopressin (DDAVP) nasal spray is a vasopressin analogue which causes rapid release of factor VIII and von Willebrand's factor from endothelial cells, hence increasing their plasma levels. It is mainly effective in women with type 1 von Willebrand's disease and mild to moderate haemophilia. A test dose is important prior to treatment to identify responders from non-responders. It is usually given in the first 2–3 days of the menstrual cycle.

The role of danazol and GnRH analogues is not well defined.

If there is a further drop in haemoglobin, she may need a blood transfusion.

Levonorgestrel IUS can be considered in the long-term management following resolution of acute bleeding.

If she has a positive pregnancy test, then appropriate management needs to be undertaken depending on the viability and location of the pregnancy.

Balen A. Chapter 14: Disorders of puberty. In: Shaw RW, Luesley D, Monga A (eds). Gynaecology (4th edn). Edinburgh: Churchill Livingstone, 2011.
Sen S and Lumsden MA. Chapter 31: Menstruation and menstrual disorder. In: Shaw RW, Luesley D, Monga A (eds). Gynaecology (4th edn). Edinburgh: Churchill Livingstone, 2011.
Letsky E, Murphy MF, Ramsay JE, Walker I. Haemorrhagic Disease and Hereditary Bleeding Disorders. London: RCOG Press, 2005.

31.17 Ruptured ectopic pregnancy management

A 28-year-old nulliparous woman presents with abdominal pain and minimal vaginal bleeding. She is discharged as the ultrasound showed a corpus luteal cyst and endometrial thickness 8 mm. Three days later, she presents with severe abdominal pain. Her last menstrual period was 4 weeks ago and a urine pregnancy test is positive. Examination reveals marked pallor, tachycardia and acute abdomen.

1. The clinical diagnosis is ectopic pregnancy. How should one manage her?   Marks (6)

2. What are the risks and additional procedures that should be explained before the operation?   Marks (6)

3. How should one counsel her before discharge, if she undergoes laparoscopic salpingectomy?   Marks (4)

4. How should one counsel her before discharge, if she were to undergo laparoscopic salpingotomy?   Marks (4)

Key points
- positive pregnancy test
- endometrial thickness 8 mm
- acute abdomen
- marked pallor
- tachycardia

Essay plan

1.

- call for help
- resuscitate
- cross-match 4 units
- inform theatre and anaesthetist
- laparotomy or laparoscopy

2.

- risks specific to surgery
- risks specific to this woman
- additional procedures
- blood transfusion

3.

- salpingectomy
- immediate risks
- future pregnancies

4.

- salpingostomy
- immediate risks and follow-up
- future pregnancies

31.17 Suggested answer

1.

- notable practice: no delay in calling for immediate help (consultant)
- commence resuscitation: if the patient collapses, insert two large bore cannulas, start two litres of intravenous fluids (crystalloids or colloids), take baseline full blood count (FBC), clotting screen, ask for urgent cross-match of 4 units
- inform theatres and the on-call anaesthetist urgently
- transfer to theatre should not be delayed because of blood or resuscitation
- Rhesus negative blood can be used for transfusion
- surgical management may be undertaken laparoscopically or by laparotomy
- laparotomy is preferred if there is significant haemodynamic compromise
- laparoscopy should be performed only if an experienced operator is available

2.

The differential diagnosis of pain and positive pregnancy test is ectopic pregnancy, unless proven otherwise.

The risks inherent to laparoscopy include bleeding, infection, injury to surrounding structures (e.g. bowel, bladder, ureter and major vessels), postoperative shoulder tip pain, abdominal pain, failure to gain entry into the abdomen and complete the procedure laparoscopically, inability to identify an obvious cause for the presenting complaint and embolism.

The additional procedures include blood transfusion, repair of any injured organs, oophorectomy and laparotomy.

3.

Salpingectomy is associated with a lower rate of persisting trophoblast and subsequent ectopic pregnancy, while having a similar intrauterine pregnancy rate in the future compared to salpingotomy. The risk of recurrent ectopic pregnancy is 10% and therefore she needs to have an ultrasound as early as 5–6 weeks of gestation in all future pregnancies to ensure that the pregnancy is intrauterine.

4.

Salpingotomy has similar intrauterine pregnancy rates to salpingectomy, while having higher rate of persistent trophoblastic tissue (4–8%) and subsequent ectopic pregnancy (20%). It is therefore necessary to treat this woman with serial beta human chorionic gonadotrophin (βhCG; βhCG is expected to fall to 25% of the pretreatment level within 4 days of surgery).

Non-sensitised women who are Rhesus negative should receive anti-D immunoglobulin.

Royal College of Obstetricians and Gynaecologists. Green-top Guideline No. 21. Management of tubal pregnancy. London: RCOG Press, 2004.
Magowan B. Churchill's Pocketbook of Obstetrics and Gynaecology (3rd edn). Edinburgh: Churchill Livingston, 2005.

31.18 Severe dyskaryosis

A 28-year-old woman, para 2, is referred to the colposcopy clinic with a referral smear report of severe dyskaryosis. She is very anxious and believes that she has cancer. She smokes, which she relates to the stress of her recent job loss.

1. What should one ask in her history?   Marks (4)

2. How would one explain the smear result and what preliminary
    investigations should be undertaken for her?   Marks (4)

3. Colposcopy is unsatisfactory but reveals cervical intraepithelial
    neoplasia (CIN3). Outline further management options for her.   Marks (6)

4. What are the complications following excision procedures of the
    transformation zone? What advice should she be given following
    the large loop excision of transformation zone (LLETZ) procedure?   Marks (6)

Key points

- 28 years old
- para 2
- anxious
- severe dyskaryosis
- smoking
- CIN3
- unsatisfactory colposcopy
- LLETZ procedure

Essay plan

1.

- menstrual history and abnormal bleeding
- contraception
- detailed smear history
- previous genital infections
- smoking

2.

- it is a precancerous condition and not cancer
- treatable and curable
- colposcopy
- cervical biopsy

3.

- LLETZ
- follow-up colposcopy and smear
- stop smoking

4.

- problems following LLETZ
- advice following LLETZ
- fertility advice

31.18 Suggested answer

1.

The history should include her last menstrual period, cycle regularity, any intermenstrual and postcoital bleeding, previous smear history and treatment for cervical smear abnormalities, contraception, e.g. combined oral contraceptive pill (COCP), previous genital tract infections, smoking history and drug and allergy history.

2.

She is very anxious and should be reassured that it is not cancer. It should be explained that the smear abnormality is likely to be a precancerous condition and if left untreated for a number of years, it may progress to cancer. Therefore it is very much a treatable and curable condition.

First of all, a special test called a colposcopy (a microscope to have a close look at the cervix, which stays outside the body) needs to be done. During this procedure, three solutions (saline, 3–5% acetic acid and Lugol iodine) are applied one after the other in sequence to highlight any abnormality on the cervix. If there is an abnormality, a cervical biopsy is taken which will be sent off to the laboratory (pathology department) for a definitive report.

The procedure may be uncomfortable and she may have some stinging sensation and mild vaginal spotting following any cervical biopsy. She will need to wear a sanitary pad and avoid sex for the next couple of days. She can go home following the above test and biopsy.

3.

There is a 50% and 75% risk of CIN2 and CIN3 progressing to cervical cancer, respectively. Therefore, she warrants treatment in the form of LLETZ. Also, the excision procedure is advised if the colposcopy is unsatisfactory in a background of severe dyskaryosis. The LLETZ procedure can be undertaken at the initial consultation or at a later date, under local anaesthesia. It can also be performed under general anaesthesia for someone who is very anxious.

Excisional procedures have a primary success rate of 95% (defined as negative smear at 6 months) and repeat therapy, when indicated, increases the success rate to 99%. Following treatment the main emphasis is on follow-up with colposcopy and cervical cytology as women still remain at increased risk of developing cervical cancer. The follow-up is at least 10 years following treatment (cervical cytology initially at 6 and 12 months and then yearly for 9 years). This may need to be reviewed in light of the introduction of human papillomavirus (HPV) testing.

She also needs to be advised about cessation of smoking as it may cause the smear abnormality to be persistent or progressive.

She can continue hormonal contraception if previously used.

4.

There are short-term and long-term complications.

Short-term complications:

- primary haemorrhage
- secondary haemorrhage
- infection

Long-term complications:

- cervical stenosis/incompetence
- unsatisfactory colposcopy
- inadequate smear
- pre-term labour

She should be informed that her fertility is unlikely to be affected. However, there is a small risk of premature labour or early rupture of membranes during pregnancy. She may need ultrasound scanning to measure the length of the cervix during pregnancy (around 20 weeks) to assess her risk of premature labour.

The cervix is a raw wet area following treatment and is therefore more prone to infection. Insertion of materials (tampons and pessaries) into the vagina should be avoided to reduce the risk of infection and to promote healing. Also there is the need to avoid sexual intercourse, swimming and baths for the next 2 weeks for the same reason.

She should expect to have some brownish discharge for 2 weeks after the LLETZ procedure but if there is any excessive bleeding (secondary haemorrhage is mainly due to infection), raised temperature or she feels unwell, she should immediately call colposcopy services or attend the emergency department. She will be seen in the colposcopy clinic in 6 months time unless there is any unexpected pathology result.

Teale G and Jordan J. Chapter 7: Lower genital tract intraepithelial neoplasia. In: Shafi MI, Luesley DM, Jordan JJ (eds). Handbook of Gynaecological Oncology. Edinburgh: Churchill Livingstone, 2001. NHS Cervical Screening Programme. Colposcopy and Programme Management. Guidelines for the NHS Cervical Screening Programme (2nd edn). Publication No 20. NHSCSP, 2010. http://www.bsccp.org.uk/docs/public/pdf/nhscsp20.pdf

31.19 Sterilisation

A 40-year-old woman, para 4, is in the day surgery unit for planned laparoscopic sterilisation.

1. What should be explained about sterilisation and what are the risks of the sterilisation operation?   Marks (6)

2. What should one ask in her history before the operation?   Marks (4)

3. On questioning she mentions unprotected intercourse on several occasions since her last menstrual period (LMP). Her periods are generally regular (every 28 days) and her last period was 3 weeks ago. Justify the management in her case.   Marks (10)

Key points

- para 4
- unprotected intercourse
- sterilisation operation
- medically fit

Essay plan

1.

- risks of laparoscopy
- risks specific to sterilisation
- alternatives

2.

- LMP and regularity of period
- contraception and exclude pregnancy
- previous surgical history
- significant family history
- last eaten
- allergies
- weight and height (and measure body mass index)

3.

- risk of luteal phase pregnancy
- risk of ectopic pregnancy with operation

31.19 Suggested answer

1.

Sterilisation is a 'keyhole' operation. The fallopian tubes are visualised and clips are applied to both the tubes to block them. It is an irreversible and permanent method of contraception which will not be reversed in the NHS under any circumstances. The risk of failure rate per 100 women years is 0.5% (1 in 200 women). If there is a failure, the risk of ectopic pregnancy is high and she should immediately report to her general practitioner for advice in the event of a missed period.

The risks inherent to laparoscopy include bleeding, infection, injury to the surrounding structures (e.g. bowel, bladder, ureter and major vessels), postoperative shoulder tip pain, abdominal pain, failure to gain entry into the abdomen and complete the procedure laparoscopically and embolism. The additional procedures include blood transfusion, repair of any injured organs and laparotomy.

Alternatives to sterilisation (and provision of an information leaflet) should have been discussed and documented in outpatients. It should be confirmed that she and her partner have considered the main alternatives of levonorgestrel IUS and vasectomy.

2.

It is important to routinely ask her about her last menstrual period, regularity of the period, most recent episode of unprotected sexual intercourse and contraception used in order to assess the risk of this woman already being pregnant. One should also measure body mass index as complications are more common with very slim and very obese women.

Previous surgical history should be obtained to assess any additional surgical risks in order to counsel the woman. It is always important to ask about her history as there may be a rare disease which may be relevant to administering anaesthesia (e.g. cholinesterase enzyme deficiency). It is also important to ask about allergies and the time she last had anything to eat or drink as there is risk of aspiration (Mendelson syndrome – pneumonia with a full stomach).

3.

Luteal phase pregnancy accounts for about 10–20% of apparent sterilisation failures. Conventionally, the practice was to do a dilatation and curettage in such women. However, this does not assure the prevention of either ectopic or intrauterine pregnancy.

If she is at mid-cycle with very recent sexual intercourse, postcoital contraception could be offered. If she is within 5 days of sexual intercourse at around presumed ovulation, an intrauterine contraceptive device (IUCD) (not an IUS) could be fitted temporarily at sterilisation.

The ideal plan is to cancel and reschedule the operation. This woman should be advised to use reliable contraception before the surgery. All the discussion and advice should be documented in the notes.

One should make sure not to yield to pressures in such situations at it may lead to litigation in view of the above complications.

Royal College of Obstetricians and Gynaecologists. Guideline: Consent Advice No. 3. Laparoscopic tubal occlusion. London: RCOG Press, 2004.
Royal College of Obstetricians and Gynaecologists. Evidence-based Guideline No. 4. Male and female sterilisation. London: RCOG Press, 2004.
Royal College of Obstetricians and Gynaecologists. Sterilisation for men and women: what you need to know (patient information leaflet). London: RCOG Press, 2004.

32.1 Acute fatty liver of pregnancy

A 32-year-old primigravida presents to the obstetric day assessment unit at 30 weeks of gestation with nausea and vomiting for 1 week. Her blood pressure on admission is 140/90. A urine test shows 3+ ketones and no protein. A cardiotocograph (CTG) is suspicious and an ultrasound scan shows the absence of amniotic fluid. The management plan is to administer corticosteroids and deliver her as soon as possible. A set of pre-eclampsia screening blood tests are taken which show normal urates and raised alanine aminotransferase (512 U/mL), bilirubin (88 µmol/L), alkaline phosphatase (530 U/L), lactate dehydrogenase (848 U/L), urea (7 mmol/L), creatinine (210 µmol/L), deranged clotting (activated partial thromboplastin time [APTT] 45 seconds and prothrombin time 15 seconds) but normal platelets and haemoglobin. Her blood glucose is 2.8 mmol/L.

1. Critically evaluate the differential diagnosis in this case.   Marks (8)

2. What is the diagnosis in this case and explain the pathophysiology
   of the disease.   Marks (3)
3. Outline a management plan for this woman.   Marks (5)

4. Describe the future implications for this woman.   Marks (4)

Normal values

Creatinine: 45–90 µmol/L for women
urea: 3–6.5 mmol/L
bilirubin: 0–20 µmol/L
lactate dehydrogenase: 140–280 U/L
APTT: 25–38 seconds
PT: 10–13 seconds
alkaline phosphatase: 44–147 IU/L

Key points

- primigravida
- 30 weeks of gestation
- nausea and vomiting
- suspicious CTG and no liquor
- absence of proteinuria in the urine
- markedly deranged liver enzymes and renal function tests
- deranged clotting
- normal platelets and urates

- increased lactate dehydrogenase (LDH)
- absent liquor

Essay plan

1.

Critically evaluate/differential diagnosis (put the most likely diagnosis first, hence evaluate):

- acute fatty liver of pregnancy (AFLP)
- pre-eclampsia
- HELLP haemolysis, elevated liver enzymes and low platelets
- haemolytic uraemic syndrome (HUS)
- thrombotic thrombocytopaenic purpura (TTP)
- liver disease

2.

- AFLP
- low blood glucose
- deranged liver function tests (LFTs) and renal function tests (RFTs)
- hyperuricaemia
- coagulopathy with normal platelets
- common in primigravida
- presents after 30 weeks gestation or at term
- male fetus
- enzyme deficiency
- presentation with nausea and vomiting

3.

- stabilise and deliver
- aggressive therapy (intravenous glucose, fresh frozen plasma [FFP] and albumin)
- multidisciplinary approach
- transfer to intensive care unit post delivery
- liver scan
- transfer to tertiary liver unit
- N-acetylcysteine
- orthotopic liver transplantation

4.

- screening for enzyme deficiency
- chances of recurrence but incidence unknown
- monitor closely LFTs during next pregnancy

32.1 Suggested answer

1.

- AFLP is rare but most common in primigravida after 30 weeks of gestation. They usually present with vomiting and abdominal pain. The blood results show markedly deranged liver enzymes (3–10-fold elevation of transaminases, bilirubin and alkaline phosphatase) and RFTs compared to HELLP syndrome. The pathognomonic features include profound hypoglycaemia, hyperuricaemia (out of proportion to the severity of pre-eclampsia) and deranged clotting profile in the presence of normal platelets. It may be associated with mild hypertension or proteinuria.

- Pre-eclampsia is most common in primigravida and can present at any time after 20 weeks of gestation. The diagnosis is made on the basis of raised blood pressure in the presence of proteinuria. However, 14% of women will go on to develop eclampsia in the absence of proteinuria. Liver and renal functions are mildly deranged in pre-eclampsia. Hyperuricaemia is not marked and platelets can be low. Placental insufficiency and fetal growth restriction are also known features

- HELLP is haemolysis, elevated liver enzymes and low platelets (<100,000). It is associated with pre-eclampsia in 5–20% of cases and a woman can present with epigastric pain and vomiting and then deteriorate very quickly. There are often signs of haemolysis on blood film and blood tests show raised lactate dehydrogenase (>600 U/L) which is suggestive of haemolysis. There will be a drop in haemoglobin due to haemolysis. Abnormal liver enzymes and coagulopathy suggest HELLP rather than TTP. Renal failure may develop in 7% of those with HELLP.

- Haemolytic uraemic syndrome (HUS) can be confused with pre-eclampsia but hypertension is less common in HUS. It occurs most commonly in the postnatal period and is associated with marked derangement of renal function and microangiopathic haemolytic anaemia, fever and thrombocytopenia.

- Thrombotic thrombocytopenic purpura (TTP) can mimic pre-eclampsia. It is associated with marked thrombocytopenia (<10,000) and renal failure. The cerebral features (headache, irritability, drowsiness, seizures and coma) are more prominent and diagnostic of TTP.

- Liver disease usually has a history of hepatitis and does not involve the kidneys.

2.

The diagnosis in this case is AFLP for the above reasons.

The exact aetiology is unclear. It is more common in primigravida after 30 weeks of gestation or at term; obese women; women carrying a male fetus; and twin pregnancy.

An enzyme deficiency of long chain 3-hydroxy-acyl-coenzyme (LCHAD) has also been described in a subgroup of population. It is considered to be a disorder of mitochondrial fatty acid oxidation. These women may succumb to AFLP or HELLP syndrome when the fetus is homozygous for beta fatty acid oxidation disorders.

3.

The optimal management for this woman is to expedite her delivery. This has been shown to improve the outcome for both mother and the baby. Coagulopathy and hypoglycaemia should be treated aggressively (50% glucose, FFP and albumin) and the use of N-acetylcysteine (an antioxidant and glutathione precursor) may be considered in women with hepatic failure. This has been shown to promote selective inactivation of free radicals.

Management in the intensive care unit in a multidisciplinary setting is crucial following delivery. It is important to liaise early with a tertiary liver unit for advice and transfer if necessary.

Patients with fulminant hepatic failure and encephalopathy should be referred urgently to a tertiary liver unit. Orthotopic liver transplantation (failed liver removed and replaced by a cadaveric liver rather than from a live donor) should be considered in women with fulminant hepatic failure and irreversible liver failure despite delivery of the fetus and aggressive therapy.

4.

There is often an improvement in symptoms and signs following delivery. Recurrence is possible and therefore liver function should be monitored in subsequent pregnancies.

Recurrence is more likely in women who are heterozygous for disorders of beta fatty acid oxidation, so screening for LCHAD deficiency is indicated.

Nelson-Piercy C. Handbook of Obstetric Medicine (4th edn). London: Informa Healthcare, 2010.
UK Obstetric Surveillance System. Acute fatty liver of pregnancy. UKOSS, 2005.

32.2 Blood transfusion

A 40-year-old woman presents to the obstetric day assessment unit with tiredness at 20 weeks of gestation. She is para 4 and has been anaemic in previous pregnancies and received a blood transfusion in her last pregnancy.

1. How should one minimise giving a blood transfusion during this pregnancy?

    Marks (7)

2. What measures are necessary if this woman needs a blood transfusion?   Marks (7)

3. What are the strategies to minimise the use of banked blood?   Marks (2)

4. How should she be managed if she refuses a blood transfusion during this pregnancy?   Marks (4)

Key points

- para 4
- anaemia
- minimise blood transfusion
- refuse blood transfusion

Essay plan

1.

- divide measures into antepartum, intrapartum and postpartum
- check mean corpuscular volume (MCV), serum iron, ferritin, B12 and folic acid
- treat anaemia
- iron deficiency – oral or parenteral iron therapy
- exclude haemoglobinopathies

- active management of third stage of labour
- check hospital blood transfusion policy

2.

- blood group and antibodies at booking (first midwife appointment) and 28 weeks of gestation
- Kell negative blood
- cytomegalovirus negative blood

3.

- pre-autologous deposit
- cell salvage

4.

- optimise pre-delivery haemoglobin (Hb)
- advance directive
- involve senior multidisciplinary team (MDT) team
- cell salvage
- early recourse to surgery to stop bleeding

32.2 Suggested answer

1.

It is important to type the anaemia with the gestation at which it presents and it should be treated as soon as it is identified. If Hb is <10.5 g/dL, consider haematinic deficiency once haemoglobinopathies have been excluded. Oral iron is the preferred route and is the first line therapy for iron deficiency anaemia. Parenteral route for iron therapy is considered only if the woman is non-compliant or intolerant to oral iron, but it needs to be commenced by the early part of the third trimester at the latest. One needs to check the hospital's transfusion policy if considering a blood transfusion.

Blood loss at delivery should be minimised. Active management of the third stage of labour is recommended to minimise blood loss, and women at high risk of haemorrhage, as is the current case, should be advised to deliver in the hospital. It is important to optimise the management of women on anticoagulants, such as low molecular weight heparin (LMWH), to minimise blood loss.

2.

Antepartum

Giving a blood transfusion antenatally depends on the clinical presentation (symptoms and signs) and gestational age at presentation rather than just the haemoglobin concentration.

All women should have their blood group and antibodies status checked at booking and at 28 weeks of gestation. Women should have a group and save sample taken as per local unit guidelines. If any blood component therapy is contemplated, a sample for group and save must be sent to the laboratory. Patients blood samples used for group and save should be kept for no more than 7 days. Only Kell negative blood should be used for transfusion in women of childbearing age. Cytomegalovirus (CMV) seronegative red cells and platelets should be used for CMV seronegative pregnant women.

The decision to perform a blood transfusion should be made on both clinical and haematological grounds. If there are no irregular antibodies, group-specific compatible blood can be provided within 10 minutes plus transport time. If irregular antibodies are found, then obtaining compatible blood may take several hours to cross-match. In an extreme situation or if the blood group is unknown, O Rhesus D negative red cells can be given.

Intrapartum

If the Hb is <7 g/dL in labour or in the immediate postpartum period, the decision to transfuse should be made according to the individual's medical history and symptoms.

Postpartum

If the Hb is <7–8 g/dL in the postnatal period, where there is no continuing or threat of bleeding, the decision to transfuse should be made on an informed choice and should be on an individual basis. In fit, healthy, asymptomatic patients there is little evidence of the benefit of blood transfusion.

3.

Pre-autologous blood deposit: in pregnancy, pre-autologous deposit is not recommended.

Intraoperative cell salvage: cell salvage is recommended for women in whom an intraoperative blood loss of more than 1500 mL is anticipated. Cell salvage should only be used by healthcare teams who use it regularly and have the necessary expertise and experience.

4.

Mortality is significantly increased in pregnant women who decline blood and blood products. The management of women who refuse a blood transfusion is similar to managing women who are Jehovah's Witnesses.

Antenatal counselling, planning and advance directive must involve a multidisciplinary team with senior input.

Considerable efforts must be made to optimise pre-delivery Hb and identify risk factors for haemorrhage.

Intrapartum techniques to avoid blood transfusion include cell salvage and early recourse to definitive surgical management in the event of massive obstetric haemorrhage.

Royal College of Obstetricians and Gynaecologists. Green-top Guideline No. 47. Management of women who decline blood and blood products during pregnancy. London: RCOG Press, 2007.

Currie J, Hogg M, Patel N, Madgwick K, Yoong W. Management of women who decline blood and blood products in pregnancy. The Obstetrician and Gynaecologist 2010; 12:13–20.

32.3 Cell-free fetal DNA

A 34-year-old woman comes in for preconception counselling. She gives a family history of genetic disease. She has brought a print-out of internet information about the free fetal DNA and asks the following questions about non-invasive free fetal DNA testing for prenatal diagnosis.

1. What is the source of free fetal DNA for prenatal diagnosis in pregnant women?   Marks (4)

2. What is the current role of free fetal DNA in prenatal diagnosis?   Marks (10)

3. What are the ethical implications of undertaking testing by using free fetal DNA?   Marks (6)

Key points

- 34 years old
- family history of genetic disease
- free fetal DNA
- source of free fetal DNA
- prenatal diagnosis
- uses of free fetal DNA
- ethical aspects

Essay plan

1.

- fetal cells
- maternal circulation
- safer option
- non-invasive
- drawback: very short half-life of free fetal DNA

2.

- Rhesus typing
- fetal sex determination
- single gene disorder detection
- detection of aneuploidy

3.

- socio-ethical implications, e.g. selective termination of pregnancy
- commercialisation
- lack of regulation
- fetal sex determination from a blood spot
- paternity testing

32.3 **Suggested answer**

1.

Current prenatal diagnosis for genetic testing or aneuploidy uses invasive diagnostic tests which carry a small but significant risk of miscarriage (chorionic villus sampling [CVS] or amniocentesis).

Fetal cells in the maternal circulation are a source of fetal DNA (identified in 1997) for a safer, non-invasive prenatal diagnosis (NIPD). However, one should bear in mind the short half-life of free fetal DNA when performing tests.

2.

Current applications do not allow complete separation and they focus on the detection or exclusion of genes not present in the mother, such as Y chromosome sequences or Rhesus D (RhD) status in RhD-negative women.

Fetal RhD typing

- since 2001, fetal RhD typing using cell-free fetal DNA has been used to direct management in RhD-negative women at increased risk of haemolytic disease of the newborn (HDN) because of a previous affected pregnancy or elevated antibody titre
- NIPD has almost completely replaced amniocentesis or CVS
- determination of other fetal RhC, c, E and Kell blood groups using cell-free fetal DNA have also been reported

Fetal sex determination

- Fetal sex can be determined by cell-free fetal DNA in maternal plasma and the identification of genes (DYS14 or SRY) on the Y chromosome.
- In the UK, it is in women at risk of X-linked disorders where early identification of a male fetus indicates a need for an invasive diagnostic test to determine whether the affected X chromosome has been inherited. No invasive test is required if the fetus is female.
- In pregnancies at risk of congenital adrenal hyperplasia (CAH), identification of female fetuses and early treatment in utero has been shown to reduce the degree of virilisation of the external genitalia. Non-invasive testing decreases the uptake of invasive diagnostic testing by nearly 50% and allows for the early cessation of dexamethasone treatment in pregnancies at risk of CAH where the fetus is found to be male.
- A recent national audit demonstrated a concordance rate of 97.8% between sex detection reported using cell-free fetal DNA performed at or after 7 weeks and sex confirmed at invasive testing or birth (testing before 7 weeks was less accurate).

Single gene disorder diagnosis

- Single gene disorders have been reported by detecting or excluding the paternal allele inherited from an affected father with an autosomal dominant condition, such as Huntington disease.

- Confirmation of Achondroplasia in a fetus presenting *de novo* with short limbs in the third trimester has also been reported.
- Currently available techniques are unsuitable for the diagnosis of X-linked and most recessive disorders.

Aneuploidy diagnosis

- Non-invasive prenatal diagnosis for Down syndrome is not feasible. Recently, Lo et al. (2007) described analysis of a cell-free fetal messenger ribonucleic acid (cell-free fetal mRNA) derived exclusively from the fetus having no maternal contribution. A gene located on chromosome 21 (PLAC4) was found to be expressed in the placenta but not in maternal blood (fetus-specific) by extracting cell-free RNA rather than cell-free DNA from maternal plasma.

3.

- the potential simplicity of performing the test and fetal sex determination where the high degree of accuracy of non-invasive prenatal diagnosis as early as 7 weeks of pregnancy carries a number of socio-ethical implications, e.g. selective termination of pregnancy
- commercialisation and patency may make this method potentially problematic to roll out to everyone
- regulation is required to avoid the above problem
- fetal sex determination from a blood spot may be possible
- paternity testing may prove easier

Royal College of Obstetricians and Gynaecologists. SAC Opinion Paper 15. Non-invasive prenatal diagnosis using cell-free DNA in maternal blood. London: RCOG Press, 2009.
Lo YM, Tsui NB, Chiu RW, Lau TK, Leung TN, Heung MM, Gerovassili A, Jin Y, Nicolaides KH, Cantor CR, Ding C. Plasma placental RNA allelic ratio permits noninvasive prenatal chromosomal aneuploidy detection. Nat Med 2007; 13:218–223.
Dennislo YM. Noninvasive prenatal diagnosis in 2020. Prenatal Diagnosis 2010; 30(7): 702–703.
Chiu RW, Akolekar R, Zheng YW et al. Non-invasive prenatal assessment of trisomy 21 by multiplexed maternal plasma DNA sequencing: large scale validity study. BMJ 2011; 342: C7401.

32.4 Choroid plexus cyst

A 36-year-old woman, para 0, attends the antenatal clinic following an anomaly scan at 19 weeks of gestation. The ultrasound report shows that the baby has a choroid plexus cyst.

1. What should this woman be told if the choroid plexus cyst is an incidental and isolated finding?   Marks (4)

2. What factors may affect the management of her case?   Marks (8)

3. Justify the management of this woman.   Marks (8)

Key points

- 36 years old
- para 0
- 19 weeks of gestation
- choroid plexus cyst

Essay plan

1.

- incidence
- isolated choroid plexus cysts are usually normal developmental findings
- the majority will resolve
- need repeat scan later in pregnancy

2.

- associated soft markers (increased nuchal thickness, pyelectasis, echogenic bowel, cardiac echogenic foci and short femur)
- associated structural defects
- review screening results (nuchal translucency [NT]/serum)
- strong family history
- maternal anxiety

3.

- isolated cyst – reassure and arrange repeat scan
- associated abnormalities – fetal medicine scan, amniocentesis, karyotyping
- abnormal karyotype – offer termination
- abnormal karyotype – if she wants to continue the pregnancy, support her with appropriate routine care
- arrange repeat scan
- provide written information
- second opinion if required
- discuss risk of recurrence in future pregnancies

32.4 Suggested answer

1.

Cystic dilatation can be seen in the choroid plexus of the lateral ventricles in 1–2% of all fetuses on routine second trimester scans. An isolated choroid plexus cyst is not a structural defect and in itself does not have major implications for the baby. The majority (90%) of cysts resolve by 26 weeks of gestation (before the end of the second trimester). However, it may be associated with a small risk of aneuploidy (5% with trisomy 18 and 1% with other karyotypic abnormalities) if there are additional factors (soft markers) or structural abnormalities on the ultrasound scan.

2.

An isolated choroid plexus cyst is not an indication for invasive testing (amniocentesis or placental biopsy). However, fetuses with bilateral choroid plexus cysts (>10 mm size) and other associated soft markers (increased nuchal thickness, pyelectasis, echogenic bowel, cardiac echogenic foci and short femur) or abnormalities have an increased risk of an abnormal karyotype and therefore should undergo karyotyping following appropriate counselling. One should specifically look for Dandy–Walker malformation.

A strong family history of chromosomal abnormalities may also warrant invasive testing in the form of amniocentesis to aid karyotyping.

In circumstances of increased maternal anxiety, such tests may be performed even in the presence of an isolated choroid plexus cyst. However, one should bear in mind the risk of miscarriage associated with amniocentesis (1%) and women should be appropriately counselled. In an isolated choroid plexus cyst, one should also review any prenatal screening tests already undertaken ('no risk' may be reassuring).

3.

The basic questions to be answered are mainly what can be done, what happens next and what happens in the future.

A detailed scan in a fetal medicine unit by a fetal medicine specialist should be arranged to identify any other associated abnormalities. These may include structural cardiac and abdominal wall defects, and soft tissue markers such as nuchal oedema and renal pelvis dilatation (features of aneuploidy). If this is the case, the woman should be managed in a fetal medicine unit and invasive testing offered (amniocentesis). If karyotyping is positive for aneuploidy, she should be offered a termination of pregnancy. Timing is important in relation to the Abortion Law and feticide may need to be considered depending on the gestation (22 weeks and above) at which termination occurs.

- On the other hand, if the woman wishes to continue the pregnancy, she should be supported throughout the pregnancy with appropriate routine care and she may need to be delivered in a tertiary centre where expertise and facilities are available to manage such fetuses and neonates.
- A repeat scan should be arranged around 26 weeks of gestation, following which she should be reviewed in the antenatal clinic.
- Written information (a leaflet) should be provided to the woman and a second opinion offered if the woman wishes.
- She should be informed about the slightly increased risk of recurrence in future pregnancies.

James D, Steer PJ, Weiner CP, Gonik B, Crowther C, Robson S (eds). High Risk Pregnancy: Management Options (4th edn). St Louis: Saunders, 2011.

32.5 Echogenic bowel

A 30-year-old woman, para 2 (both normal vaginal deliveries), booked (attended her first midwife appointment) at 12 weeks of gestation during this pregnancy. She is currently at 22 weeks of gestation and has been referred to the antenatal clinic as her fetal scan revealed hyperechogenic bowel.

1. Define echogenic bowel.   Marks (2)

2. What are the causes of echogenic fetal bowel and what is its significance?   Marks (8)

3. How should this woman be managed in view of the current findings and why?   Marks (10)

Key points

- 30 years old
- 22 weeks of gestation
- echogenic bowel in fetus

Essay plan

1.

- definition of echogenic bowel

2.

- soft marker for aneuploidy
- associated with cystic fibrosis (CF) and other anomalies listed below
- association with hypoxia/ischaemia and poor pregnancy outcome
- most babies have normal outcome

3.

- screen parents for CF
- karyotyping for aneuploidy
- maternal serum for cytomegalovirus (CMV) IgM
- serial scans for growth
- paedtric alert

32.5 Suggested answer

1.

Fetal bowel is defined as hyperechogenic if it appears similar to or more echogenic than the surrounding bone in the same machine settings (appears white on scan).

2.

The underlying cause is considered to be bowel ischaemia and this may reflect poor placental function. It is a marker of aneuploidy and may be associated with other soft marker or fetal abnormalities.

Echogenic bowel is associated with meconium ileus, trisomy 21, CMV infection, CF, fetal growth restriction, fetal death and necrotising enterocolitis in the newborn. However, most babies will have a normal outcome.

Echogenic fetal bowel is a soft marker and can be a normal finding (67% cases) in most fetuses. However, it can be associated with an abnormal karyotype with increased association with other soft markers (choroid plexus cyst, echogenic cardiac foci) or abnormal serum screening. Women with such findings on scan should therefore be counselled by an appropriate specialist.

3.

Screening for the above possible causes is important in order to plan management during pregnancy. The following tests are suggested:

- A scan by a fetal medicine specialist to confirm the above findings and rule out any other associated fetal abnormalities. It should be differentiated from calcifications caused by bowel obstruction, fetal infection and meconium peritonitis.
- the woman should be appropriately counselled by a fetal medicine specialist.
- Written information should be provided in case the woman wants some time to think about the problem. She should also be offered a second opinion if she wishes to have one.
- CF screening of both parents should be performed and, if positive, invasive testing (amniocentesis) should be offered to find out whether the baby is affected (amniotic fluid can be used for DNA mutation analysis). Delta F 508 mutations are responsible for more than 90% of cases.
- Karyotyping for trisomies should be offered in the presence of other soft markers, fetal abnormalities or abnormal or suspicious serum screening.
- The risk of a 1% miscarriage rate with amniocentesis should be explained.
- Screening for any recent maternal flu-like symptoms and a blood test for serum IgM for CMV should be arranged.
- In the presence of an abnormal karyotype, she should be offered a termination of pregnancy or she should be supported appropriately if she wants to continue the pregnancy.
- Serial growths scans are recommended as this condition is associated with an increased risk of fetal growth restriction and fetal death. The timing and frequency of scans should be left to the discretion of the fetal medicine specialist.
- Paediatricians should be informed earlier during pregnancy and at delivery as it is associated with bowel problems at birth which can be fatal.

James D, Steer PJ, Weiner CP, Gonik B, Crowther C, Robson S (eds). High Risk Pregnancy: Management Options (4th edn). St Louis: Saunders, 2011.

32.6 Eclampsia

A 40-year-old primigravida presents to the labour ward at 37 weeks of gestation with headache and flashes of light. Her blood pressure is 170/110 mmHg and urine shows 3+ proteinuria. Vaginal examination reveals closed cervix with Bishop score of 5. She has her first eclamptic fit on admission to the labour ward.

1. What are the initial steps in her management?   Marks (4)
2. What are the key steps in her further management?   Marks (8)
3. How should she be counselled about the future?   Marks (8)

Key points

- primigravida
- 37 weeks of gestation
- symptoms of severe pre-eclampsia (headache and visual symptoms)
- first eclamptic fit
- Bishop score

Essay plan

1.

- airway, breathing and circulation – ABC
- call for help or obstetric crash call 2222
- follow eclampsia protocol on the labour ward
- pre-eclampsia (PET) blood test and group and save
- Foley's catheterisation of the bladder with an hourly urine bag

2.

- control of seizures
- control of hypertension
- delivery following stabilization
- fluid restriction and balance
- strict input/output chart
- close monitoring of vitals and urine output
- continue magnesium sulphate ($MgSO_4$) 24 hours post delivery or the last fit, whichever occurs later

3.

- risk of developing chronic hypertension in the future
- risk of developing hypertensive disorder in the next pregnancy
- risk of recurrent pre-eclampsia in the next pregnancy
- risk of recurrent eclampsia in the next pregnancy
- risk of pre-eclampsia in family members
- regular monitoring of blood pressure (BP) during the next pregnancy
- start aspirin as soon as she is pregnant in the future

32.6 Suggested answer

1.

- Obstetric crash call as it is an obstetric emergency (2222). This call includes an obstetric consultant, registrar, senior house officer, anaesthetist, labour ward coordinator and matron, labour ward ODA, pathology technician, haematology on-call doctor, porter, site manager, paediatric registrar and paediatric matron.
- Immediately secure the airway and position the patient in the left lateral position to prevent aspiration.
- Secure two large bore cannulas once she stops fitting and take blood to test for haemoglobin, platelet count, liver function tests, renal function tests (urea and creatinine), urates and clotting profile (international normalised ratio, prothrombin time and activated partial thromboplastin time [APTT]) and group and save.
- Loading dose of intravenous $MgSO_4$ of 4 g should be administered to prevent further fits.

2.

- Follow eclampsia protocol on the labour ward.

- Once loading dose of MgSO$_4$ is given, a maintenance dose of 1 g per hour should be started.
- Adequately control BP to prevent stroke or cardiac failure secondary to hypertension. If the mean arterial pressure is persistently high (≥125 mmHg) intravenous antihypertensives should be initiated to control BP quickly. The drug of choice depends on the local protocol. When using hydralazine, preloading with 250–500 mL of gelofusin is preferred to prevent a sudden drop in BP to avoid fetal cardiac abnormalities or bradycardia. Labetalol should be avoided in women who are known asthmatics.
- Restrict crystalloid intravenous fluids to a total of 85 mL/hour to prevent fluid overload and pulmonary oedema.
- Strict input and output chart (hourly) is crucial. Pre-eclampsia affects every organ in the body. Renal damage can lead to oliguria. One should watch for signs of MgSO$_4$ toxicity as it is excreted in urine.
- The woman should be nursed in a high dependency unit (HDU) with one-to-one care.
- Close monitoring (every 15 minutes) of respiratory rate, BP, oxygen saturation, deep tendon reflexes and urine output is important to identify signs of MgSO$_4$ toxicity.
- One should also repeat the PET blood tests almost every 6 hours in women with severe pre-eclampsia.
- Invasive monitoring (central venous pressure) is indicated in women with renal damage (oliguria or anuria with rising urea and creatinine), pulmonary oedema and cardiac failure.
- Once she is stabilised, she should be delivered. If there are no contraindications she can be induced with vaginal prostaglandins, but if the cervix is unfavourable a caesarean section may be preferred in a primigravida.

3.

- Monitor BP at the general practitioner centre during the postpartum period as she may go on to develop chronic hypertension.
- Avoid the combined oral contraceptives pill (COCP).
- Start aspirin (75 mg once daily) as soon as she is pregnant the next time.
- Start oral labetalol if she develops raised BP in the next pregnancy.
- Arrange a uterine artery Doppler ultrasound scan at 20 weeks gestation in the next pregnancy. The presence of uterine artery notches increase the risk of having pre-eclampsia and fetal growth restriction.
- The risk of developing chronic hypertension is 23% on average.
- The risk of hypertensive disorder in a subsequent pregnancy is 33%.
- The rate of recurrence of pre-eclampsia is around 10% if she had pre-eclampsia at term in her first pregnancy.
- The incidence of eclampsia is 4.9 in 10,000 pregnancies but the incidence of recurrent eclampsia is approximately 10%.
- Eclampsia carries a risk of 1.8% maternal mortality.
- The risk of neonatal death is 34 in 1000 live births.
- Thirty-eight per cent of eclamptic fits occur before hypertension and proteinuria are documented.

- There is increased risk of family members developing pre-eclampsia (siblings).

Royal College of Obstetricians and Gynaecologists. Green-top Guideline No. 10a. The management of severe pre-eclampsia/eclampsia. London: RCOG Press, 2010.

Managing Obstetric Emergencies and Trauma. The MOET Course Manual (2nd edn). MOET, 2007.

Magowan B. Churchill's Pocketbook of Obstetrics and Gynaecology (3rd edn). Edinburgh: Churchill Livingston, 2005.

Hernandez-Diaz S, Toh S, Cnattingius S. Risk of pre-eclampsia in first and subsequent pregnancies: prospective cohort. BMJ 2009; 338:b2255; discussion http://www.medscape.com/viewarticle/704801_4

James D, Steer PJ, Weiner CP, Gonik B, Crowther C, Robson S (eds). High Risk Pregnancy: Management Options (4th edn). St Louis: Saunders, 2011.

32.7 Epilepsy

A 20-year-old woman is referred to the preconception clinic. She has a history of epilepsy and is planning for pregnancy.

1. What should she be asked in her history?   Marks (4)

2. What are the maternal and fetal risks if she gets pregnant and what measures should be taken to reduce them?   Marks (8)

3. How should her pregnancy be managed?   Marks (8)

Key points

- 20 years old
- preconception clinic
- history of epilepsy
- planning for pregnancy
- maternal and fetal risks
- reduce risks
- management

Essay plan

1.

- detail history about epilepsy
- medication
- contraception – current and planned
- previous pregnancies and outcome
- other medical history
- family history and support

2.

- effect of pregnancy on epilepsy
- effect of epilepsy and medication on mother and fetus during pregnancy

3.

- management during antenatal period (first, second and third trimesters)
- management during labour
- management during puerperium

32.7 Suggested answer

1.

A detailed history about the woman's epilepsy is important. It should include duration and frequency of fits and their onset, type of fit, control, fit-free interval, and type and dose of medication used for epilepsy treatment.

There is no relation to the seizure type or course of epilepsy during previous pregnancies. However, women with multiple seizure types are more likely to experience an increase in seizure frequency during pregnancy.

It is important to assess other medical co-morbidities which need appropriate planning or treatment, family history and the support she has at home.

Enquire about current and future contraceptive use.

2.

Maternal risks include increased risk of miscarriage, increase in seizure frequency (10–30%) during pregnancy, labour and puerperium, risk of aspiration during seizure and increased maternal mortality, e.g. (sudden unexpected death in epilepsy [SUDEP]).

Fetal risks include a 2–3-fold increase in congenital malformations (neural tube defects, cardiac defects and orofacial defects) and stillbirths. Risk of the child developing epilepsy later in life is also increased (4–5% if either parent has epilepsy and 15–20% if both parents have epilepsy). If there is an affected sibling, the risk would be 10%.

Measures to reduce risks

It is advisable to use contraception until the seizures are adequately controlled. If she is on hepatic enzyme inducing drugs (primidone, phenytoin, carbamazepine, phenobarbitone) she should be warned about requiring higher doses of oestrogen to attain adequate contraception.

Hospital-led care in a joint neurology and obstetric clinic is the ideal situation.

Folic acid supplementation of 5 mg should be taken from preconception as most antiepileptic drugs have an antifolate action and are teratogenic. If there is good control with the current medication, it is important not to change the medication to another drug.

It is advisable to use a single drug if possible, and at the lowest possible antiepileptic medication dose to control seizures and minimise fetal risks. Medication can be stopped in joint consultation with neurologists, if the seizure-free interval is more than 2 years.

Educate the woman regarding the need for a good sleep pattern, avoidance of stress, bath usage when alone and driving alone. Family members should also be educated regarding the recovery position during seizures to prevent aspiration.

It is important to offer an epidural early in labour to avoid pain which can precipitate a seizure. She should be advised against water and home births.

3.

She should be managed in a joint neurology and/or obstetric clinic. The main aim is to achieve adequate seizure control with a minimal dose of antiepileptic medication. Folic acid supplementation (5 mg) is important to prevent some of the side effects of antiepileptic medication (neural tube defects). An early pregnancy scan and nuchal screening is important to detect any fetal abnormalities, so that termination can be offered if necessary. A 20 week detailed anomaly scan is very important to rule out major structural abnormalities.

She should be warned that seizures may increase, decrease or remain unchanged during pregnancy. If there is any increase in seizure frequency, she will need a modification to the dose of antiepileptic medication and this should be based on clinical grounds.

During the second trimester, a fetal cardiac scan should be arranged to exclude any cardiac abnormalities and fetal growth scans should be arranged if necessary.

The use of vitamin K in pregnancy is controversial.

In labour she should be offered an early epidural in order to be pain free. There is no contraindication to vaginal delivery and caesarean section is indicated only for obstetric complications. During puerperium, she should be encouraged to breastfeed the baby and it should be explained to her that the secretion of most antiepileptic drugs (carbamazepine, sodium valproate and phenytoin) in breast milk is low.

She should be educated about safe bathing (keeping the door open and avoiding baths when alone) and safe driving.

Nelson-Piercy C. Handbook of Obstetric Medicine (4th edn). London: Informa Healthcare, 2010.
Walker SP, Permezel M, Berkovic SF. The management of epilepsy in pregnancy. BJOG 2009; 116:758–767.

32.8 Fetal cardiac arrhythmia

A low-risk primigravida visits her midwife for a routine check at 28 weeks of gestation. On abdominal examination, the uterus is large for dates and the fetal heart rate is irregular. She is referred to the hospital obstetric day assessment unit. A forty minute cardiotocograph (CTG) in the hospital is normal. She attends for an ultrasound examination the next day which shows the fetal heart rate of 220 beats/minute (bpm). A diagnosis of supraventricular tachycardia is made. Also noted are fetal ascites and the presence of bilateral pleural effusions. All her booking (her first midwife appointment) blood tests were normal.

1. What are the initial steps in the management of this woman?   Marks (8)

2. One week later, the fetal CTG reveals a heart rate of 180 bpm and similar findings on the ultrasound scan as before. How should she be managed further?   Marks (8)

3. How should she be counselled about the future?   Marks (4)

Key points

- primigravida
- low risk
- large for dates
- supraventricular tachycardia
- fetal heart rate 220 bpm
- ascites
- pleural effusion

Essay plan

1.

- identify the problem
- fetal tachyarrhythmia
- likely supraventricular tachycardia
- non-immune hydrops secondary to fetal tachyarrhythmia
- review by a fetal medicine specialist
- repeat ultrasound scan by a fetal medicine specialist
- flecainide to mother or baby
- inform paediatricians
- review in 1 week

2.

- second line therapy
- consider corticosteroids for lung maturity
- inform paediatricians
- review in 1 week
- consider delivery if still resistant to treatment
- *in utero* transfer to tertiary unit
- delivery by caesarean section
- treat baby in neonatal intensive care unit (NICU)
- debrief mother

3.

- recurrence unknown
- monitor baby in future pregnancy

32.8 Suggested answer

1.

One should consider the following factors while managing fetal tachycardia: gestational age, signs of hydrops, type and mechanism of tachycardia, and risks and benefits of maternally administered drugs.

In this case, it is important to identify the problem, which is non-immune hydrops caused by cardiac failure secondary to fetal tachyarrhythmia. She should be urgently referred to a fetal medicine specialist for review as well as a repeat scan to confirm the findings.

An urgent fetal echocardiogram should be performed to determine the cardiac rate and rhythm and rule out any structural abnormalities (a cardiac abnormality is found in 30% of cases of non-immune hydrops). The prognosis is better in the absence of structural cardiac abnormalities.

In utero, the treatment of the fetus should be initiated with maternal administration of flecainide to treat fetal arrhythmia (most fetal medicine units prefer to use this drug). Both mother and baby should be monitored by electrocardiogram (ECG) and CTG, respectively while receiving the loading dose of the drug.

The poor prognosis and risk of intrauterine death if the fetus does not respond to treatment should be explained to the mother. A follow-up should be arranged in 1 week to see a fetal medicine specialist to reassess the fetal heart rate and rhythm. Paediatricians should be informed in case she needs delivery so that they can plan further management.

2.

The fetal heart rate is 180 beats/minute (still high) and is considered to be not completely responding to treatment. Therefore one should consider second line therapy. If rapid control of tachycardia is required, intravenous amiodarone or oral sotalol can be used. Due to the risk of hypothyroidism with amiodarone, it is not recommended for long-term use.

Adenosine can be (directly) administered into the umbilical vein to terminate supraventricular tachycardia but is associated with a high rate of recurrence.

Verapamil and propranolol can cause maternal hypotension and compromise fetal cardiac function as well as causing fetal growth restriction.

Digoxin is not considered first line therapy in a hydropic baby.

The paediatricians should be informed and corticosteroids administered if delivery is imminent. The mother and the baby should be reviewed in 1 week by a fetal medicine specialist and delivery considered if the fetus does not respond to maternal therapy. The mother should be warned about the guarded prognosis and risk of neonatal death.

Delivery should be by caesarean section and consent for the caesarean including classical approach should be taken. A consultant should perform the caesarean and a consultant paediatrician should be available in the theatre at the time of delivery.

A cot should be reserved in the NICU before delivery. If the facilities and expertise are not available in the current hospital to manage this baby, the woman should be transferred out to a tertiary centre for delivery. The baby should be treated by paediatricians at birth and a fetal echocardiogram repeated to rule out any abnormalities.

The mother should be debriefed about the events.

3.

The risk of recurrence is unknown in the absence of any structural abnormalities in the baby.

Increased anxiety of the woman is expected in future pregnancies.

Future pregnancies should be monitored closely.

James D, Steer PJ, Weiner CP, Gonik B, Crowther C, Robson S (eds). High Risk Pregnancy: Management Options (4th edn). St Louis: Saunders, 2011.

32.9 Genetic disorder

A 28-year-old woman, para 0, attends the antenatal clinic at 12 weeks of gestation for a review of her blood test results. She is very anxious as her sister's first child died at the age of 15 years. He had worsening muscle weakness and was wheelchair bound at the age of 11 years.

1. What is the diagnosis of her sister's child and why? How does one diagnose this condition?   Marks (10)

2. What is the risk to her current child and how does one explain this? How should her pregnancy be managed this time? What are the implications to family members?   Marks (10)

Key points

*   28 years old
*   para 0
*   12 weeks of gestation
*   anxious
*   sister's son died
*   muscle weakness

Essay plan

1.

*   Duchenne muscular dystrophy (DMD)
*   confirm diagnosis: history, examination and investigation

2.

*   assess the risk
*   maternal risk of carrier
*   fetal risk of disease
*   fetal risk of being a male
*   sex determination
*   DMD gene mutation testing
*   role of termination
*   risk to the family

32.9 Suggested answer

1.

The most common cause is muscular dystrophy.

The diagnosis of this child is most likely to be Duchenne muscular dystrophy (DMD). It can be confirmed by reviewing the medical records of her sister's first child or by gene studies for the patient.

DMD is the most common cause of childhood muscular dystrophy. The gene for DMD is located on the short arm of the X chromosome and therefore is X-linked. This condition mainly affects males, with an incidence of 1 in 3500 male births in the UK. The females are carriers of one abnormal gene and one normal gene and are usually normal. The mother is not affected and is well.

Affected males are normal at birth but walking is delayed. Muscle weakness is progressive and most of them will be wheelchair bound. Life expectancy average is about 20 years. Early mortality most often due to respiratory complications.

The diagnosis can be confirmed by reviewing her sister's first child's medical records, testing the patient and testing the patient's sister. Family history is important as there is a high risk of recurrence in family members. Serum shows high levels of creatinine phosphokinase (CPK) and the history is typical of progressive muscle weakness. Ambulatory milestones are delayed.

This disorder is caused by a mutation in the dystrophic gene, located in humans on the X chromosome (XP21). In about two thirds of cases, an affected male inherits the mutation from his mother, who carries one altered copy of the DMD gene. The other one third of cases probably result from new mutations. Gene testing can be used to diagnose the condition in males after birth or by prenatal diagnosis.

2.

She should be managed in a fetal medicine unit by a fetal medicine specialist.

This woman has a family history as her sister's son died with progressive muscle weakness. The mother of this woman is obviously a carrier as she has passed on the mutation to her daughter. There is a chance that this woman is a carrier of the DMD mutant gene (she has a 1 in 2 chance of carrying the DMD gene). The risk that this pregnancy is affected with DMD is 1 in 8 (her carrier risk multiplied by her chance of passing on the mutant gene by the chance of a male pregnancy [1 in 2 × 1 in 2 × 1 in 2]).

This woman can be tested for DMD mutations to establish whether she is a carrier because it has implications for transmission to other offspring and will help in genetic counselling and prenatal diagnosis. If she is a definitive carrier, the risk that the fetus will be affected is 1 in 4. Fetal sex can now be established by non-invasive testing of maternal blood using free fetal DNA (ff-DNA).

If positive, then termination can be offered. If the fetus is male and the carrier status is not identified, some women may still want to terminate the pregnancy.

If the fetus is female, the woman should be reassured as the fetus will be normal but may be a carrier.

There is a risk that other family members may be carrying the DMD gene mutation. Carrier testing will therefore be necessary in the family and if positive for DMD gene mutation, they should be referred to a regional genetics centre.

Connor JM. Section 2: Common genetic conditions in obstetrics and gynaecology. Medical Genetics for the MRCOG and Beyond. London: RCOG Press, 2005.

32.10 Herpes simplex infection

A 33-year-old woman, para 3, at 30 weeks of gestation presents to the day assessment unit with severe vulval pain. Clinical examination reveals multiple vesicular lesions suggestive of primary herpes simplex.

1.	What should be the immediate management for this woman?	Marks (8)
2.	What are the risks to the fetus?	Marks (4)
3.	How should the rest of her pregnancy be managed?	Marks (8)

Key points
- 30 weeks of gestation
- severe vulval pain
- herpes simplex

Essay plan

1.

- confirm diagnosis
- supportive – analgesia
- acyclovir
- screen for other sexually transmitted infections (STIs)

2.

- risk to fetus
- morbidity
- mortality

3.

- antepartum
- intrapartum
- postpartum
- neonate

32.10 Suggested answer

1.

Management is purely supportive or symptom control (analgesics and sitz baths). If urinary retention occurs catheterisation may be necessary. Oral acyclovir (after 20 weeks gestation) is advised to alleviate the severity of the symptoms and duration of viral shedding. If there is secondary infection of the skin, antibiotic cover may be needed.

She should be told to report immediately if unwell (specifically for symptoms and signs of encephalitis and disseminated infection), and in the event of the development of disseminated infection, she should be admitted and may need to be managed jointly with an infectious disease specialist if necessary.

A referral to the genito-urinary medicine clinic is important to exclude other sexually transmitted infections.

The herpes virus can be detected by sampling the fluid from the vesicle after deroofing or taking a swab from an ulcerative lesion. An type-specific herpes infection screen with IgG antibody testing may be considered to differentiate primary from secondary infection but it is not recommended.

2.

Both type 1 and type 2 herpes virus can cause neonatal infection, but only following vaginal delivery; transplacental infection does not occur. It can affect the neurological, cutaneous, oral and ocular system (in isolation or combination). Disseminated infection in the neonate is associated with severe morbidity and mortality as high as 30% (only after primary infection).

It is noted that passive transfer of immunity from mother to fetus does not prevent the neurogenic virus spreading to the brain of the neonate (which is low risk after recurrent episodes).

3.

The fetus is at risk of developing herpes (30–60% fetal transmission of infection) especially if the woman develops a primary herpes infection within 6 weeks of the expected date or at delivery. Therefore a planned caesarean section is recommended for all such women. However, in women with a primary herpes infection in the first and second trimester, caesarean delivery is not recommended as the risk to the fetus is low.

In the current case, this woman is more than 6 weeks from her expected date of delivery. Although evidence is not strong, suppressive therapy with acyclovir may be considered for the last 4 weeks of pregnancy before the delivery date to reduce the chance of a recurrence of the herpes infection.

This woman can undertake a vaginal delivery. However, she should be thoroughly counselled about the risks and benefits of vaginal delivery versus caesarean section. During labour, one should carefully consider avoiding or delaying artificial rupture of membranes and invasive procedures on the fetus (e.g. fetal blood sampling [FBS], fetal scalp electrode [FSE] and ST waveform analysis [STAN] monitoring).

Women with spontaneous rupture of membranes should be delivered as soon as possible because undertaking a caesarean section beyond 4 hours following the rupture of membranes does not offer much benefit.

Recurrent herpes during the antenatal period is not an indication for caesarean section as the risk of neonatal herpes is low (3%). However, this should be discussed with the woman and a caesarean section can be performed if the woman wishes after balancing the risk of caesarean section versus the risk of fetal transmission of infections.

Women with recurrent genital herpes lesions and confirmed rupture of membranes at term should be advised to have delivery expedited by appropriate means.

Paediatricians should be involved from the beginning and have a plan for management of the neonate, e.g. close observation of the neonate for signs of herpes infection or intravenous acyclovir to the neonate if the mother opts to have vaginal delivery and had primary genital herpes within six weeks of delivery.

Royal College of Obstetricians and Gynaecologists. Green top Guideline No. 30. Management of genital herpes during pregnancy. London: RCOG, 2007.

32.11 Interventional radiology in obstetrics and gynaecology

A 40-year-old woman, para 4, presents to the labour ward at 39 weeks of gestation with spontaneous labour. She progresses quickly and has a spontaneous vaginal delivery. Fifteen minutes later, the placenta is delivered by controlled cord traction by a senior midwife. She then starts bleeding vaginally due to atonicity. The local protocol for the management of postpartum haemorrhage (PPH) is followed and all medical resources are exhausted. She is still bleeding and the estimated blood loss so far is 2.5 L.

1. Describe the indications for the use of interventional radiology techniques in both elective and emergency clinical situations in obstetrics.   Marks (12)

2. What are advantages of uterine artery embolisation (UAE) when used in the treatment of PPH? What are the complications of UAE following treatment of PPH?   Marks (8)

Key points

- para 4
- massive PPH
- interventional radiology
- indications for using interventional radiology: obstetrics
- side effects of interventional radiology
- pregnancy outcomes following interventional radiology

Essay plan

1.

- UAE
- the role of UAE in this case
- emergency indications in obstetrics
- elective indications in obstetrics
- vascular malformations in obstetrics

2.

- advantages of UAE: easy identification of bleeding site, preservation of fertility, decreased rebleeding rate and success rate of 94.9%

- complications of UAE (8.7%): low grade fever, pain, failure of embolisation requiring hysterectomy, pelvic infection, groin haematoma, iliac artery perforation, transient buttock ischaemia, transient foot ischaemia and bladder gangrene

32.11 Suggested answer

1.

UAE is a safe and effective alternative to hysterectomy in the management of PPH. It has been used to reduce or totally stop bleeding, both in obstetrics and gynaecology. It is now routinely included as part of the protocol in the management of PPH in hospitals in the UK. If resources and expertise are available, this is an effective method to stop the bleeding in this case.

Emergency indications: Obstetrics

It has a definitive role in atonic as well as traumatic PPH in obstetrics. This can occur following normal or prolonged labours and delivery with or without caesarean section (surgical complications or uterine tears at the caesarean section). It also has a role when the bleeding occurs postoperatively in the recovery room or in the ward following caesarean section or normal delivery. It has been used in the management of bleeding due to coagulopathy following obstetric hysterectomy.

Elective indications: Obstetrics

It has been included in care plans for placenta praevia and accreta. These conditions can be present in a scarred uterus (placenta praevia and accreta on a previous caesarean section scar) as well as an unscarred uterus.

UAE is the most effective management tool for haemorrhage caused by vascular malformations in the uterus (e.g. uterine artery malformations, arteriovenous fistula, arteriovenous malformations and pseudo aneurysm formation due to failure to secure the apex of a lateral extension at caesarean section). The usual presentation is painless, profuse secondary postpartum haemorrhage and can be difficult to diagnose clinically. A Doppler ultrasound scan ('to and fro' phenomenon) and angiography are helpful in making this diagnosis.

In such cases, one should remember not to rush to evacuate the uterus as this may worsen the bleeding.

2.

The advantages of UAE include easy identification of the bleeding site, preservation of the uterus and fertility, and decreased rebleeding from collaterals with more distal occlusion of the bleeding vessels. The reported success rate of UAE is 94.9%.

There is a risk of developing complications following UAE when used for treatment of PPH (8.7% of women develop complications). The common ones reported in the literature include low grade fever and pain, while the rarer ones include failure of embolisation requiring hysterectomy, pelvic infection, groin haematoma, iliac artery perforation, transient buttock ischaemia, transient foot ischaemia and bladder gangrene.

The return of menses and pregnancies have been reported following UAE for treatment of PPH. Ensure women are advised to use contraception if they do not want to conceive in the future.

Royal College of Obstetricians and Gynaecologists. Good Practice Guideline No. 6. The role of emergency and elective interventional radiology in post partum haemorrhage. London: RCOG Press, 2007.
Royal College of Obstetricians and Gynaecologists. Green-top Guideline No. 27. Placenta praevia and placenta praevia accreta: Diagnosis and management. London: RCOG Press, 2005.
Steer PJ. The surgical approach to postpartum haemorrhage. The Obstetrician & Gynaecologist 2009; 11:231–238.
Abu-Ghazza O, Hayes K, Chandraharan E, Belli A-M. Vascular malformations in relation to obstetrics and gynaecology: diagnosis and treatment. The Obstetrician & Gynaecologist 2010; 12:87–93.
Vedantham S, Goddwin SC, McLucas B, Mohr G. Uterine artery embolization: an underused method of controlling pelvic hemorrhage. Am J Obstet Gynecol 1997; 176:938–948.
Badaway SZA, Etman A, Singh M, Murphy K, Mayelli T, Philadelphia M. Uterine artery embolization: the role in obstetrics and gynecology. J Clin Imaging 2001; 25:288–295.

Note

The complications of UAE following treatment for fibroids are different from the complications of UAE following treatment for PPH (except low grade fever, pain and infection).

The complications of UAE following treatment of uterine fibroids include embolisation syndrome (women present with abdominal pain, low grade fever, vaginal discharge, nausea and vomiting), ischaemic pain, expulsion of the infarcted fibroid, sepsis (<1%), amenorrhoea and ovarian failure (5%). Therefore one should possibly avoid its use in non-pregnant women who wish to conceive in the future.

Future pregnancy implications following UAE for treatment of uterine fibroids include miscarriage (as high as 35.8%), pre-term delivery (16.1%), fetal growth restriction (7.3%), malpresentation (10.4%), postpartum haemorrhage (13.9%) and increased risk of caesarean delivery (67.2%). More studies would be necessary to assess the effects of UAE on pregnancy and fertility.

Homer H and Saridogan E. Pregnancy outcomes after uterine artery embolisation for fibroids. The Obstetrician & Gynaecologist 2009; 11:265–270.
Homer H and Saridogan E. Uterine artery embolization for fibroids is associated with an increased risk of miscarriage. Fertil Steril 2010; 94:324–330.
Kunde D and Khalaf Y. Alternatives to hysterectomy for treatment of uterine fibroids. The Obstetrician & Gynaecologist 2004; 6:215–221.

32.12 Maternal resuscitation

A 40-year-old woman is requesting her second lower segment caesarean section (LSCS). Her first LSCS was for placenta praevia and she wants to have at least five children.

1. What does she really need to know for the future. Two years later, she is a 42-year-old woman, para 4 (all LSCS), presenting with abdominal pain and severe shock at 34 weeks of gestation. Her routine 20 week scan showed major placenta praevia. An elective caesarean section was booked for 37 weeks of gestation. Thirty minutes later, she becomes unresponsive with an unrecordable pulse and blood pressure.

Marks (6)

2. What is the diagnosis and what would be the steps in her management?   Marks (7)

3. What are the principles in managing this woman?   Marks (7)

Key points
- 40 years old
- previous caesarean section
- major placenta praevia
- shock
- diagnosis
- management
- principles of management

Essay plan

1.

- placenta praevia
- placenta accreta
- increased morbidity and mortality
- increased caesarean section complications\
- ruptured uterus

2.

- intraperitoneal bleeding secondary to rupture uterus and placental bleeding (shock in the absence of vaginal bleeding)
- resuscitation (blood and blood products)
- perimortem caesarean section
- 2222 emergency calls (including major obstetric haemorrhage and cardiac arrest call)

3.

- resuscitation and delivery simultaneously
- time is crucial
- team approach to management
- mother comes first and baby next

32.12 Suggested answer

1.

- the risk of placenta praevia (PP) and placenta accreta (PA) increases proportionately with each previous caesarean section (0.26% in an unscarred uterus to 10% in women with four or more previous caesarean sections). The risk of placenta accreta also increases in association with placenta praevia and a previous caesarean section (5% in an unscarred uterus to 67% with previous four caesarean sections)
- other risk factors which increase the risk of placenta accreta in her case include advanced maternal age, placenta praevia and multiparity

- increased damage to the bowel, bladder and ureters due to adhesions secondary to previous surgeries
- increased maternal morbidity and mortality

2.

- the diagnosis is intraperitoneal bleeding. It may be secondary to rupture uterus or placenta accrete
- 2222 – always specify the nature of the call, hospital zone and exact location
- 2222 – cardiac arrest call
- 2222 – major obstetric haemorrhage call
- 2222 – obstetric emergency call
- resuscitation and delivery: remember the airway, breathing and circulation (ABC) routine
- perimortem caesarean section is recommended after 4 minutes

3.

- start thinking when you get a cardiac arrest or emergency call in obstetrics
- identify that this is an obstetric and medical emergency
- mother comes first and baby comes next. Do not worry about the baby, the ultimate goal is to save the mother
- time is the crucial factor to save this woman
- a synchronised team approach is essential for a better outcome
- perimortem caesarean section is recommended after 4 minutes
- aggressive resuscitation with a haematologist's input
- close monitoring in the intensive care unit after delivery

Managing Obstetric Emergencies and Trauma. The MOET Course Manual (2nd edn). MOET, 2007.
Magowan B. Churchill's Pocketbook of Obstetrics and Gynaecology (3rd edn). Edinburgh: Churchill Livingston, 2005.
Clark SL, Koonings PP, Phelan JP. Placenta previa/accreta and prior caesarean section. Obstet Gynecol 1985; 66:89–92.

32.13 Non-immune hydrops

A 30-year-old woman, para 2, attends the obstetric day assessment unit for reduced fetal movements at 27 weeks of gestation. Clinical examination reveals large for dates and a growth scan on the same day shows the fetus with generalised oedema and ascites. The blood group is Rhesus B positive and shows an absence of red cell antibodies.

1. What is the diagnosis? What are the possible causes?   Marks (6)

2. What should this woman be told?   Marks (6)

3. How should she be managed at this stage?   Marks (8)

Key points

- para 2
- reduced fetal movements

- large for dates
- ascites in fetus
- Rhesus positive
- absence of red cell antibodies

Essay plan

1.

- non-immune hydrops
- causes: haematological, structural (e.g. cardiac), infections, chromosomal, metabolic and idiopathic
- causes: maternal, fetal or placental

2.

- explain the diagnosis
- possible causes
- prognosis depends on the cause
- need further investigations to answer all the questions
- may need *in utero* blood transfusion

3.

- history
- examination
- investigation
- diagnosis
- management depends on the cause

32.13 Suggested answer

1.

The diagnosis in this case is non-immune hydrops (incidence is 1 in 1000). In one third of cases, the cause is idiopathic.

Other common causes include:

- chromosomal abnormalities (15%): especially trisomies, triploidy and Turner syndrome
- pulmonary (5%): diaphragmatic hernia and congenital pulmonary adenomatoid malformations
- cardiac (30%): structural abnormalities with tachyarrhythmias and congenital heart block
- renal abnormalities (3%): bladder neck obstruction
- haematological: α-thalassaemia, and G6PD deficiency
- infection (10%): parvovirus B19, cytomegalovirus, syphilis, rubella and toxoplasmosis
- tumours: sacrococcygeal teratoma
- twin to twin transfusion
- placental and cord lesions: chorioangioma

2.

It is important to involve her family and partner and give information about support groups to help her to understand the condition and make an informed choice. She should also see a counsellor in the hospital for further counselling and support through the pregnancy.

The prognosis depends on the cause and is usually poor if non-immune hydrops is discovered before 30 weeks of gestation. The risk of a chromosomal abnormality is high and therefore karyotyping will be offered.

Fetal blood transfusion is the treatment for hydrops secondary to anaemia.

In the case of parvovirus B19 infection, an *in utero* blood transfusion with 'O' Rhesus negative and cytomegalovirus irradiated red cells can be given to treat anaemia in severe cases. In mild cases which show improvement with further scans, no intervention or treatment may be necessary.

Fetal *in utero* surgery in the form of shunts (for pleural effusion or ascites) may be offered if all the investigations are normal or before planned delivery. It may also be appropriate to consider a termination of pregnancy with the detection of major anomalies and extreme prematurity. If the woman opts not to have a termination, she should be supported and delivery should be accomplished in a tertiary centre. The options can be either vaginal delivery or caesarean section but most often delivery is performed by caesarean section as it can be difficult to deliver a severely hydropic baby vaginally. She should be informed that caesarean section will not alter the outcome.

3.

She should be referred to a specialist fetal medicine unit (tertiary centre) for a detailed ultrasound scan (for detailed anatomic survey, fetal echocardiogram and Doppler) and other investigations.

The woman should be asked about any flu-like symptoms, recent infection, contact with infection, personal and family history of congenital or chromosomal abnormalities and family history of any rare metabolic disorders, e.g. Gaucher disease, gangliosidosis and G6PD deficiency.

Fetal karyotyping (fetal blood sampling or amniocentesis) should be offered as the risk of chromosomal abnormalities is high (but only if >22 weeks). The other tests that can be carried out with fetal blood sampling include full blood count (FBC), blood group and direct Coombs test, serology for viral infection (e.g. parvovirus B19 IgG and IgM antibodies to detect recent infection) and haemoglobin electrophoresis.

Peak systolic velocity of the middle cerebral artery should be arranged and if found to be high indicates fetal anaemia. This is an indication for cord blood sampling. If severe anaemia is detected, *in utero* transfusion is indicated especially with parvovirus infection (spontaneous resolution occurs in 1 in 3 cases).

A fetal echocardiogram should be arranged to determine the heart rate and rhythm and to rule out cardiac abnormalities. The prognosis is poor with congenital heart block if associated with structural abnormalities (because the abnormality is usually severe). The outcome is variable (if hydropic <50% survive and if not hydropic they are usually fine) or good if the fetus is structurally normal. *In utero* treatment with maternal administration of steroids has been associated with resolution in some cases. Tachyarrhythmias can be treated by giving transplacental therapy (through the mother) or direct fetal therapy (flecainide).

Maternal serum screening for infection (toxoplasma, rubella, cytomegalovirus, herpes simplex and syphilis), FBC and electrophoresis (haemoglobinopathies), and anti-Ro and anti-La antibodies (congenital heart block) should be performed to identify respective causes.

Twin-to-twin transfusion can be treated by ablating the connecting vessels.

The neonatal team should be involved early in both counselling the mother and management of the baby.

A termination of pregnancy can be offered if major anomalies are detected or in case of extreme prematurity. If the mother opts to continue the pregnancy, delivery should be arranged at the tertiary centre.

James D, Steer PJ, Weiner CP, Gonik B, Crowther C, Robson S (eds). High Risk Pregnancy: Management Options (4th edn). St Louis: Saunders, 2011.

32.14 Obstetric cholestasis 1

A 35-year-old primigravida attends the obstetric day assessment unit at 34 weeks of gestation with itchy palms and soles of her feet for the previous 2 weeks. It is worse at night and not relieved with the local application of an emollient. Clinical examination reveals no rash on the body.

1. What is the aetiology of obstetric cholestasis (OC)?   (3 marks)

2. How would one confirm the diagnosis of obstetric cholestasis in this woman?   (3 marks)

3. Enumerate the risks to the fetus.   (4 marks)

4. Enumerate the risks to the mother.   (2 marks)

5. Critically discuss the use of drug therapy in this case. When would one deliver this woman and why?   (8 marks)

Key points
- primigravida
- 34 weeks of gestation
- itchy palms and soles
- absence of rash
- obstetric cholestasis

Essay plan
1.

- aetiology
- multifactorial

- oestrogens
- ethnic origin
- genetic

2.

- diagnosis is by exclusion
- past and family history
- liver function test and bile acids
- tests for hepatitis B and C
- cytomegalovirus
- Epstein–Barr virus
- autoimmune screen
- liver ultrasound scan for gallstones, fatty liver and cirrhosis

3.

- fetal risks
- premature delivery
- intrauterine death
- meconium staining of amniotic fluid
- fetal distress
- intracranial haemorrhage

4.

- maternal risks
- unable to sleep
- poor quality of life
- postpartum haemorrhage
- depletion of vitamin K dependent clotting factors

5.

- symptomatic relief – emollients, antihistamines
- ursodeoxycholic acid unlicensed during pregnancy
- cholestyramine
- vitamin K
- delivery at 37 weeks of gestation (no evidence to refute or accept)

32.14 Suggested answer

1.

OC is multifactorial and oestrogen appears to be the main culprit involved. The levels of oestrogen are highest in the third trimester and this is the time most women will present with this condition. A similar condition is seen in women taking combined oral contraceptive pills (COCPs).

The mechanism by which oestrogen acts is unclear. It is postulated that oestrogen causes disruption of the membrane transport mechanisms in the hepatocytes and bile ducts leading to an altered cholesterol:phospholipid ratio.

Family history is positive in 33–50% of patients and there is a possible suggestion of an autosomal dominant inheritance pattern. Geographically, the highest rates have been reported in South America, especially in Chile (12–22%) and the lowest in Europe (0.2%).

2.

The diagnosis is one of exclusion. Information regarding family history, similar symptoms with use of the COCP, and previous pregnancies should be obtained.

Other conditions including liver disease, alcohol abuse, drug history (methyldopa) and viral hepatitis should be excluded.

Liver function is altered in this condition. The typical abnormality is a 2–4-fold rise in the serum transaminases. The bile acid shows a 10–100-fold increase in levels. This is particularly helpful when the transaminase levels are normal.

Finally, other causes of cholestasis should be excluded. The investigations include ultrasound (to exclude gall stones), hepatic serology (A, B, C, Epstein–Barr virus and cytomegalovirus) and screening for autoimmune liver disease such as chronic active hepatitis (anti-smooth muscle antibodies) and primary biliary cirrhosis (anti-mitochondrial antibodies).

3.

The risks to the fetus are a higher rate of intrauterine death, stillbirth, perinatal death, meconium staining of the liquor, intrapartum fetal distress, spontaneous or iatrogenic pre-term delivery and intracranial haemorrhage due to vitamin K deficiency.

4.

The risk to the mother is decreased absorption of fat-soluble vitamins (especially vitamin K). This will lead to the depletion of vitamin K-dependent clotting factors (II, VII, IX, X) and therefore increased risk of postpartum haemorrhage (PPH).

Lack of sleep due to severe itching may result in a poor quality of life.

5.

Symptomatic relief is the first step in the management.

Antihistamines (chlorpheniramine, promethazine) have been routinely used in the hope of relieving itching. This may not be helpful in all cases.

Topical emollients are safe but their efficacy is unknown.

An exogenous bile acid, ursodeoxycholic acid, is increasingly used during pregnancy in the management of OC. It has been shown to improve the pruritus symptoms and liver function but whether it improves perinatal mortality and morbidity is unknown. It is currently unlicensed in pregnancy.

Other drugs which have been used in the treatment include S-adenosylmethionine, dexamethasone and cholestyramine. Cholestyramine causes steatorrhoea and deficiency of fat-soluble vitamins.

The use of water-soluble vitamin K (menadiol sodium phosphate) in doses of 5–10 mg daily is indicated when the prothrombin time is prolonged. If the prothrombin time is normal, water-soluble vitamin K (menadiol sodium phosphate) in low doses should be used only after careful counselling about the likely benefits. Postnatal vitamin K must be offered to babies in the usual way.

The Royal College of Obstetricians and gynaecologists (RCOG) recommends induction of labour after 37 weeks of gestation in patients with a biochemical abnormality (raised transaminases and bile acids). The patient should be informed of the increased risk of perinatal morbidity and maternal morbidity with early intervention (induction). They should also be informed about the inability to predict stillbirth if the pregnancy continues. Due to associated fetal risks, close monitoring is advised during labour. Active management of the third stage of labour is advocated in view of the increased risk of PPH.

Anthony K and Nelson-Piercy C. Obstetric Cholestasis. Personal assessment in continuing education. Reviews, questions and answers. Volume 3. London: RCOG Press, 2003: 48–49.
Royal College of Obstetricians and Gynaecologists. Green-top Guideline No. 43. Obstetric cholestasis. London: RCOG Press, 2011.

32.15 Obstetric cholestasis 2

A 35-year-old woman, para 2 (spontaneous vaginal deliveries), presents to the obstetric day assessment unit at 29 weeks of gestation with severe generalised itching.

1. What questions should one ask this woman in her history and what investigations should one recommend and why?   Marks (8)

2. She attends the day assessment unit 1 week later and the blood test confirms OC. How would you manage her and why?   Marks (8)

3. She has a normal vaginal delivery following an induction of labour at 38 weeks of gestation. Her alanine aminotransferase is 100 IU/L and bilirubin 16 μmol/L at the time of delivery. She feels well and wants to be discharged. What should be discussed and recommended to her and give the reasoning.   Marks (4)

Key points
- para 2
- 29 weeks of gestation
- generalised itching
- obstetric cholestasis

Essay plan
1.
- details of itching
- previous history of OC
- past history of similar symptoms while on the combined oral contraceptive pill (COCP)
- family history

- skin diseases and rash
- drug history
- liver enzymes
- liver scan
- rule out other liver pathology (hepatitis and autoimmune)

2.

- symptomatic and supportive therapy
- drug therapy
- delivery at 37–38 weeks of gestation

3.

- no long-term effects
- generally symptoms resolve after delivery
- need for repeat liver function tests (LFTs) in 10 days after delivery to check resolution
- risk of recurrence in future pregnancy
- risk of recurrence of symptoms with COCP use, therefore avoid COCP
- risk of other family members suffering with similar symptoms

32.15 Suggested answer

1.

History

The most likely diagnosis in a woman presenting with itching in the third trimester is OC. However, it is a diagnosis of exclusion. The nature of itching is generalised or confined to the palms of the hands and the soles of the feet which is often the case in OC. The woman notices that it is often worse at night, affecting her quality of life due to the irresistible itching. There may also be mild jaundice, pale stools and dark urine with OC.

It is important to ask if this woman had similar symptoms in her previous two pregnancies as OC tends to recur in subsequent pregnancies.

One needs to exclude other causes of itching during pregnancies, e.g. chronic skin conditions such as eczema, bullous skin condition pemphigoid and polymorphic eruption of pregnancy.

The new concept of genetic association of OC now requires asking whether similar symptoms are present in members of the family.

Any history is not complete without a drug history as drug reactions can lead to skin rash and also itching.

Investigations

OC is a diagnosis of exclusion.

Baseline LFTs, especially serum transaminases and bile acid levels, are important and these have been found to be raised in OC.

Other causes for deranged LFT and liver pathology should be ruled out by doing the following tests:

- blood test for autoimmune screen, e.g. anti-smooth muscle antibody, anti-mitochondrial antibody
- blood test for hepatitis A, B, C and E, Epstein–Barr virus and cytomegalovirus
- liver ultrasound scan for gallstones, fatty liver and cirrhosis

2.

Management is mainly symptomatic and supportive.

The woman's quality of life is affected with severe itching. Antihistamines should be liberally prescribed and advised to be taken, especially during night-time. If taken during the day, the woman should avoid driving.

Emollients for local application are also important to avoid skin dryness and to break the itch-scratch-itch cycle.

The use of water-soluble vitamin K (menadiol sodium phosphate) in doses of 5–10 mg daily is indicated when prothrombin time is prolonged (there is a theoretical risk of postpartum haemorrhage (PPH) and haemorrhagic disease in the newborn of women with OC).

Most maternity units prescribe ursodeoxycholic acid (UDCA) as it has been shown to improve symptoms but has no effect on fetal outcome. However, the woman needs to be told that it is unlicensed for pregnancy and may not improve fetal outcome.

If LFTs are normal and the symptoms persist, LFTs should be repeated at least weekly.

The woman should be asked about fetal movements at every visit.

Most maternity units ask the woman to come in for fetal monitoring in the form of a weekly cardiotocograph (CTG) and to arrange scans for umbilical artery Doppler. However, this is not evidence-based and has no predictive value.

A plan should be made for time, mode and place of delivery.

Most maternity units deliver these women at 37–38 weeks of gestation. However, there is no evidence to accept or refute this management. Such management is in practice due to the risk of unexplained stillbirth in women with OC. The woman should be informed about the increased risk of perinatal and maternal morbidity with early intervention.

She should obviously be delivered in the hospital with close fetal monitoring during labour. OC is not a contraindication for vaginal delivery and caesarean section is indicated only for obstetric complications.

Active management of the third stage of labour may be used due to theoretical risk of PPH.

3.

OC does not have long-term effects on the mother and symptoms normally resolve following delivery. The Royal College of Obstetricians and Gynaecologists (RCOG) recommends a repeat follow-up LFT on day 10 post delivery to check if the liver function tests have returned to normal.

The woman should be warned that this condition may recur in subsequent pregnancies and she should be screened for this condition at 28 weeks of gestation or earlier if symptomatic. She should be advised to avoid the oestrogen-containing COCP as it may cause similar conditions. She should also be warned that other members of the family are at risk of developing this condition in view of the genetic association.

Anthony K and Nelson-Piercy C. Obstetric Cholestais. Personal assessment in continuing education. Reviews, questions and answers. Volume 3. London: RCOG Press, 2003: 48–49.
Royal College of Obstetricians and Gynaecologists. Green-top Guideline No. 43. Obstetric Cholestasis. London: RCOG Press, 2011.

32.16 Operative vaginal delivery

A 32-year-old woman, para 0, is induced at 41 weeks of gestation for pre-eclampsia. She has made good progress in labour and has been fully dilated for the last 140 minutes. She has been actively pushing for 80 minutes and now feels tired and needs assistance. She is contracting four in 10 minutes on abdominal palpitation and on vaginal examination the cervix is fully dilated with the fetal head in the occipito-transverse position. The station of the fetal head is below spines (+1) with minimal caput and moulding.

1.   What are the prerequisites for safe instrumental vaginal delivery?   Marks (8)

2.   The woman chooses to have only ventouse delivery. What serious risks should be discussed before undertaking delivery?   Marks (4)

3.   What additional procedures should one discuss with this woman undergoing ventouse delivery and why?   Marks (8)

Key points
- prolonged second stage
- maternal exhaustion
- need for instrumental delivery

Essay plan

1.

- pre requisites
- full dilatation
- absence of membranes
- bladder empty
- assessment of correct fetal position
- lithotomy position
- cephalic – less than one fifth palpable per abdomen
- analgesia
- skill of operator
- presence of paediatrician

2.

- maternal risks
- fetal risks

3.

- episiotomy and suturing
- manual rotation
- caesarean section
- suturing of third- and fourth-degree tears
- manoeuvres for shoulder dystocia
- blood transfusion

32.16 Suggested answer

1.

A careful assessment in relation to the clinical context, examination (abdominal and vaginal) and clear communication with the mother are essential before undertaking operative vaginal delivery.

The essential prerequisites before operative vaginal delivery include:

- fetal head – less than one fifth palpable per abdomen
- full dilatation of the cervix and absence of membranes
- vertex presentation and determination of the exact position which helps the correct use of the type of instrument and application of the instrument
- good analgesia, e.g. perineal infiltration and pudendal block
- aseptic techniques
- empty the bladder or remove the indwelling catheter
- operator skills and knowledge in using the instruments with a backup plan in case of failure of the instrumental delivery
- paediatrician should be present for delivery

2.

The serious maternal and fetal risks include:

- third- and fourth-degree tears (1–4 in 100)
- extensive vaginal and vulval tear (1 in 10)
- subgaleal haematoma (3–6 in 1000)
- intracranial haemorrhage (5–15 in 10,000)
- facial nerve palsy

3.

The following additional procedures need to be discussed with the woman:

- episiotomy – performed with instrumental deliveries to increase the space and assist delivery (5–6 out of 10 ventouse deliveries)
- manoeuvres for shoulder dystocia – operative vaginal delivery is one of the risk factors for shoulder dystocia and should be anticipated in advance

- blood transfusion – instrumental delivery can be associated with extensive vaginal and vulval tear resulting in traumatic postpartum haemorrhage (PPH). There may also be an element of atonic PPH (1–4 in 10 instrumental deliveries)
- repair of perineal tear – instrumental delivery is associated with third- and fourth-degree perineal tears (1–4 in 100 ventouse deliveries)
- manual rotation – prior to ventouse delivery
- caesarean section – in case of failure of ventouse delivery

Royal College of Obstetricians and Gynaecologists. Consent Advice No. 11. Operative vaginal delivery. London: RCOG Press, 2010.
Royal College of Obstetricians and Gynaecologists. Guideline No. 26. Operative vaginal delivery. London: RCOG Press, 2005.

32.17 Perinatal mental health

A 29-year-old woman, para 1, attends her antenatal booking (her first midwife appointment) visit at 14 weeks of gestation. She lives alone as she is separated from her partner. She had severe postnatal depression following her last pregnancy.

1. How can mental illness be predicted in a pregnant woman?   Marks (4)

2. What are the risk factors for postnatal depression?   Marks (4)

3. What are the effects of depression on the mother?   Marks (6)

4. What are the effects of maternal depression and treatment on the fetus? Marks (6)

Key points

- mental illness
- pregnant
- risk factors and postpartum depression
- effects of depression on mother
- effects of depression on fetus
- effects of maternal treatment on fetus

Essay plan

1.

- self-reporting
- current history
- past history
- fixed questionnaire

2.

- risk factors
- postpartum depression

3.

- physical
- mental

4.

- prenatal
- neonatal
- childhood

32.17 Suggested answer

1.

It can be self-reported by the patient or the health professional can ask specific questions at first contact, e.g. (a) During the past month, have you often been bothered by feeling down, depressed or hopeless? (b) During the past month, have you often been bothered by having little interest or pleasure in doing things?

A simple questionnaire for depression is part of routine antenatal care in the UK.

Elicit her history about current or past mental illness, past history of treatment by a mental health team and family history of perinatal mental illness.

2.

The risk factors for postpartum depression include: personal and family history of mental illness, depression in current pregnancy, medical disorders during pregnancy, multiple problems with pregnancy, previous history of postpartum depression and sometimes there are no risk factors.

3.

These women are more likely to self-harm, eat less, take less personal care, fail to attend the antenatal clinic regularly, and more likely to smoke and take recreational drugs. Their interpersonal relationships with other people can be stressful and emotional. Physical bonding with the baby can be disrupted.

Their quality of life is diminished with increased personal suffering and this leads to increased morbidity during pregnancy and an increased likelihood of attempting suicide.

The use of higher doses of venlafaxine is associated with raised blood pressure.

There is an increased risk of gestational diabetes and weight gain with the use of olanzapine.

4.

The fetal effects during pregnancy include pre-term birth, low birth weight and low apgar scores. Increased serum cortisol and catecholamine levels may induce adverse changes in placental function by altering uterine blood flow and inducing uterine irritability.

The potential prenatal side effects on the fetus include physical malformations or anomalies (Ebstein anomaly with lithium, cleft palate with benzodiazepines and omphalocele with paroxetine and sertraline), fetal growth restriction and intrauterine death. The neonatal problems include withdrawal symptoms with almost all antidepressants (usually mild and self-limiting), respiratory distress although mild, tremors, jitteriness, decreased muscle tone, low blood sugar, behavioural problems and, rarely, seizures.

Clozapine is associated with agranulocytosis in the fetus and breastfed infants.

Children born to depressed mothers are more likely to have behavioural problems and/or disruption in cognitive and emotional development.

National Institute of Health and Clinical Excellence. Antenatal and postnatal mental health: clinical management and service guidance (CG45). NICE, 2007.

Louik C, Lin AE, Werler MM, Hernández-Díaz S, Mitchell AA. First-trimester use of selective serotonin-reuptake inhibitors and the risk of birth defects. N Engl J Med 2007; 356:2675–2683.

Alwan S, Reefhuis J, Rasmussen SA, Olney RS, Friedman JM. Selective serotonin-reuptake inhibitors and risk of persistent pulmonary hypertension of the newborn. N Engl J Med 2007; 356:2684–2692.

Chambers CD, Hernández-Díaz S, Van Marter LJ, et al. Bupropion-SR, sertraline, or venlafaxine-XR after failure of SSRIs for depression. N Engl J Med 2006; 354:579–587.

Department of Health. http://www.dh.gov.uk

32.18 Polyhydramnios

A 40-year-old multiparous woman attends her antenatal appointment at 28 weeks of gestation. As her uterus measures 34 cm, she is sent for a scan, which reveals polyhydramnios and a single intrauterine fetus. Her booking (first midwife appointment) blood tests are normal and a dating scan shows a single intrauterine pregnancy with a normal nuchal fold translucency.

1. Define polyhydramnios and describe the principal causes.   Marks (6)

2. One week later she attends the antenatal clinic with the results of the investigations. All the investigations are normal (an infection screen for TORCH [**T**oxoplasmosis; **O**ther infections – syphilis, Varicella-Zoster virus, parvovirus B19 and hepatitis B; **R**ubella; **C**ytomegalovirus; **H**erpes simplex virus], a detailed scan for fetus in the fetal medicine unit and an oral glucose tolerance test). What are the risks associated with polyhydramnios?   Marks (4)

3. What is the diagnosis in this case and how should she be managed and why?   Marks (10)

Key points
- 40 years old
- measures 34 cm (therefore clinically large for dates)
- single intrauterine pregnancy
- polyhydramnios

Essay plan

1.

- define polyhydramnios
- causes of polyhydramnios

2.

- risk of polyhydramnios: pressure symptoms, maternal risks, fetal risks

3.

- diagnosis in this case: idiopathic polyhydramnios as all investigations are normal
- outline management and justify why that is being done

32.18 Suggested answer

1.

Polyhydramnios is defined as an amniotic fluid index (AFI) above the 95th centile which can be divided into mild, moderate and severe depending on the depth of the liquor:

- Maternal causes: idiopathic or maternal diabetes
- Fetal causes: congenital anomalies of the gut which affect fetal swallowing (muscular dystrophies, anencephaly and intestinal obstruction including oesophageal), fetal infections (TORCH), fetal anaemia leading to cardiac failure (parvovirus infection and alloimmunisation), Rhesus isoimmunisation and sacrococcygeal teratoma

2.

For the mother, risks include pressure symptoms due to abdominal distension (abdominal discomfort, pain and difficulty in breathing), pre-term labour, pre-term premature rupture of membranes, cord prolapse, abruption and postpartum haemorrhage (PPH). There is also a risk of an unstable lie of the baby which may require caesarean section for delivery.

Mirror syndrome is a rare condition affecting pregnant women that is characterised by maternal oedema, albuminuria and pre-eclampsia (there is an unusual association of fetal hydrops with maternal pre-eclampsia) and fetal hydrops (fetal symptoms are related to fluid retention due to ascites and polyhydramnios).

3.

The diagnosis in this case is idiopathic polyhydramnios as all investigations are normal. The aims of management are maternal comfort and prolonging the pregnancy.

If the woman is asymptomatic and presenting with mild polyhydramnios, no further treatment is necessary; if she is symptomatic with moderate or severe polyhydramnios, therapeutic amnioreduction may be necessary to relieve maternal pressure symptoms. This may also improve the perinatal outcome. Repeated taps may be necessary due to reaccumulation of the amniotic fluid. She should be thoroughly counselled as this procedure is associated with risks which include pre-term premature rupture of membranes, chorioamnionitis, membrane detachment and placental abruption.

Conventionally, various medical treatments have been tried. Salt restriction has not shown any proven benefit and diuretics are harmful as they can reduce the uteroplacental perfusion. Indomethacin has been used and shown to reduce liquor volume. However, one should be cautious and stop the drug by 34 weeks of gestation as it can cause premature closure of the ductus arteriosus and impaired renal function in the fetus.

Maternal corticosteroids should be considered if delivery is anticipated soon. In moderate to severe polyhydramnios, elective induction of labour and the controlled artificial rupture of membranes in theatre (ideal) should be considered as there is an increased risk of cord prolapse and abruption with spontaneous rupture of membranes. The pregnancy is considered high risk for labour and continuous fetal monitoring is advised during labour in view of the high risk of cord prolapse. Unstable lie of the baby may necessitate a caesarean section as the mode of delivery.

James D, Steer PJ, Weiner CP, Gonik B, Crowther C, Robson S (eds). High Risk Pregnancy: Management Options (4th edn). St Louis: Saunders, 2011.

32.19 Postdated pregnancy

A 39-year-old woman, para 0, attends the antenatal clinic at 41 weeks of gestation. She has good fetal movements and the fundal height measures 39 cm.

1. What are her management options and why? Marks (6)

2. What are the complications of induction of labour (IOL) and how can they be prevented or managed? Marks (6)

3. She chooses expectant management beyond 42 weeks of gestation. How should one monitor her? What are the risks of going beyond 42 weeks of gestation? Marks (8)

Key points
- postdated
- 41 weeks of gestation
- induction of labour

Essay plan

1.

- expectant
- membrane sweep
- IOL

2.

- uterine hyperstimulation
- fetal distress
- failed IOL
- cord prolapse
- uterine rupture

3.

- increased antenatal monitoring
- twice weekly cardiotocograph (CTG)
- ultrasound examination of maximum pool depth
- weekly umbilical artery Doppler
- monitor fetal movements
- no method of fetal monitoring is predictive of future wellbeing
- meconium staining of liquor
- intrauterine fetal death and stillbirth
- placental insufficiency
- intrapartum asphyxia of fetus
- increased risk of long labour, failed induction, epidural anaesthesia, instrumental delivery and shoulder dystocia

32.19 Suggested answer

1.

Most women will go into labour by 41 weeks of gestation. Expectant management is therefore not an unreasonable option.

Membrane sweeping promotes the onset of spontaneous labour and hence reduces the need for formal IOL. However, she should be warned about the discomfort and vaginal spotting following the procedure.

IOL should be offered between 41 and 42 weeks as the risks outweigh the benefits beyond 42 weeks. She should be informed about when, where and how the IOL is carried out, pain relief, method of induction, options if she does not want IOL or if IOL fails. The woman's preferences and local circumstances should also be taken into account.

2.

Complications of IOL are listed below.

Uterine hyperstimulation

Uterine hyperstimulation is a known complication with prostaglandin use for IOL. Tocolysis should be considered if this occurs during IOL.

Failed IOL

If IOL fails, the woman should be supported and reassured. Fetal monitoring with CTG should be used to assess fetal wellbeing. A second attempt of IOL can be made or she can be offered a caesarean section. This entirely depends on the woman's wishes or the clinical circumstances.

Cord prolapse

Artifical rupture of the membranes should be avoided if the presenting part is high in the pelvis or there is cord presentation.

Uterine rupture

If uterine rupture is suspected, the baby should be delivered by emergency caesarean section.

Also, check for placental location by reviewing the 20 week scan in order to avoid membrane sweep or IOL in women with a low-lying placenta.

3.

A pregnancy extended to or beyond 42 weeks of gestation is termed a prolonged pregnancy. It occurs in 10.3% of pregnant women. Certain complications are common with a prolonged pregnancy and these include meconium aspiration, fetal compromise (perinatal morbidity) and fetal death (perinatal mortality). As the baby continues to grow there is also an increased risk of shoulder dystocia and the need for an operative delivery. For the woman, there is an increased need for IOL and oxytocin stimulation of labour.

Fetal surveillance and IOL are the two strategies employed that may reduce the risk of an adverse outcome. If the woman declines IOL, the National Institute of health and Clinical Excellence (NICE) recommends twice-weekly CTG and measurement of amniotic fluid depth by ultrasound.

Daily fetal movement assessment should be initiated beyond 41 weeks. At 42 weeks of gestation a nipple stimulation contraction stress test and biophysical profile are suggested but not used in UK practice. However, opinion regarding the effectiveness of fetal surveillance methods, ideal methods and timing and frequency of methods is not clear.

National Institute of Health and Clinical Excellence. Induction of labour (CG70). NICE, 2008. www.nice.org.uk/CG070FullGuideline
Jetti A, Poovali S, Stanley PK. Prolonged pregnancy. Obstet Gynaecol Reprod Med 2008; 18:7–11.

32.20 Postpartum haemorrhage

A 40-year-old woman, para 5, delivered vaginally 1 hour ago, complains of increased vaginal bleeding with clots.

1. What is primary postpartum haemorrhage (PPH)? What are the risk factors for primary PPH?
    What are the main causes of primary PPH?   Marks (7)

2. What are your steps in the initial management of uterine atony in this woman?   Marks (6)

3. What is secondary PPH? What are the causes of secondary PPH? How should a woman with secondary PPH be managed?   Marks (7)

Key points

- 40 years old
- para 5
- vaginal delivery

- primary PPH
- uterine atony
- secondary PPH

Essay plan

1.

- primary PPH: <24 hours after delivery (>500 mL)

Risk factors

- grand multiparity
- obesity
- macrosomia
- increased maternal age
- antepartum haemorrhage
- previous PPH
- prolonged labour
- operative delivery

Causes

- uterine atony
- retained placenta
- partially retained placental bits or membranes
- placenta accreta
- vaginal tears
- coagulopathy

2.

- obstetric crash call 2222

Management

- resuscitation (airway, breathing and circulation [ABC])
- oxygen mask
- rub up contractions
- bladder empty
- oxytocin infusion
- ergometrine intravenously or intramuscularly
- carboprost intramuscularly (Hemabate)
- transfer to theatre

3.

- secondary PPH: >24 hours after delivery
- most common cause: infected products
- caesarean section incision
- vessels in the placental bed (arteriovenous malformations)
- hydatidiform mole
- choriocarcinoma

Management

- vaginal swab
- intravenous antibiotics
- resuscitation
- evacuation of the uterus under general anaesthesia

32.20 Suggested answer

1.

Primary PPH was one of the major causes of maternal mortality reported during 2000–2002, according to the Confidential Enquiry into Maternal and Child Health (CEMACH) report.

Primary PPH is defined as blood loss >500 mL within 24 hours following delivery.

The risk factors for primary PPH include increased maternal age, increased maternal parity, obesity, macrosomic fetus, antepartum haemorrhage, previous PPH, prolonged labour, and operative vaginal or abdominal delivery.

The main causes of primary PPH include:

- uterine atony (90% of cases)
- retained placenta
- retained bits of placenta or membranes
- placenta accreta and praevia
- genital tract trauma
- coagulopathy

The mnemonic to remember is four Ts:

- tone – atony
- tissue – retained tissue
- trauma – genital trauma
- thrombin – coagulation disorder

2.

If there is excessive vaginal bleeding post delivery one should ask for more help (obstetric crash call 2222). A large bore cannula should already be *in situ* and she should be on oxytocin infusion for active management of the third stage of labour. Another large bore cannula should be instituted and 2 L of crystalloids started followed by a colloid. Blood should be cross-matched and transfused appropriately. There should be an allotted person to write down the times treatment was initiated, the type of treatment given, blood loss, amounts of fluids given, vital signs and urine output. An oxygen mask should be placed over the patient's face.

The obstetrician should lead the scene. The initial step is to rub up contractions, expel blood clots and ensure that the bladder is empty. Oxytocin infusion should be continued and ergometrine 500 µg should be administered intravenously or intramuscularly depending on the amount of bleeding. If the bleeding continues, the contractions should be rubbed up and intramuscular haemobate 250 µg should be administered every 15 minutes – a maximum dose of 2 mg can be given. However, after two doses, one should be cautious and a decision should be made to transfer the woman to theatre. Further management should be undertaken under general anaesthesia, e.g. uterine balloon insertion, B Lynch suture, internal iliac artery ligation and hysterectomy.

A consultant obstetrician should be called for help by the time 2 litres of blood is lost.

3.

Secondary PPH is defined as any excessive bleeding after 24 hours following delivery.

The most common cause is infected retained products. A vaginal swab should be taken for culture and sensitivity before commencing intravenous broad spectrum antibiotics which are effective against anaerobic and aerobic organisms. The woman should be appropriately resuscitated if necessary and an evacuation of the uterus performed under general anaesthesia. This can be postponed to 12–24 hours post antibiotics to prevent septicaemia unless there is excessive vaginal bleeding which is uncontrollable.

Other causes include:

- bleeding from the caesarean section incision
- bleeding from the placental bed
- hydatidiform mole
- choriocarcinoma
- uterine artery malformations
- arteriovenous fistula and arteriovenous malformations
- pseudo aneurysm formation due to failure to secure the apex of a lateral extension at caesarean section

The last three conditions are rare and the usual presentation is painless, profuse secondary PPH which is difficult to diagnose clinically. A Doppler ultrasound scan ('to and fro' phenomenon) and angiography are helpful in making a diagnosis. Uterine artery embolisation or a hysterectomy will be necessary to stop the bleeding.

If the bleeding is related to a molar pregnancy, advice from a regional trophoblastic centre should be sought (Charing Cross, Sheffield and Dundee in the UK).

Letsky E, Murphy MF, Ramsay JE, Walker I. Haemorrhagic Disease and Hereditary Bleeding Disorders. London: RCOG Press, 2005.

32.21 Recurrent urinary tract infection

A 34-year-old primigravida presents to the obstetric day assessment unit at 28 weeks of gestation with symptoms of urinary tract infection (UTI). She had previously had two episodes of proven UTI during this pregnancy and was treated with antibiotics.

1. What should she be asked in her history?   Marks (6)

2. Critically evaluate the investigations that should be arranged for her.   Marks (7)

3. How should she be managed and why?   Marks (7)

Key points

- 34 years old
- primigravida
- 28 weeks of gestation
- UTI
- history
- investigation
- management

Essay plan

1.

- symptoms (bladder, kidney and stone)
- signs (unwell, raised temperature)
- rule out diabetes
- systemic lupus erythematoses (SLE)
- stones
- kidney anomalies and disease

2.

- urine dipstick
- midstream urine
- renal ultrasound (KUB)
- blood sugar/glucose tolerance test (GTT)
- urea and electrolytes
- full blood count (FBC) and C-reactive protein (CRP)
- obstetric ultrasound scan for fetal growth and wellbeing
- cardiotocograph (CTG) and/or umbilical artery Doppler

3.

- current management: treatment with antibiotics
- future management: prophylactic antibiotic till delivery

32.21 Suggested answer

1.

A detailed history of symptoms should be asked regarding suprapubic pain, renal pain, renal colic pain, frequency of micturition, painful micturition, haematuria and raised temperature (rigors and shivering episodes).

One should rule out a history of diabetes, SLE, past history of renal stones, renal anomalies (horseshoe-shaped kidneys, double ureter and pelvic kidney) and other renal diseases such as polycystic kidneys.

Also ask history regarding uterine contractions, spontaneous rupture of membranes (SROM) and fetal movements as women with UTI are at risk of going into pre-term labour.

2.

Urine dipstick is not sufficiently specific to detect UTI. Urine culture and sensitivity is important as this will provide the information regarding the antibiotic sensitivity of the organism. The urine sample (MSU) should be a clean catch sample of the mid-stream urine. Otherwise, it is associated with the risk of contaminated samples and this may prevent growing the specific organism causing the UTI.

Blood cultures should be performed if there are systemic signs of infection.

Renal ultrasound is important in women with recurrent UTI to exclude renal stones, kidney disease (renal scarring, hydronephrosis, pyonephrosis and polycystic kidney disease) and renal anomalies (horseshoe-shaped kidneys, double ureter and pelvic kidney).

Blood sugar can be done to rule out diabetes but it may be better to perform a GTT.

A baseline renal function test (urea, creatinine) should be performed. These can be deranged in kidney disease. Blood tests for electrolytes (to correct imbalance), FBC and CRP are indicated and improvement in these markers may indicate a response to medical therapy.

It is important to assess the fetal wellbeing. A CTG can be performed and an obstetric ultrasound arranged for growth and liquor.

3.

Current management

Her previous MSU reports should be reviewed for antibiotic sensitivity before initiation of a further course of antibiotic treatment. If there is any doubt, one should consult the microbiologist regarding initiation of the type of antibiotics. Once the current MSU culture results are available, specific antibiotics should be added or excluded depending on the sensitivity of the organism to the antibiotics. If the woman does not respond to any of these therapies, one should contact the microbiologist for further advice.

If it is just simple cystitis and there are no systemic signs of infection, she can be treated with oral antibiotics and sent home to be followed up in the antenatal clinic in 1 week.

If there are systemic signs of infection and the woman is unwell, she should be admitted, intravenous antibiotics administered to treat the infection, regular paracetamol given for normalising her temperature and intravenous fluids given to correct dehydration. Once stabilised, she could be switched to oral antibiotics for 5–7 days and then followed up in the antenatal clinic in 1 week. A repeat MSU after the completion of the treatment would be useful to ensure the infection has been completely treated.

She should be referred to a urologist if indicated.

It is important to assess the fetal wellbeing. A CTG should be performed and an obstetric ultrasound arranged for growth and liquor.

Future management

Since this woman is getting recurrent UTIs during this pregnancy, she is at risk of developing a further episode of UTI, pyelonephritis and permanent kidney damage due to scarring. The other risks include fetal growth restriction and premature labour. Paediatricians should be informed regarding her condition and she should be admitted to hospital as appropriate.

To prevent her from getting a further recurrent UTI, she should be started on long-term prophylactic oral antibiotics until delivery, depending on the sensitivity of the organism. These sensitivities can change from time to time and therefore a repeat MSU should be performed if the woman presents with symptoms of UTI while on prophylactic antibiotics.

Trimethoprim (200 mg once daily) can be given during the later stages of pregnancy but it is absolutely contraindicated in the first trimester as it has an antifolate action.

Nitrofurantoin should be avoided after 36 weeks of gestation due to the risk of haemolytic anaemia in the baby.

Cephalexin is not a broad spectrum antibiotic and therefore there is the possibility of developing resistance quickly.

Amoxicillin is a good choice but cannot be given to women with a penicillin allergy.

One should follow the local hospital antibiotic policy.

Nelson-Piercy C. Handbook of Obstetric Medicine (4th edn). London: Informa Healthcare, 2010.

32.22 Renal transplant

A 25-year-old woman, gravida 2 para 1, attends the antenatal clinic at 8 weeks of gestation. She had a renal transplant 2 years ago and wishes to continue this pregnancy.

1. What are the factors in this woman's history that would promote graft survival in the current pregnancy?   Marks (6)

2. What are the common complications one could expect in this pregnancy?   Marks (4)

3. Critically discuss her management during this pregnancy.   Marks (10)

Key points

- 8 weeks of gestation
- renal transplant 2 years ago
- wishes to continue pregnancy
- graft survival

Essay plan

1.

- wellbeing for post renal transplant
- absence of proteinuria, hypertension or other medical diseases
- stable renal function
- lowest maintenance dose of drug therapy
- steroids
- immunosuppressive drugs
- antihypertensives
- no evidence of graft rejection

2.

- complications
- maternal
- fetal

3.

- management during antenatal period
- management during labour and delivery
- management during postpartum period

32.22 Suggested answer

1.

The following factors are important for graft survival in the current pregnancy and at 5 years post renal transplant:

- good health for approximately 2 years post renal transplant
- absence or minimal proteinuria
- absence of hypertension or well-controlled hypertension
- absence of any underlying medical diseases, e.g. systemic lupus erythematoses (SLE), scleroderma and polyarteritis nodosa (often associated with hypertension)
- no evidence of graft rejection
- absence of pelvicaliceal dilatation on ultrasound examination
- stable renal function with serum creatinine <180 µmol/L (preferably <125 µmol/L)
- lowest maintenance dose of drug therapy (prednisolone 15 mg or less per day, azathioprine 2 mg/kg or less per day and cyclosporin 5 mg/kg or less per day)

2.

Maternal complications

Renal function is augmented in most women during pregnancy with a 15% risk of permanent renal impairment and a 5% risk of graft rejection. There is a 35% chance of spontaneous miscarriage before the end of the first trimester, 30% risk of developing hypertension, pre-eclampsia or both, 40–60% risk of pre-term delivery and 20–40% risk of intrauterine growth restriction. Therefore close monitoring of the mother and fetus is important during this pregnancy.

Fetal complications

The risks to the fetus include respiratory problems (respiratory distress syndrome), leucopenia, thrombocytopenia, adrenocortical insufficiency and infection.

3.

Management during antenatal period

An uncomplicated pregnancy outcome relates to the degree of functional renal impairment and the presence or absence of hypertension rather than the nature of underlying renal condition.

Women are classified into three categories according to the degree of renal impairment:

- mild impairment (serum creatinine <125 µmol/L) and absent or well-controlled hypertension
- moderate renal impairment (serum creatinine 125–250 µmol/L) and moderate hypertension
- severe renal impairment (serum creatinine >250 µmol/L) and severe hypertension

She should be seen by a senior obstetrician in a joint antenatal clinic with a nephrologist. Close regular monitoring for renal function (to diagnose renal impairment and graft rejection), anaemia (full blood count), infection (blood for cytomegalovirus and herpes and urine for culture and sensitivity), blood pressure (weekly) and growth of the baby (serial growth scans to detect fetal growth restriction) are important to manage the above complications. It also helps to decide on the time of delivery and counselling of the woman with regards to the pregnancy outcome.

Management during labour and delivery

- pelvic location of the kidney is not a contraindication to vaginal delivery
- caesarean section should be reserved for obstetric indication only
- close monitoring of the mother (including fluid input and urinary output) and continuous fetal monitoring during labour is advised

Management during postpartum period

- women need to be thoroughly counselled about future pregnancies and their outcomes (repeated pregnancies do not adversely affect transplant function or fetal development)
- breastfeeding should be avoided as the drugs used for immunosuppression are excreted in breast milk
- contraception should also be discussed
- thromboprophylaxis needs to be reviewed (women with significant proteinuria are prone to develop thromboembolism)
- counselling for the increased risk of developing malignancy including female genital tract malignancy due to her immunosuppressive treatment and the importance of being up to date with her cervical smears

Davison JM. Chronic renal disease in pregnancy. Personal assessment in continuing education. Reviews, questions and answers. Volume 3. London: RCOG Press 2003; pp. 48–49
Nelson-Piercy C. Handbook of Obstetric Medicine (4th edn). London: Informa Healthcare, 2010.

32.23 Retained placenta

A 40-year-old woman who is 36 weeks pregnant delivers in the car park. She is now transferred to the labour ward and the placenta remains undelivered 40 minutes post delivery.

1. What information should one want to know about this woman and why? Marks (4)

2. What initial management steps should one ask the senior house office to do? Marks (2)

3. How should this woman be managed? Marks (6)

4. Describe the principles of manual removal of placenta. Marks (8)

Key points
- spontaneous vaginal delivery
- retained placenta

Essay plan

1.

- clinically stable or unstable
- bleeding or not bleeding
- vital signs
- what oxytocic drugs used

2.

- intravenous access
- full blood count (FBC) and group and serum storage
- nil by mouth
- consent

3.

- clinically stable – try controlled cord traction, oxytocin infusion in the umbilical vein
- clinically unstable or placenta undelivered – manual removal of placenta

4.

- regional or general anaesthesia
- asepsis
- long gloves
- if right-handed, use the right hand to remove the placenta
- the left hand is used as a fundal guard to prevent perforation
- avoid inadvertent pulling on the cord as this may lead to uterine inversion
- prophylactic antibiotics at induction of the anaesthesia
- oxytocics following delivery of the placenta
- keep bladder empty – catheterise

32.23 Suggested answer

1.

One needs information to decide the urgency of the operation. This includes:

- the haemodynamic stability of the mother (vital signs including pulse and blood pressure)
- whether the woman is bleeding actively and how much blood has been lost so far
- whether the bladder is empty

2.

A venous access should be secured with blood taken for the FBC and group and save. The woman should be kept nil by mouth and warned about the need for the manual removal of the placenta if undelivered with all the measures or if she starts bleeding heavily.

3.

Most of the time the placenta is separated and held back beyond the cervix. Therefore a further attempt to remove the placenta in the form of controlled cord traction (CCT) should be made before undertaking manual removal of the placenta (MROP). If the woman is haemodynamically stable, oxytocin infusion (20 units in 20 mL of normal saline) through the umbilical cord (vein) can be tried as it promotes placental separation. If this method fails or there is excessive vaginal bleeding, manual removal of the placenta should be undertaken in theatre.

4.

Informed written consent should be taken after explaining the procedure and the risks (including excessive bleeding, blood transfusion, perforation of the uterus and morbidly adherent placenta). The procedure is performed under regional or general anaesthesia and this depends on the haemodynamic stability of the woman. It is usually done under antibiotic cover to reduce the risk of infection (prophylactic intravenous antibiotic).

The procedure should be done under sterile conditions plus personal precautions taken to avoid soaking the arms with blood (long elbow length gloves [gonlets] and wearing an appropriate length gown).

One should go along the umbilical cord with the dominant hand and find a cleavage between the uterus and the placenta. This allows a step-by-step separation of the placenta with the right hand. Concurrently, measures should be taken to avoid uterine perforation and inversion of the uterus by keeping the left hand on the fundus (the left hand is supposed to act as a fundal guard, stabilise the uterus and prevent the use of excessive force with the right hand) and also to avoid inadvertent pulling on the placenta before separation.

Once the placenta is out, explore the uterine cavity to ensure it is empty. This can be done digitally or with the use of an ultrasound scan. The final step is to keep the uterus contracted to avoid (a) an atony and further bleeding, and (b) uterine inversion. This can be achieved by starting oxytocin 40 units drip in 500 mL Hartmann solution and/or the use of misoprostol (800 µg) per rectally.

The woman should be closely observed for the next couple of hours in recovery. She should be monitored for any excessive bleeding and then can be transferred to the postnatal ward.

National Institute for Health and Clinical Excellence. Intrapartum care. Care of healthy women and their babies during childbirth. Chapter 17: Complicated labour: third stage (CG55). NICE, 2008.

32.24 Sickle cell disease

A 20-year-old Afro-Caribbean woman is referred to the preconception clinic for counselling because she is planning to conceive. She has been diagnosed with sickle cell disease on her recent admission to the medical ward with a sickle cell crisis for the first time.

1. What information should one provide that is relevant to her condition prior to planning pregnancy and why? Marks (8)

2. What assessments should be arranged to exclude any chronic disease complications during preconception? Marks (6)

3. Nine months later, she presents to the labour ward with mild contractions at 37 weeks of gestation. How should she be managed during labour and delivery? Marks (6)

Key points
- preconception counselling
- sickle cell disease
- asessments before pregnancy
- counselling before pregnancy
- management during labour and delivery

Essay plan

1.

- sickle cell crisis
- hyperemesis
- infection
- anaemia
- acute chest syndrome
- intrauterine fetal growth restriction
- fetal distress
- fetal affection by sickle cell disease
- induction of labour (IOL)/caesarean section
- screen for end-organ damage

2.

- echocardiography
- blood pressure and urine analysis

- liver function tests
- retinal screening
- serum ferritin
- red cell antibodies

3.

- thromboembolic stockings and hydration
- avoid hypoxia, acidosis and hypothermia
- prevent infection
- avoid dehydration
- anaesthetic review and pain relief
- inform haematologist
- fetal monitoring
- regional anaesthesia for caesarean section
- caesarean section for obstetric indications
- breast feeding not contraindication
- prophylactic low molecular weight heparin (LMWH)
- maintain O2 saturation: 94%
- fetal assessment for sickle cell disease and antibodies
- contraception

32.24 Suggested answer

1.

One should provide information regarding how sickle cell disease affects pregnancy and how pregnancy affects the disease as well as how these outcomes can be improved.

She is at risk of developing anaemia, infection, sickle cell crisis, acute chest syndrome and thromboembolism.

She should avoid factors which can precipitate a sickle cell crisis and these include dehydration, infection, hypoxia, cold, over-exertion and stress. The common conditions such as hyperemesis should be treated appropriately.

Influenza vaccine should be offered if not administered within the last year.

If necessary, prophylactic penicillin antibiotics should be offered as there is a risk of pneumococcal septicaemia due to a non-functioning spleen.

She will need regular screening for anaemia (haemoglobin and serum ferritin) and infection (especially urinary tract infection [UTI]) and treated appropriately. Folic acid supplementation (5 mg) should be started during preconception and continued throughout the pregnancy. The anaemia itself should be treated with iron tablets or if necessary exchange transfusion if indicated.

Fetal growth restriction is common and therefore growth scans every 4 weeks are indicated. There is an increased risk of the baby being affected by sickle cell disease if she or her partner is affected or if both are carriers. This can be tested early during the pregnancy by doing an invasive test (chorionic villus sampling [CVS] or amniocentesis) or after the birth of the baby if they decline these tests.

Caesarean section may be necessary for fetal distress during labour.

One should screen her for end-organ damage such as retinopathy, nephropathy, pulmonary hypertension, liver dysfunction and red cell antibodies.

2.

Screening for end-organ damage before conception is important as morbidity and mortality is increased in the presence of these conditions.

The presence of pulmonary hypertension increases the risk of maternal mortality and therefore echocardiography should be performed if this has not been performed within the last year. A tricuspid regurgitant jet velocity >2.5 m/s is associated with an increased risk of pulmonary hypertension.

Blood pressure and urine analysis should be performed to identify women with hypertension and proteinuria. Liver function and renal function tests should be performed annually to identify liver dysfunction and nephropathy.

Proliferative retinopathy is common in women with sickle cell disease and this may lead to loss of vision. The Royal College of Obstetricians and Gynaecologists (RCOG) recommends preconception screening for retinopathy for women with sickle cell disease.

The patient should be screened for iron overload. T2 cardiac magnetic resonance imaging should be arranged for women with high serum ferritin levels or who have had multiple blood transfusions in the past. Iron chelation therapy is recommended before conception for women with a high iron overload.

Screening for red cell antibodies should be performed as they increase the risk of haemolytic disease of the newborn. Knowledge of this helps monitoring during pregnancy and informs the paediatrician when planning the appropriate management of the newborn baby at birth. One should also inform the haematologist as planning is necessary if this woman needs a blood transfusion during pregnancy or labour.

3.

The principles of management are same during pregnancy or labour.

One should avoid hypoxia, acidosis, infection, cold, dehydration, stress and pain to prevent a sickle cell crisis. She should be adequately oxygenated with oxygen saturation maintained at least at 94%. She should be well hydrated and provided with TED stockings during labour to prevent thromboembolism. Pethidine should be avoided but other opiates can be given for pain relief. Regional anaesthesia is recommended during labour and for caesarean section.

The anaesthetist, haematologist and paediatrician should be informed of the admission of this woman to the labour ward for delivery. Continuous fetal monitoring is recommended to monitor the baby in view of the increased risk of fetal distress.

Vaginal delivery is not contraindicated and caesarean section should be performed only for obstetric indications.

The above principles apply following delivery to prevent a sickle cell crisis. LMWH prophylaxis for 7 days after vaginal delivery and for 6 weeks following caesarean section is recommended to prevent thromboembolism.

Fetal assessment should be undertaken to exclude sickle cell disease if indicated or for anaemia and antibodies if the mother is positive for red cell antibodies.

Breastfeeding is not contraindicated during puerperium.

Progestogens (cerazette, medroxyprogesterone acetate and levonorgestrel IUS) should be used as first line contraception as these are safe and effective while oestrogen-containing pills (low dose) should be used as second line contraception.

Royal College of Obstetricians and Gynaecologists. Green-top Guideline No. 61. Management of sickle cell disease in pregnancy. London: RCOG Press, 2011.

32.25 Spontaneous rupture of membranes at term

A 30-year-old woman, para 0, presents to the obstetric day assessment unit at 39 weeks of gestation with spontaneous rupture of membranes (SROM).

1. Describe the initial assessment of this woman.   Marks (8)

2. What are her management options?   Marks (4)

3. Critically evaluate her management options.   Marks (8)

Key points
- primigravida
- 39 weeks of gestation
- SROM
- initial assessment
- management options
- critically assess management

Essay plan
1.

- history (well or unwell, duration of SROM, colour and odour of liquor, temperature and contractions)
- examination (general, abdominal, speculum)
- investigation (high vaginal swab, full blood count [FBC], C-reactive protein [CRP])
- cardiotocograph (CTG)

2.

- expectant
- immediate induction of labour (IOL)
- IOL after 24 hours
- augmentation of labour

3.

- signs of infection – need immediate IOL
- no signs of infection – expectant management
- other obstetric indication for delivery – need immediate IOL
- no other obstetric indication – expectant management

32.25 Suggested answer

1.

One should ask about the history of SROM (gush of fluid or trickle all along the legs), the duration of SROM (<24 hours or >24 hours), colour of the liquor (meconium or clear), odour (smelly or offensive), fetal movements, whether she is well or unwell or has any fever, abdominal pain and contractions.

Examination to confirm SROM is the next most important step. A speculum examination to check for SROM, colour and offensiveness is necessary before initiation of treatment. On abdominal examination, assess for presentation, tenderness and contractions. It is also important to assess the fetal condition (CTG).

Vital signs give a lot of information about the woman (temperature, pulse and blood pressure). A raised temperature and pulse may indicate a uterine infection when there is no other source of infection.

A high vaginal swab should be taken and this may help to gain sensitivity of the organisms in case the woman develops an infection. FBC and CRP are not routinely indicated. They should be performed when there are symptoms or signs of infection and in the presence of prolonged SROM.

2.

The management options to be discussed include:

- expectant management
- immediate IOL
- IOL after 24 hours
- augmentation of labour immediately or when she goes into labour

3.

- All options should be discussed with the woman and it is ultimately an informed choice made by the woman regarding management. Everything should be clearly documented in the notes.
- If there is a clear history with confirmed SROM and the woman is well, she can be managed expectantly and an IOL booked after 24 hours. During this period she should be urged to be admitted if she feels unwell or develops a raised temperature or spontaneous labour. The risk of infection (uterine, fetal and distant sepsis) should be explained to the woman with prolonged SROM and therefore she should be asked to return in the next 24 hours for IOL.

- If there are symptoms and signs of infection (fever, unwell, raised temperature, tachycardia, uterine tenderness and offensive liquor), an IOL should be offered immediately and its importance should be explained to the woman. She and her baby should be closely monitored during labour and intravenous broad spectrum antibiotics administered in order to treat infection. FBC, CRP and blood cultures should be performed and if necessary the microbiologist should be contacted for advice. Where necessary, delivery should be expedited if there is maternal or fetal compromise.
- Meconium-stained liquor is another indication for immediate IOL especially if there is thick meconium. With thick meconium, theoretically there is more risk of fetal distress, therefore it would be better to augment with oxytocin rather than induce with prostaglandin.
- If the woman comes in with spontaneous labour following expectant management and is still in early labour, it is good practice to augment labour with prolonged SROM (the risk of infection increases with the duration of SROM). If progress is slow, it may suggest that her forewaters are intact and will need artificial rupturing.
- Last but not least, if there are other obstetric indications for immediate induction of labour (e.g. raised blood pressure, pre-eclampsia, reduced fetal movements, intrauterine fetal growth restriction [IUGR]), she should be offered immediate IOL. Cephalic presentation should be confirmed in all circumstances before induction or augmentation of labour.

National Institute for Health and Clinical Excellence. Induction of labour (CG70). NICE, 2008. www.nice.org. uk/CG070FullGuideline

32.26 Thrombocytopaenia

A 25-year-old woman attends the antenatal clinic for a review of her booking (her first midwife appointment) blood results at 24 weeks of gestation. All her booking blood results were normal except her platelets count which was 90×10^9/L.

1. What are the causes of low platelets during pregnancy?   Marks (6)

2. How should she be investigated?   Marks (4)

3. What are the fetal implications and what precautions one should take during labour? How should she be managed during this pregnancy?   Marks (10)

Key points
- 25 years old
- 24 weeks of gestation
- low platelets
- causes
- investigations
- fetal implications
- management

Essay plan

1.
- diagnosis is one of exclusion

- gestational
- pre-eclampsia
- haemolysis, elevated liver enzymes and low platelets (HELLP)
- immune
- idiopathic autoimmune thrombocytopaenia
- drug-related
- human immunodeficiency virus (HIV) infection
- disseminated intravascular coagulation (DIC) rare
- antepartum haemorrhage
- sepsis

2.

- history
- examination
- repeat platelet count
- blood film

3.

- fetal thrombocytopaenia
- management depends on cause
- monitor platelets
- steroids
- intravenous immunoglobulin
- liaise with haematologist
- liaise with paediatricians

32.26 Suggested answer

1.

The overall incidence of maternal thrombocytopenia is 6–7%. Gestational thrombocytopenia of pregnancy is the most common cause of maternal thrombocytopenia (74%) followed by hypertensive disorders (21%: pre-eclampsia and HELLP) and immune causes (4%).

Idiopathic autoimmune thrombocytopenia is the most common immune-related cause of thrombocytopenia followed by drug-related and some associated with HIV infection.

DIC is a rare cause and is usually due to pre-eclampsia, placental abruption, amniotic fluid embolism and retention of dead fetus.

2.

Diagnosis is one of exclusion by systematically taking history, examination, investigation and follow-up.

History of any platelet disorder (past, personal or family), medical disorders (hypertension), fetal movements, easy bruising and vaginal bleeding is important.

Check for any bruises and petechial haemorrhages. Check for raised blood pressure and urine dipstick for proteins and arrange baseline blood tests to rule out pre-eclampsia and HELLP (full blood count [FBC], liver function tests [LFTs], renal function tests [RFTs] and urates).

The platelet count should be repeated to confirm the results are correct. A blood film should also be requested to exclude the platelet count being low due to cell clumping.

Platelet antibodies is not a sensitive test to diagnose an immune cause or to predict fetal outcome.

3.

The maternal platelet count or platelet antibody is of no proven value in predicting the fetal or neonatal platelet count. However, there is a risk of neonatal thrombocytopenia due to maternal autoantibodies. In view of this, one should avoid fetal scalp electrode, fetal blood sampling and ventouse delivery.

Ideally, the woman should be managed in a joint obstetrics and haematology clinic. The management obviously depends on the cause. Gestational thrombocytopenia usually starts in the second trimester and is usually more marked near the delivery time. It is a diagnosis of exclusion but is probably due to haemodilution and increased non-immune platelet destruction. It does not affect adversely the mother or fetus and returns to normal by 6 weeks after delivery. Management mainly involves monitoring the platelets and avoiding unnecessary interventions.

Hypertensive disorders account for 21% of cases of maternal thrombocytopenia and 50% of women with pre-eclampsia develop thrombocytopenia. It is usually mild but it can sometimes be severe. Generally it correlates to the severity of the pre-eclampsia. In mild cases, one needs to monitor the platelet count but if the pre-eclampsia is severe or develops HELLP, the woman will need stabilisation and delivery.

Immune thrombocytopenia: the British Committee for Standards in Haematology on behalf of the British Society for Haematology recommend the following steps in managing such women.

If the maternal platelet count >50 × 10⁹/L:

- monitor the platelet count twice weekly
- allow vaginal delivery

If the platelet count is < 80 × 10⁹/L:

- avoid epidural analgesia

If the platelet count is <50 × 10⁹/L:

- The risk of bleeding at delivery is increased
- Increase the platelets to >50 × 10⁹/L to allow vaginal delivery
- Increase the platelets to >80 × 10⁹/L for caesarean section
- If the platelet count falls to <20 × 10⁹/L or there is bleeding, treatment may be required earlier during the pregnancy

The treatment includes either steroid therapy or intravenous immunoglobulin. Steroids inhibit the reticuloendothelial system and hence inhibit destruction of antibody-coated platelets. They also decrease antibody synthesis. At this stage, this woman does not need any therapy except monitoring of the platelet count twice weekly. If the platelet count falls ($<50 \times 10^9$/L), then prednisolone may be used (starting at a dose of 1 mg/kg/day). It should be maintained at the lowest dose that helps to maintain platelets to prevent bleeding.

If the patient needs long-term steroids or very high doses to maintain platelets, one should consider intravenous immunoglobulin. The response rate is quoted to be 80% and the duration of response is 2–3 weeks. Platelet top-ups can be administered to maintain the count before delivery and to avoid bleeding.

Caesarean section is recommended only for obstetric indications.

Invasive fetal monitoring including fetal scalp electrode, fetal blood sampling, and ST waveform analysis (STAN) monitoring and ventouse delivery should be avoided. A cord sample should be taken after delivery to check the baby's platelet count and it should be monitored closely for 1 week.

If the low platelet count is drug-related, one should stop the drug and this should resolve the problem most of the time.

If related to APH or DIC, management is with the use of appropriate blood components (fresh frozen plasma [FFP] and platelet transfusion).

Letsky E, Murphy MF, Ramsay JE, Walker I. Chapter 3: Maternal and fetal thrombocytopaenia. Haemorrhagic disease and hereditary bleeding disorders. London: RCOG Press, 2005.
Myers B. Thrombocytopaenia in pregnancy. The Obstetrician & Gynaecologist 2009; 11:177–183.

32.27 Thromboembolism during pregnancy

A 36-year-old woman, para 0, had a deep venous thrombosis (DVT) 3 years ago while she was on the combined oral contraception pill (COCP). She was initially treated with Enoxaparin sodium and later commenced on warfarin for 6 months. Currently she is 6 weeks pregnant and presents to the early pregnancy assessment unit for mild vaginal spotting. A transvaginal scan (TVS) reveals a single viable intrauterine pregnancy with a crown rump length (CRL) corresponding to 6 weeks of gestation.

1. What factors increases the risk of thromboembolism during pregnancy?   Marks (6)

2. How should this pregnancy be managed and why?   Marks (11)

3. What advice should she be given about the future?   Marks (3)

Key points

- 36 years old
- previous DVT
- 6 weeks of gestation
- single viable intrauterine pregnancy
- COCP

Essay plan

1.

- pre-existing risk factors
- current transient risk factors

2.

- review previous notes
- take a detailed past and family history
- allergy
- make a consultant appointment in a joint high-risk obstetric and haematology clinic
- screen for thrombophilia
- start antenatal low molecular weight heparin (LMWH) prophylaxis
- thromboembolic stocking
- multidisciplinary input
- avoid transient risk factors during labour
- anaesthetic input during labour
- role of protamine sulphate
- role of unfractionated heparin
- postpartum LMWH for 6 weeks
- breastfeeding not contraindicated

3.

- increased risk of recurrence of thromboembolism during future pregnancies
- need for antenatal and postnatal LMWH during future pregnancies
- avoid COCP

32.27 **Suggested answer**

1.

Thromboembolism remains the commonest cause of direct maternal death in the UK. The risk factors can be pre-existing or current.

The pre-existing factors that increase the risk of thromboembolism during pregnancy include: age>35 years, body mass index >30 kg/m^2, parity >3, previous thromboembolism, history of thrombophilia, paraplegia, gross varicose veins, sickle cell disease and nephrotic syndrome.

The transient factors that increase the risk of thromboembolism during pregnancy include any condition leading to dehydration (hyperemesis, prolonged labour) or immobilisation (long-haul travel, prolonged labour), infection, ovarian hyper stimulation syndrome ovarian hyperstimulation syndrome (OHSS), surgical procedure, pre-eclampsia and excessive blood loss. The risk is highest during the puerperium.

2.

A detailed history about the previous episode of DVT should be taken including the site, extent, treatment and the duration of the treatment.

Since her previous episode of thrombosis was oestrogen-related, she should be started on antenatal LMWH prophylaxis. The prophylaxis should start as early as possible and should continue throughout the pregnancy and 6 weeks postpartum. She should be advised to wear TED stockings antenatally and postnatally for 6 weeks as per the Royal College of Obstetricians and Gynaecologists (RCOG) guidelines.

If previously allergic to LMWH (skin allergy or thrombocytopaenia), an alternative drug, Danaparoid, can be used for thromboprophylaxis. A baseline platelet count and urea and creatinine should be performed before commencing therapy with LMWH.

A personal and family history of thrombophilia and thromboembolism is vital information for managing her during pregnancy.

She should be managed as high risk for pregnancy, labour and puerperium. Therefore it should be hospital-led care and she should see a consultant soon in the joint high-risk obstetric and haematology clinic for multidisciplinary input regarding her management.

A thrombophilia screen should be arranged if she has not had one in the past. However, the results should be interpreted carefully during pregnancy and by an appropriate person in view of the changes in clotting factors during pregnancy.

She should have a risk of venous thromboembolism (VTE) assessment at booking (her first midwife appointment) and this should be reviewed when admitted antenatally, in labour and postnatally. One should avoid transient risk factors such as dehydration and immobilisation during pregnancy, labour and puerperium as these increase the risk of thrombosis.

The anaesthetist should be informed when this woman is admitted to the labour ward so as to plan pain relief. If she is on prophylactic LMWH, an epidural should be avoided 12 hours from the last dose. However, if she develops a VTE during the current pregnancy and is currently on therapeutic LMWH, an epidural should be avoided for 24 hours from the last dose.

If she has received an epidural during labour for pain relief, LMWH should be withheld until 4 hours after the insertion or removal of the epidural catheter.

One should also be aware of the antidote protamine sulphate, in case she receives LMWH inadvertently during labour.

If she is at high risk of bleeding following delivery (e.g. postpartum haemorrhage [PPH]), she should be started on unfractionated heparin for thromboprophylaxis.

Breastfeeding is not contraindicated with the use of heparin.

3.

She should be informed about the increased risk of the recurrence of thromboembolism in all her future pregnancies and therefore the need for antenatal and postnatal LMWH thromboprophylaxis. She should avoid COCP for contraception and alternatives should be discussed during the puerperium.

Royal College of Obstetricians and Gynaecologists. Green-top Guideline No. 37. Reducing the risk of thrombosis and embolism during pregnancy and puerperium. London: RCOG Press, 2009.
Calderwood CJ and Thanoon OI. Thromboembolism and thrombophilia in pregnancy. Obstet Gynaecol Reprod Med 2009; 19:339–343.

32.28 Umbilical cord blood

A 38-year-old Asian woman attends the antenatal clinic at 20 weeks of gestation following her anomaly scan which is normal. She had a child with a genetic disease who died at the age of 5 years in a different country and therefore details are not available. She wants to know more about umbilical cord blood banking and its uses so that she can make a decision to save fetal umbilical cord blood for the future following her delivery.

1. What are the uses of umbilical cord blood banking?   Marks (4)

2. What does umbilical cord blood contain?   Marks (4)

3. Critically evaluate the time of collection of umbilical cord blood.   Marks (6)

4. What are the advantages and disadvantages of umbilical cord blood
    for stem cell therapy?   Marks (6)

Key points
*   umbilical cord blood banking
*   uses of umbilical cord blood
*   critically evaluate time of collection
*   advantages of umbilical cord blood for stem cell therapy
*   disadvantages of umbilical cord blood for stem cell therapy

Essay plan
1.

*   metabolic diseases
*   immunological diseases
*   haematological diseases
*   genetic diseases
*   degenerative diseases
*   research

2.

*   contents of umbilical cord blood, e.g. stem cells

3.

*   time of collection, e.g. immediately following delivery
*   crucial time for care of mother and baby, e.g. obstetric emergency and resuscitation for the baby
*   mother and baby care should not be compromised
*   a separate allotted person should collect the cord blood outside the labour room

4.

- advantages over standard stem cell therapy, e.g. bone marrow transplant
- disadvantages over standard stem cell therapy

32.28 Suggested answer

1.

The uses of umbilical cord blood include its use in metabolic disorders, genetic diseases, immunological disorders and haematological disorders (mainly by autologous or related cord blood stem cell transplantation) in children and adults. It has also been tried to improve or cure degenerative diseases and is a potentially powerful tool for research.

In the future, cord blood might be a useful source of stem cells other than haemopoietic precursors (they may have the capacity to develop into many different lineages including cartilage, fat cells, hepatic and cardiac cells).

Storage of cord blood for therapeutic purposes will require a licence from the Human Tissue Authority under the terms of the Human Tissue Act.

2.

Cord blood contains haemopoietic stem cells (HSC). At collection they are relatively few in number compared to the cells obtained from bone marrow or peripheral blood HSC donation (approximately one log less), but have greater proliferative potential and colony-forming capacity. They are more responsive to some growth factors as they are more 'naïve' than proliferative cells from bone marrow, and they seem to produce fewer complications associated with some aspects of HSC transplantation.

3.

The timing of umbilical cord blood collection is crucial. It is usually undertaken during the third stage of labour while the placenta remains *in situ* or shortly thereafter. This is the time when there can be potential obstetric emergencies such as postpartum haemorrhage (PPH) and collapse (the mother and baby need one-to-one care). Therefore, there should be an allotted person to collect this blood who is not involved in the other aspects of delivery.

In premature babies, early cord clamping can be disadvantageous as these babies are at risk of anaemia and haemodynamic instability (there is some evidence that a delay of 30–120 seconds is associated with fewer transfusions for anaemia and fewer intraventricular haemorrhages).

A cord around the neck may need to be released or cut early to allow delivery. There should be no pressure on attendants to avoid cutting the cord.

During a caesarean section, it is routine practice to clamp the cord immediately and pass the infant to an attendant after delivery of the baby. Following this, the placenta is delivered by controlled cord traction. Sometimes the placenta is removed manually and the uterine incision is closed quickly to avoid excessive bleeding. Undue delay to effect collection or any delay where there is an increased risk of haemorrhage would be inappropriate.

Good practice is that used by NHS Cord Blood Bank, where cord blood is collected aseptically after delivery of the placenta by trained National Blood Service (NBS) staff within the delivery unit but outside the delivery room (which does not interfere with either the care of the mother or the baby).

Donor mothers are interviewed antenatally to obtain written informed consent to use the cord blood for any patient who needs it, for testing for microbiological markers both current and future, and to ensure the mother meets with specific donor-selection criteria set by expert advisory groups.

4.

The advantages of umbilical cord blood for stem cell therapy include:

- cord blood transplantation will tolerate a mismatch of tissue types between donor and the recipient greater than is acceptable with bone marrow or peripheral blood
- lower incidence and severity of graft versus host disease
- lower incidence of viral transmission: in particular, cytomegalovirus and Epstein–Barr virus
- lack of donor attrition: bone marrow donors may change their mind over time or may no longer be available
- low numbers of haemopoietic progenitor cells and stem cells in each cord blood donation

Disadvantages include:

- delayed engraftment
- lack of availability of subsequent donations of stem cells and/or lymphocytes from the graft donor in graft failure or disease relapse

Royal College of Obstetricians and Gynaecologists. Standard setting to improve women's health. Scientific Advisory Committee Opinion Paper 2. London: RCOG Press, 2006.

32.29 Uterine inversion

A 26-year-old woman, para 1, suddenly has a lump coming out of her vagina while trying to deliver the placenta. This is noticed by the midwife who pulls the emergency buzzer. Examination reveals uterine inversion.

1. What is uterine inversion and what is the most common cause for it? What is the aetiology of uterine inversion?　　Marks (2)

2. Describe the complications of uterine inversion.　　Marks (4)

3. What are the differential diagnoses of uterine inversion following delivery?　　Marks (4)

4. Describe the non-surgical methods one would use to rectify the uterine inversion in this woman and the principles behind them.　　Marks (10)

Key points

- lump in vagina
- placenta *in situ*
- uterine inversion
- common cause
- aetiology
- complications
- differential diagnosis
- non-surgical management

Essay plan

1.

- definition: uterine inversion
- inadvertent pulling on the cord
- unknown
- spontaneous in 50% of cases
- Credé's method of expressing the placenta

2.

- haemorrhage: most common
- shock
- neurogenic shock
- severe abdominal pain
- infection

3.

- uterine atony and postpartum haemorrhage (PPH)
- genital tract lacerations and PPH
- coagulopathy
- retained placenta without separation of the placenta
- uterovaginal prolapse
- prolapse of large submucous fibroid

4.

- identify the condition
- call for help
- resuscitation
- manual replacement
- hydrostatic method

32.29 Suggested answer

1.

Uterine inversion is a rare but serious obstetric emergency (incidence in the UK is 1 in 28,000 deliveries). It is defined as inversion of the fundus into the uterine cavity.

The most common cause of this condition is inappropriate management of the third stage of labour in the form of inadvertent pulling on the umbilical cord before separation of the placenta.

The exact aetiology remains unknown. It can be spontaneous (40–50%) and occur following the pulling of the placenta from below or pushing from above (Credé's method of expression of placenta) and various other associated factors.

2.

- haemorrhage is the most common presentation (seen in 94% of patients)
- sudden cardiovascular collapse or shock (39% of patients) – the woman may present initially with neurogenic shock and later haemorrhagic shock
- infection
- severe abdominal pain
- prolapse of uterus through the vagina

3.

These differential diagnoses are for postpartum collapse and lumps in the vagina:

- uterine atony and PPH
- genital tract lacerations and PPH
- coagulopathy
- retained placenta without separation of the placenta
- uterovaginal prolapse
- prolapse of large submucous fibroid

4.

The key step to management is the same as for any other obstetric emergency:

- call for help
- secure airway, breathing and circulation (ABC)
- treatment of the condition

The two non-surgical methods described include: (a) manual replacement and (b) hydrostatic method.

Manual replacement

Manual replacement of the uterus or Johnson manoeuvre alone (first described by AB Johnson in 1949) or with tocolysis is tried as a primary procedure.

As Johnson stated in 1949, the principle behind this manoeuvre is that 'the uterus has to be lifted into the abdominal cavity above the level of umbilicus before reposition can occur. It is thought that then the passive action of uterine ligaments will rectify the inversion.'

Johnson mentioned that the whole hand including two thirds of the forearm is to be placed in the vagina. Holding the fundus in the palm and keeping the tips of the fingers at the uterocervical junction, the fundus is raised above the level of umbilicus. This places the uterine ligaments under tension. The pressure generated relaxes and widens the cervical ring and facilitates the reposition of the fundus through the ring, thus correcting the inversion.

The placenta should only be removed after the repositioning of the uterus and complete correction of the inversion in order to avoid shock and torrential bleeding.

If repositioning takes place before the oedema of the uterus and contraction ring develops, the procedure is relatively easy to perform.

If manual reposition fails with tocolysis, halogenated anaesthesia can be used for good uterine relaxation. Once the manual replacement is successful, the uterus should be held in place for a few minutes and uterotonics administered to promote contraction of the uterus and prevent re-inversion.

Hydrostatic methods

In 1945 JV O'Sullivan published the first report of two cases describing the hydrostatic replacement of the uterus following acute uterine inversion.

With this method, the uterus is placed in the vagina and warm sterile water or isotonic sodium chloride solution is rapidly instilled into the vagina via a rubber tube, while the accoucheurs hand block the introitus. The fluid distends the vagina and pushes the fundus upwards into its natural position by hydrostatic pressure. The bag of fluid should be elevated about 100–150 cm above the level of the vagina to ensure sufficient pressure for insufflation. The only problem with this method is the difficulty in maintaining a tight water seal at the introitus.

Depending on the patient's general condition the procedure can be performed with tocolysis or general anaesthesia using halothane if the contraction ring is already formed. The advantage of general anaesthesia is that in addition to maternal pain relief it promotes uterine relaxation.

The problem of maintaining a tight water seal at the introitus may be overcome with the use of a silastic ventouse cup, though a hand may still be necessary to improve the tight seal.

The possible complications are infection and failure of the procedure.

Bhalla R, Wuntakal R, Odejinmi F, Khan RU. Acute inversion of the uterus. The Obstetrician & Gynaecologist 2009; 11:13–18.

Johnson AB. A new concept in replacement of the inverted uterus and report of nine cases. Am J Obstet Gynecol 1949; 57:557–562.

Kochenour NK. Intrapartum obstetric emergencies. Crit Care Clin 1991; 7:851–864.

Berkeley C, Bonney V, Macleod D. The Abnormal in Obstetrics. London: Arnold, 1938.

Samarrae K. Puerperal inversion of the uterus, with reference to pregnancy following Spinelli operation. J Obstet Gynecol 1965; 72:426–429.

O'Sullivan J. Acute inversion of the uterus. BMJ 1945; 2:282–283.

Abouleish E, Ali V, Jouma B, Lopez M, Gupta D. Anaesthetic management of acute puerperal uterine inversion. BJOA 1995; 75:486–487.

Mehra U and Ostapowicz F. Acute puerperal inversion of the uterus in a primipara. Obstet Gynecol 1976; 47:S30–S32.

Calder A. Emergencies in operative obstetrics. Baillieres Best Pract Clin Obstet Gynaecol 2000; 14:43–55.

32.30 Uterine rupture

A 28-year-old woman, para 1 (previous baby delivered by lower segment caesarean section [LSCS] for breech presentation), comes to the labour ward with a loss of fetal movement at 38 weeks of gestation. An ultrasound scan confirms intrauterine death (IUD). She wishes to have a vaginal delivery. She is given mifepristone and sent home. The next day she comes to the labour ward with contractions and a vaginal examination reveals a 1 cm cervical dilatation. She does not wish to have a postmortem.

1. How should she be managed at this stage?   Marks (6)

2. After an anaesthetic review she was provided with patient controlled analgesia (PCA). Four hours later she was started on oxytocin (5 units) to augment her labour as she was still 1 cm dilated. How should she be managed at this stage?   Marks (4)

3. Four hours after the oxytocin (currently 12 mL/h), she is contracting one in 10 minutes and has made no progress from her previous findings. The midwife states that the woman's pulse is 108 beats/minute and her blood pressure (BP) 78/40 mmHg and therefore she wants to start 1 L of Hartmann solution. The woman also has gush of fresh red vaginal loss. What is the diagnosis and and why? How should she be managed now?   Marks (10)

Key points
- previous LSCS
- 38 weeks of gestation
- vaginal birth after caesarean (VBAC)
- intrauterine device (IUD)
- oxytocin usage

Essay plan

1.

- offer sympathy
- offer support
- offer pain relief
- send the blood for full blood count (FBC), clotting and group and save
- do screening blood tests for IUD
- discuss risks of VBAC
- close monitoring in labour
- reassess in 4 hours

2.

- risk of rupture uterus with oxytocin
- close monitoring in labour
- short trial of labour
- if no progress, need for emergency LSCS

3.

- diagnosis: scar dehiscence or uterine rupture
- urgent review

- stop oxytocin
- inform the on-call consultant
- inform theatres
- inform the on-call anaesthetist
- major obstetric haemorrhage call
- consent for laparotomy and hysterectomy
- delivery of the baby and suturing of the uterus if feasible
- blood and blood products transfusion
- intensive therapy unit (ITU) care
- debrief
- bereavement counsellor
- arrange follow-up in 6 weeks
- risk of future uterine rupture unknown
- elective LSCS in next pregnancy

32.30 Suggested answer

1.

There are two aspects related to her management. One is management of IUD and the second is management of VBAC.

One should be sympathetic and offer her support during labour and post labour. She should be pain free (anaesthetist involved) and the number of professional people visiting her in the labour ward should be minimised by providing one-to-one care.

Screening blood tests for an IUD should be performed as per the unit protocol. A baseline FBC, clotting profile and group and save should be sent and a large bore intravenous cannula inserted. She should be informed about the risk of disseminated intravascular coagulation (DIC) with an IUD, successful VBAC (71–76%), risk of uterine rupture with VBAC (<1%), additional risk of blood transfusion or endometritis and peripartum hysterectomy (1 in 1300 women with previous one LSCS).

One should make a clear plan about monitoring during the labour (pulse and BP every 15 minutes), the timing of the vaginal assessment for progress (reassess in 4 hours) and what happens if there is no progress at the next vaginal examination (e.g. oxytocin augmentation).

2.

One should discuss that the risk of uterine rupture increases by three times when oxytocin is used.

A clear plan should be made regarding the rate and duration of oxytocin to be used and the next vaginal assessment. A short trial of oxytocin is reasonable (6 hours) and if there is no progress, an emergency caesarean section should be offered. Close monitoring of the labour should continue with vital signs every 15 minutes, observing bloody red vaginal loss, contractions and pain despite analgesia.

3.

The diagnosis in her case is one of uterine rupture. The pointers to the diagnosis of uterine rupture in a woman with previous LSCS include poor contractions despite a maximum rate of oxytocin, tachycardia, low BP and red fresh vaginal bleeding.

The first step is to stop the oxytocin, examine the woman (abdominal and vaginal examination), inform the on-call consultant, anaesthetist and theatres and obtain her consent for laparotomy including hysterectomy.

A major obstetric haemorrhage call should be put out and 4 units of blood cross-matched. Laparotomy should be performed by the consultant. A uterine repair is done if it is feasible or one should proceed to hysterectomy if she continues to bleed and uterine repair is not feasible. One should leave a Robinson intraperitoneal drain and Foley's catheter with an hourly urometer.

She should be closely monitored and nursed in the ITU or high dependency unit during the postoperative period to watch for any further bleeding. Blood and blood products should be transfused as necessary.

The woman should be debriefed about the events and future pregnancies and mode of delivery should also be discussed. One should clearly explain that the risk of recurrent uterine rupture is unknown in women with previous uterine rupture but theoretically there is likely to be an increased risk. Therefore, it is advisable to have an elective caesarean section during the next pregnancy (the timing of delivery is debatable).

She should have counselling with a bereavement midwife regarding the fetal loss and a 6-week clinic appointment arranged with her consultant.

The community midwife and general practitioner should be informed about her condition.

Royal College of Obstetricians and Gynaecologists. Green-top Guideline No. 45. Birth after previous caesarean section. London: RCOG Press, 2007.

32.31 Vaginal breech delivery

A 36-year-old primigravida woman presents to the antenatal clinic at 37 weeks of gestation with a breech presentation and wishes to have a vaginal breech delivery.

1. What options should be discussed before counselling the woman for vaginal breech delivery and why?   Marks (8)

2. What factors are regarded as unfavourable for vaginal breech delivery?   Marks (6)

3. How should her labour be managed?   Marks (6)

Key points
- primigravida
- 37 weeks of gestation
- vaginal breech delivery

Essay plan

1.

- external cephalic version (ECV)
- elective caesarean section
- reduced fetal morbidity with caesarean section
- increased fetal morbidity with vaginal breech delivery

2.

- footling breech
- increased estimated fetal weight
- decreased estimated fetal weight
- hyperextended fetal neck
- lack of experience of the operator
- associated obstetric complications
- previous caesarean section

3.

- experienced person available to conduct breech delivery
- avoid augmentation with oxytocin
- early recourse to lower segment caesarean section (LSCS) in case of non-descent of breech in the second stage of labour
- caesarean section facilities available
- continuous fetal monitoring
- fetal blood sampling from buttocks not recommended
- epidural analgesia not routinely advised

32.31 Suggested answer

1.

External cephalic version (ECV) should be offered to all women with a breech presentation at term (after 36 weeks) unless it is contraindicated. The aim is to increase the likelihood of a vaginal birth, and delivery of the baby with cephalic presentation is much safer. The risk of fetal distress and emergency caesarean with ECV is <1%.

The woman should be informed about the risks and benefits of a planned caesarean section versus a planned vaginal delivery for breech presentation at term, both for the current and for future pregnancies.

In the light of term breech trial, elective caesarean section should be advised to women where ECV fails or the woman declines ECV. A planned caesarean section at term is associated with reduced perinatal and neonatal mortality and early neonatal morbidity compared to a planned vaginal breech delivery at term. However, long-term morbidity for the mother following a planned caesarean section is not increased.

If women choose to have an elective caesarean section, it should be done at 39 weeks to reduce the risks of respiratory problems in the neonate (National Institute for Health and Clinical Excellence guidelines).

2.

- large baby (>3800 g) and clinically inadequate pelvis: expect slow labour, difficulties with delivery and emergency caesarean section
- footling or kneeling breech presentation: high risk for cord prolapses
- growth-restricted baby (<2000 g): expect increased risk of fetal hypoxia during labour
- hyperextended fetal neck in labour (diagnosed with ultrasound): expect difficulty in delivery of the after coming head
- lack of presence of trained clinical expertise in vaginal breech delivery
- past history of caesarean section
- other obstetric conditions (e.g. growth restricted babies, placenta praevia)

3.

Delivery should be undertaken by an obstetrician experienced in doing vaginal breech deliveries and should take place in the hospital where facilities with immediate recourse to emergency caesarean section are available. The labour should ideally start spontaneously and progress normally. Women should have a choice of analgesia during vaginal breech and epidural analgesia should not be routinely advised but should be considered and encouraged.

Continuous electronic fetal heart rate monitoring should be offered to all women having vaginal breech delivery in view of the increased risk of cord prolapse (7%). It is not advisable to do fetal blood sampling from the buttocks during labour.

Augmentation of labour is not recommended and a caesarean section should be considered for non-descent of breech at any point in the second stage of labour.

Royal College of Obstetricians and Gynaecologists. Green-top Guideline No. 20a. External cephalic version and reducing the incidence of breech presentation. London: RCOG Press, 2006.

Index

Note: Page numbers in **bold** refer to tables.